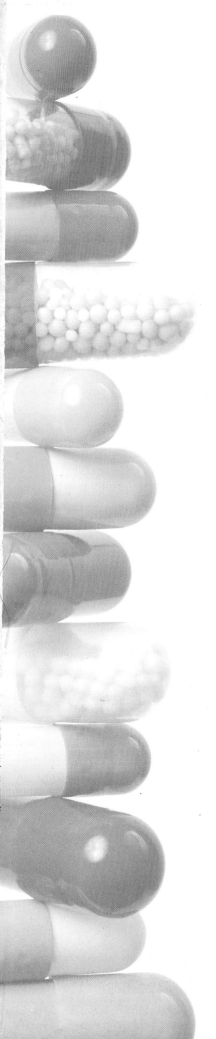

CALCULATING DRUG DOSAGES

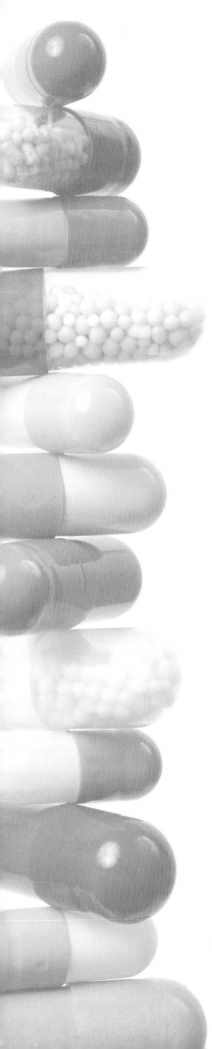

CALCULATING DRUG DOSAGES

A Patient-Safe Approach to Nursing and Math

Sandra Luz Martinez de Castillo, RN, MA, EdD
Professor Emeritus
Contra Costa College Nursing Program
San Pablo, California

Maryanne Werner-McCullough, RN, MS, MNP
Professor Emeritus
Contra Costa College Nursing Program
San Pablo, California

F.A. Davis Company • Philadelphia

F. A. Davis Company
1915 Arch Street
Philadelphia, PA 19103
www.fadavis.com

Printed in the United States of America

Last digit indicates print number: 10 9 8 7 6 5 4 3 2 1

Senior Acquisitions Editor, Nursing: Megan Klim
Senior Content Project Manager: Elizabeth Hart
Electronic Project Editor: Sandra Glennie
Design and Illustration Manager: Carolyn O'Brien

As new scientific information becomes available through basic and clinical research, recommended treatments and drug therapies undergo changes. The author(s) and publisher have done everything possible to make this book accurate, up to date, and in accord with accepted standards at the time of publication. The author(s), editors, and publisher are not responsible for errors or omissions or for consequences from application of the book, and make no warranty, expressed or implied, in regard to the contents of the book. Any practice described in this book should be applied by the reader in accordance with professional standards of care used in regard to the unique circumstances that may apply in each situation. The reader is advised always to check product information (package inserts) for changes and new information regarding dose and contraindications before administering any drug. Caution is especially urged when using new or infrequently ordered drugs.

Library of Congress Cataloging-in-Publication Data

Names: Martinez de Castillo, Sandra Luz, author. | Werner-McCullough,
    Maryanne, author.
Title: Calculating drug dosages : a patient-safe approach to nursing and math
    / Sandra Luz Martinez de Castillo, Maryanne Werner-McCullough.
Other titles: Calculating drug dosages (2017)
Description: Philadelphia : F.A. Davis Company, [2017]
Identifiers: LCCN 2015039660 | ISBN 9780803624962
Subjects: | MESH: Pharmaceutical Preparations—administration &
    dosage—Nurses' Instruction. | Mathematics—Nurses' Instruction.
Classification: LCC RS57 | NLM QV 748 | DDC 615.1/401513—dc23 LC record available at
http://lccn.loc.gov/2015039660

To my parents, Miguel and Blanca, who said that I could.

— Sandra

To Ron, who understands.

— Maryanne

Preface

Dear Students:

It is our pleasure to present *Calculating Drug Dosages: A Patient-Safe Approach to Nursing and Math*. Patient safety in medication administration has provided the foundation and motivation for the development of each chapter. Therefore, in addition to demonstrating how to solve a drug dosage problem, we have included medication administration situations encountered in clinical practice. Each chapter is unique and designed to build your confidence in drug dosage calculation.

In the chapters you will find:

- A choice of one of four methods of calculation.
- Math tips that are related to medication administration in clinical practice.
- Clinical situations that demonstrate issues regarding medication administration.
- Simulated physician's orders and electronic medication administration records.
- Excerpts from drug references that apply to the calculation of dosages.
- Practice problems that will help you to develop math competency.
- Situations that promote clinical reasoning and decision making.

Developing competency in drug dosage calculations takes practice. We encourage you to practice solving drug dosage problems every day and to always follow recommended guidelines when administering medications. Taking the time to practice demonstrates professional growth and commitment to patient safety.

This book, combined with your consistent practice of drug dosage calculations, is designed to be a valuable resource to prepare you for error-free medication administration.

To the Instructor:

Thank you for using *Calculating Drug Dosages: A Patient-Safe Approach to Nursing and Math* to teach students how to calculate drug dosages accurately and with confidence. In the development of this book we have emphasized the importance of safety in the total process of medication administration, from reading the physician's order to the calculation of the dose and documentation of the medication.

Key features of the book include:

- Drug dosage problems solved in four methods: Linear Ratio and Proportion, Fractional Ratio and Proportion, Dimensional Analysis, and the Formula Method.
- Drug dosage problems that require the use of critical thinking and clinical reasoning.
- Simulated physician's orders and electronic medication administration records.
- Excerpts from drug references that apply to the calculation of dosages.
- Apply Learned Knowledge activities that reinforce the mathematical drug dosage concepts presented.
- Developing Competency drug dosage problems at the end of each chapter.
- Additional drug dosage problems available online that reinforce the content of each unit.

- Emphasis on the implementation of safe practices appropriate to the situation.
- Advocacy for applying a "Vigilant Process" in medication administration for the older adult.

We hope that this book becomes a valuable resource for you and that your students develop the competency needed in the administration of medications.

Sandra and Maryanne

Reviewers

Barbara W. Allerton, MSN, RN
Professor Emeritus
Boise State University
Boise, Idaho

Ceanne Alvine, PhD, RN
Instructional Faculty/Advisor
Pima Community College
Tucson, Arizona

Robert Auch, MSN, RN
Faculty
Ridgewater College
Willmar, Minnesota

Terry L. Bichsel, BSN, RN
Practical Nursing Coordinator
Moberly Area Community College
Moberly, Missouri

Connie J. Booth, MSN, RN
Nursing Program Chair
Des Moines Area Community College
Boone, Iowa

Jeanie Burt, MSN, MA, RN, CNE
Assistant Professor
Harding University Carr College of
   Nursing
Searcy, Arkansas

Marilyn J. Cady, BS, RN
Associate Professor Nursing
Iowa Western Community College
Council Bluffs, Iowa

Debra L. Carter, EdD, MSN, RN, FNP
Associate Professor of Nursing
The University of Virginia's College at Wise
Wise, Virginia

Lisa Cooley, MSN, RN
Nursing Department Chair
Jefferson Community College
Watertown, New York

Natalie O. DeLeonardis, MSN, RN
Coordinator of Practical Nursing
Pennsylvania College of Technology North Campus
Wellsboro, Pennsylvania

Marian T. Doyle, MSN, MS, RN
Associate Professor of Nursing
Northampton Community College
Bethlehem, Pennsylvania

Maria C. Farber, MSN, RN, BC, OCN
Nursing Instructor
Middlesex Community College
Edison, New Jersey

Abimbola Farinde, PharmD, MS
Clinical Pharmacist Specialist
Clear Lake Regional Medical Center
Webster, Texas

Clara Garrett, MSN, BSN
Professor of Nursing
Big Sandy Community and Technical College
Prestonsburg, Kentucky

Ruth Gladen, MS, RN
Director of RN Program; Associate Professor
North Dakota State College of Science
Wahpeton, North Dakota

Annette M. Gunderman, DEd, MSN, RN
Associate Professor of Nursing
Bloomsburg University
Bloomsburg, Pennsylvania

Terry Harper, MSN, RN
Associate of Science in Nursing Instructor
Southwest Georgia Technical College
Thomasville, Georgia

Rosemary Hasenmiller, MS, RN, CNM
Assistant Professor
St. Ambrose University
Davenport, Iowa

Jill Holmstrom, EdD, RN, CNE
Associate Professor
Concordia College
Moorhead, Minnesota

Deborah Hunt, PhD, RN
Assistant Professor of Nursing
The College of New Rochelle
New Rochelle, New York

Teresa V. Hurley, DHEd, RN
Associate Professor of Nursing
Mount Saint Mary College
Newburgh, New York

Vicki L. Imerman, MSN, RN
Nursing Professor
Des Moines Area Community College
Boone, Iowa

Sheri Lynn Jacobson, MSN, RN, APRN
Assistant Professor
Winston-Salem State University
Winston-Salem, North Carolina

Maryanne Krenz, MA, RN
Associate Professor Nursing
Brookdale Community College
Lincroft, New Jersey

Maxine G. Kron, BOE, RN Diploma
District Director Practical Nursing
Hinds Community College
Jackson, Mississippi

Kathleen N. Krov, PhD, RN, CNM, CNE
Assistant Professor
Raritan Valley Community College
North Branch, New Jersey

Mary Kulp, MSN, RN
Associate Professor of Nursing
Jefferson Community and Technical
    College
Louisville, Kentucky

Amy Lankford, MSN, RN
Director of Nursing
Wilkes Community College
Wilkesboro, North Carolina

Amy Ma, DNP, FNP-BC
Associate Professor, Director of Graduate
    Program
Long Island University, Brooklyn
Brooklyn, New York

Maggie Mackowick, MS, RN
Assistant Professor
North Dakota State University
Fargo, North Dakota

Phyllis Magaletto, MS, RN, BC
Professor
Cochran School of Nursing
Yonkers, New York

Camella G. Marcom, MSN, RN
Associate Degree Nurse Instructor
Vance-Granville Community College
Henderson, North Carolina

Mary Alice Maze, BSN, RN
Adjunct Faculty
Galen College of Nursing–Cincinnati
Cincinnati, Ohio

Lindsay McCrea, PhD, RN, FNP
Professor
California State University, East Bay
Hayward, California

Maria A. Medina, MSN, RN
Nursing Instructor
Trinidad State Junior College
Alamosa, Colorado

Bethany Mello, DNP, NP-c
Assistant Professor
University of Jamestown
Jamestown, North Dakota

April Rowe Neal, MS, RN
Assistant Professor
Luther College
Decorah, Iowa

Sharon M. Nowak, EdD, MSN, RN
Professor of Nursing
Jackson College
Jackson, Michigan

Emily Dawn Orr, MSN, RN, CCRN
Associate Degree Nursing Faculty Member
Wilkes Community College
Wilkesboro, North Carolina

Michelle D. Pearson-Smith, MSN, RN
Assistant Professor
Lewis-Clark State College
Lewiston, Idaho

Irish Patrick Williams, PhD, MSN, RN, CRRN
Nursing Instructor
Hinds Community College
Jackson, Mississippi

Jean Ann Wilson, RN
Nurse Practitioner Coordinator, Norton Campus
Colby Community College
Norton, Kansas

Sandra Reed Wilson, MSN, RN
Program Coordinator
Crowder College
Cassville, Missouri

Jean Yockey, MSN, FNP-BC, CNE
Associate Professor, Nursing
University of South Dakota
Vermillion, South Dakota

Tara Zacharzuk-Marciano, MA, RN
Nurse Educator
SUNY Ulster Community College
Stone Ridge, New York

Acknowledgments

The authors wish to acknowledge and thank the companies who allowed the reproduction of their drug labels and medication equipment images:

Abbott Laboratories

B. Braun Medical, Inc.

Baxter Healthcare Corporation

Bayer Corporation

Becton, Dickinson and Company

Covis Pharmaceuticals, Inc.

Eli Lilly & Company

GlaxoSmithKline

Novo Nordisk, Inc.

Pfizer, Inc.

   Pfizer Labs Division of Pfizer Inc.

   Pharmacia & Upjohn Co. Division of Pfizer Inc.

   Parke-Davis Division of Pfizer Inc.

PDC Healthcare

Retractable Technologies, Inc.

Sagent Pharmaceuticals, Inc.

Smiths Medical

Teva Pharmaceuticals USA Inc.

   Barr Laboratories Inc.

West-Ward Pharmaceutical Corp.

We owe so much to all the staff at F. A. Davis. Sincere thanks to Tom Ciavarella, Liz Hart, Lisa Thompson, Sandy Glennie, and Meghan Ziegler for your wisdom and insight during the writing and editing process. Your support and collaboration made this textbook happen.

Special thanks to the students for teaching us what we needed to teach.

Table of Contents

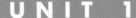

UNIT 1

Safety in Medication Administration

Safe medication administration requires the collaborative effort of all healthcare providers to initiate, evaluate, and contribute to practices that promote patient safety. This unit provides you with information that emphasizes safe medication administration practice, from the initial reading of a medication order and drug label to the application of the Six Rights of Medication Administration.

 APPLICATION TO NURSING PRACTICE

The nurse uses the patient's medication administration record and the drug label to ensure that the correct drug and dose is administered to the patient.

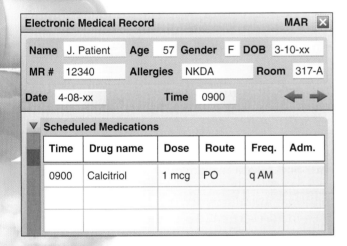
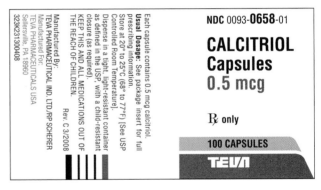

In applying safe medication administration practice, the nurse must understand the information on the drug label to answer questions such as:

- Is this the right drug?
- What is the dosage strength of the drug?
- What is the recommended route of administration?
- Is this a controlled substance?

1

Safety in Medication Administration

LEARNING OUTCOMES

Discuss safe practices that help to prevent medication administration errors.

Identify safe medication practices that assist patients and families in taking greater responsibility for the management of their medication therapy.

Discuss how the Six Rights of Medication Administration promote safe practice.

Safety in medication administration involves the collaborative effort of healthcare professionals, drug manufacturers, healthcare organizations, ongoing scholarly research, and informed patients and families. Safety in medication administration is everyone's responsibility, from the establishment of national standards for the manufacturing and monitoring of drugs, to standard guidelines for prescribing and administering medications, to assisting patients in assuming greater responsibility for the management of their medication.

The prominent report *To Err Is Human: Building a Safer Health System* (1999), published by the Institute of Medicine, brought attention to the number of annual deaths in hospitals that were attributed to preventable medical errors. Medical errors that cause harm to the patient, including medication errors, are costly and have devastating effects for patients, families, and society.

To consistently work toward minimizing errors, healthcare organizations are encouraged to establish a ***"culture of safety."*** Organizations that embrace a culture of safety promote activities that create a continuous awareness for patient safety and encourage collaboration among healthcare staff from all levels to seek solutions to problems. An integral component of the culture of safety is the concept of ***"just culture."*** First introduced in 2001 by attorney David Marx, the concept focuses on identifying and analyzing factors and the sequence of actions that lead to a patient error. This careful analysis of the error recognizes that situations or processes within the healthcare system may lead the individual to make an unintentional error. This nonpunitive approach allows healthcare professionals to discuss the error or situations that may cause possible errors without fear of punishment. The culture of safety also recognizes that healthcare professionals need to be held accountable for errors that occur due to at-risk behaviors (i.e., not using two patient identifiers prior to giving medications, not double-checking medications per institutional policy) or reckless behaviors (i.e., taking shortcuts such as not following the Six Rights of Medication Administration). The primary focus of this analysis is to learn how best to prevent similar errors in the future.

There are many government and nongovernment agencies that address healthcare and patient safety issues, for example: the U.S. Food and Drug Administration, the U.S. Department of Health and Human Services, the American Society of Health-System Pharmacists, and the National Coordinating Council for Medication Error Reporting and Prevention. Because of the research with medication safety and the implications of the findings and recommendations to nursing practice, the Institute of Medicine and the Institute of Safe Medication Practices will be discussed.

The Institute of Medicine

The Institute of Medicine (IOM), an independent, nonprofit organization established in 1970, serves to inform government policy makers and the public sector on national healthcare issues. Through national research studies, the IOM provides reliable information and makes recommendations for best practices. In the July 2006 IOM report *Preventing Medication Error: Quality Chasm Series*, the IOM indicated that medication errors can occur at every phase of the medication process, from prescribing and dispensing to administering and monitoring for the effects of the drug. However, based on the report, medication errors occur most frequently at the prescribing and administering phases. The prevention of harm to a patient is of priority. To this end, the IOM strongly advocates that the first and foremost intervention for safety in the use of medications is the establishment of a partnership between the patient and the healthcare provider. The goal of this partnership is to facilitate the process for the patient to take more responsibility in the management and in the monitoring of his or her medications.

Table 1-1 lists the recommendation identified in the IOM report. More information on the report may be obtained at the Web site http://www.iom.edu/~/media/files/report%20files/2006/preventing-medication-errors-quality-chasm-series/medicationerrorsnew.pdf.

The implications for nursing practice in Table 1-1 serve as a reminder of the importance of teaching patients and families so that they can take a more active role in monitoring their medications.

Table 1-1. Institute of Medicine Recommendations for Reducing Medication Errors

IOM RECOMMENDATIONS	IMPLICATIONS FOR NURSING PRACTICE
Patients/families need to take greater responsibility for monitoring their medications and reporting changes.	Communicate and provide ongoing patient teaching regarding drug therapy, with a focus on the individual needs of the patient, his or her culture, and lifestyle.
	Encourage the use of reliable resources for obtaining drug information. Ensure the patient knows whom to contact for questions regarding his or her drug therapy.
Patients/families need to maintain accurate records of all medications.	Review list of all medications, educate, consult, and listen to patient's concerns and questions.
Openness regarding errors and problems	Communicate openly with the patient and family when errors occur, explain consequences and interventions to correct the problem.

The Institute of Safe Medication Practices

The Institute of Safe Medication Practices (ISMP) is a nonprofit agency established in 1975 with the primary purpose of identifying the causes of medication errors and of recommending evidence-based strategies for the prevention of these errors. An invaluable resource, ISMP keeps healthcare professionals, healthcare facilities, the pharmaceutical industry, and other government agencies informed of medication safety issues (http://www.ismp.org). The research, resources, and services provided by the ISMP have had a strong influence in changing medication practices across all healthcare settings. In 2003, the ISMP published a list of abbreviations, symbols, and dose designations (the way medication doses are written) that were prone to cause medication errors if misread or misinterpreted. Table 1-2 highlights some of the ISMP recommended changes in the use of abbreviations, symbols, and dose designations with examples for correct use. The recommendations made by the ISMP were supported by national patient safety organizations and have become standard practice. The complete list of Error-Prone Abbreviations, Symbols and Dose Designations published by ISMP is found in the Safe Dosage Resources on Davis*Plus*.

HIGH ALERT MEDICATION LIST

The ISMP also provides a listing of high-alert medications; these are medications that have an increased risk of causing significant patient harm (see Safe Dosage Resources on Davis*Plus*). All drugs have the potential for side effects and adverse effects; however, drugs identified as "high alert" indicate that the drug has an increased potential for patient harm, and signifies the need for healthcare professionals to be vigilant in the preparation of the ordered dose, the administration of the drug to the patient, and the monitoring of

Table 1-2. The Institute of Safe Medication Practices: Example of Potentially Dangerous Abbreviations, Symbols, and Dose Designations

DANGEROUS ABBREVIATIONS, SYMBOLS, AND DOSE DESIGNATIONS	EXAMPLE
Do not use trailing zeros.	Write 5 mg, never 5.0 mg
Use leading zeros for doses less than one measurement unit.	Write 0.3 mg, never .3 mg
Place adequate space between the drug name, dose, and unit of measure.	Write calcitriol 0.5 mcg, never calcitriol 0.5mcg
Spell out the word "units." Never use "U," which easily can be mistaken as a zero, causing a 10-fold overdose.	Write 30 units, never 30 u
Do not use a period after abbreviations such as "mg." or "mL." (Write "mg" or "mL" without the period.)	Write mL, mg, mcg, g, etc. Never mL., mg., mcg., or g.
Use the abbreviation "mcg" for microgram. Do not use the Greek letter μ to represent "micro" in healthcare.	Write 4 mcg or 4 micrograms, never 4 μg, because "μg" could be misread as mg
For the abbreviation of milliliter, use mL (lower/uppercase). Do not use "cc," which has been misread as "U" or the number 4.	Write 10 mL, never 10 cc
Include properly spaced commas for dose numbers expressed in thousands (e.g., 5,000 units). Use the word "thousand" for larger doses in the hundreds of thousands (e.g., 150 thousand rather than 150,000).	Write heparin 5,000 units, never heparin 5000 units
Use the word "million" for doses expressed in millions (e.g., 1 million units) to avoid possible misplacement of commas and misreading the dose if the commas are not seen correctly with such large numbers.	Write penicillin 1.5 million units, never penicillin 1,500,000 units

Modified from the complete listing available at http://www.ismp.org/Tools/errorproneabbreviations.pdf

the patient for the drug's effects. Drug references prominently identify high alert drugs (Fig. 1-1).

CONFUSED DRUG NAMES LIST

There are several drug names that, when spoken or written, look alike and sound alike. These drug names have the potential to be confused with each other and may lead to a medication error. Figure 1-2 provides an example of drug name pairs that look alike and sound alike. The ISMP publishes a listing of drugs names that **look alike** or **sound alike** (Confused Drug Names). This listing is found at the Web site www.ismp.org/tools/confuseddrugnames.pdf, and is included in the Safe Dosage Resources on Davis*Plus*.

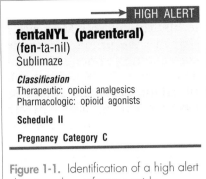

Figure 1-1. Identification of a high alert drug in a drug reference guide.

To minimize errors, it is recommended that the nurse become familiar with look-alike and sound-alike drug names, double-check the drug name against the doctor's order and the patient medication record, and know why the patient is receiving the drug. More information regarding look-alike and sound-alike drugs can be found in Chapter 2, The Drug Label.

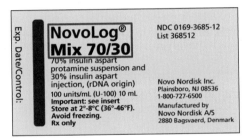
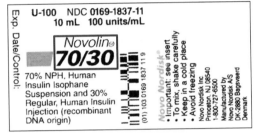

Figure 1-2. Examples of confused drug name pairs from the ISMP listing.

THE JOINT COMMISSION

The Joint Commission, the national healthcare accrediting organization, developed a "Do Not Use" list of abbreviations as a national safety patient goal, emphasizing the importance of eliminating the use of several abbreviations. The list from The Joint Commission includes some abbreviations found in the ISMP's list of Error-Prone Abbreviations, Symbols, and Dose Designation. The Joint Commission's official list can be found in the Safe Dosage Resources on Davis*Plus* and on the Web site http://www.jointcommission.org/assets/1/18/Do_Not_Use_List.pdf.

More Safety Practices

TALL MAN LETTERING

In its continuous effort to promote safety in medication administration and to reduce the risk of errors, the Office of Generic Drugs of the U.S. Food and Drug Administration (FDA) recommends that drug manufacturers use tall man lettering in writing the names of specific drugs. **Tall man lettering** is the use of mixed-case letters (lower- and uppercase) in a drug name with the specific purpose of highlighting a section of the drug name, therefore making the name more noticeable on the packaging and on the drug label. This helps distinguish the drug from another drug with a similar name (Fig. 1-3).

RISK EVALUATION AND MITIGATION STRATEGY

In 2007, the U.S. Food and Drug Administration was granted the authority to implement the **Risk Evaluation and Mitigation Strategy (REMS)** program to watch over the use of certain drugs, such as opioids, prescribed primarily in the management of moderate to

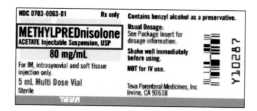 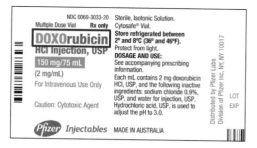

Figure 1-3. Examples of drug names with tall man lettering.

severe pain. The REMS is a risk management program that helps to ensure that the benefits of a specific drug or drug class outweigh the risks. When a drug or drug class is under the REMS program, drug manufacturers are mandated to comply with specific requirements, such as the development of a plan for monitoring the drug for as long as the drug is on the market, safety strategies that address training for healthcare providers, and development of patient information that identifies the drug's risks and benefits. As part of the safety strategies, manufacturers need to provide a medication guide or package insert to be issued by the pharmacist each time the drug is dispensed.

The medication guide needs to include FDA-approved information to help the consumer become aware of serious adverse effects. The desired outcome of the REMS program is improved patient safety. Box 1-1 contains an example of a medication guide available from the FDA Web site www.fda.gov/Drugs/DrugSafety/ucm085729.htm.

Box 1-1. Example of a REMS Medication Guide Approved by the FDA

Medication Guide
MS CONTIN® (MS-KON-tin)
(morphine sulfate controlled-release) Tablets, CII
MS CONTIN is:

- A strong prescription pain medicine that contains an opioid (narcotic) that is used to treat moderate to severe around-the-clock pain.

Important information about MS CONTIN:

- Get emergency help right away if you take too much MS CONTIN (overdose). MS CONTIN overdose can cause life-threatening breathing problems that can lead to death.
- Never give anyone else your MS CONTIN. They could die from taking it. Store MS CONTIN away from children and in a safe place to prevent stealing or abuse. Selling or giving away MS CONTIN is against the law.

Do not take MS CONTIN if you have:
- severe asthma, trouble breathing, or other lung problems.
- a bowel blockage or narrowing of the stomach or intestines.

Before taking MS CONTIN, tell your healthcare provider if you have a history of:

- head injury, seizures
- liver, kidney, thyroid problems
- problems urinating
- pancreas or gallbladder problems
- abuse of street or prescription drugs, alcohol addiction, or mental health problems

Tell your healthcare provider if you are:

- pregnant or planning to become pregnant. MS CONTIN may harm your unborn baby.
- breastfeeding. MS CONTIN passes into breast milk and may harm your baby.
- taking prescription or over-the-counter medicines, vitamins, or herbal supplements.

Box 1-1. **Example of a REMS Medication Guide Approved by the FDA—cont'd**

When taking MS CONTIN:

- do not change your dose. Take MS CONTIN exactly as prescribed by your healthcare provider.
- take each dose at the same time every day. If you miss a dose, take MS CONTIN as soon as possible and then take your next dose 8 or 12 hours later as directed by your healthcare provider. If it is almost time for your next dose, skip the missed dose and go back to your regular dosing schedule. Do not take more than 1 dose in 8 hours.
- swallow MS CONTIN whole. Do not cut, break, chew, crush, dissolve, or inject MS CONTIN.
- **Call your healthcare provider if the dose you are taking does not control your pain.**
- **Do not stop taking MS CONTIN without talking to your healthcare provider.**

While taking MS CONTIN Do Not:

- drive or operate heavy machinery, until you know how MS CONTIN affects you. MS CONTIN can make you sleepy, dizzy, or light-headed.
- drink alcohol or use prescription or over-the-counter medicines that contain alcohol.

The possible side effects of MS CONTIN are:

- constipation, nausea, sleepiness, vomiting, tiredness, headache, dizziness, abdominal pain. Call your healthcare provider if you have any of these symptoms and they are severe.

Get emergency medical help if you:

- have trouble breathing; shortness of breath; fast heart beat; chest pain; swelling of your face, tongue, or throat; extreme drowsiness; or if you are feeling faint

These are not all the possible side effects of MS CONTIN. Call your doctor for medical advice about side effects. You may report side effects to the FDA at 1-800-FDA-1088. **For more information, go to http://dailymed.nlm.nih.gov.**

Manufactured by: Purdue Pharma L.P., Stamford, CT 06901-3431, www.purduepharma.com or call 1-888-726-7535.
This Medication Guide has been approved by the U.S. Food and Drug Administration. Issue: July 2012
Modified from www.fda.gov/Drugs/DrugSafety/ucm085729.htm

Drug references identify medications under the REMS program by adding the REMS acronym to the drug information (Fig. 1-4). The nurse can use the medication guide to help teach the patient and family about the drug.

BLACK BOX WARNINGS

Black box warnings have been included on the label of specific prescription medications to advise the healthcare professional and the patient about serious potential risks and side effects related to the use of the drug. Figure 1-5 on page 8 provides an example of the black box warning from the package insert for the drug metoclopramide. Notice the accompanying directions on the drug label.

Healthcare professionals need to make a concerted effort to read drug labels carefully, consult the pharmacist, and seek reliable drug references and Web sites for current information and FDA recommendations. More information regarding black box warnings on drug labels can be found in Chapter 2.

→ REMS | HIGH ALERT

morphine (mor-feen)
Astramorph PF, AVINza, ✽Doloral, Duramorph PF, Embeda, ✽Epimorph, Infumorph, Kadian, ✽M-Eslon, ✽Morphine H.P, ✽M.O.S, ✽M.O.S.-S.R, MS Contin, ✽Statex

Classification
Therapeutic: opioid analgesics
Pharmacologic: opioid agonists

Schedule II

Pregnancy Category C

Figure 1-4. Morphine identified as part of the REMS program

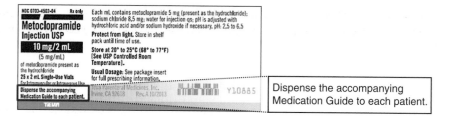

Metoclopramide Injection USP
Package Insert
4502
Rx only

WARNING: TARDIVE DYSKINESIA

Treatment with metoclopramide can cause tardive dyskinesia, a serious movement disorder that is often irreversible. The risk of developing tardive dyskinesia increases with duration of treatment and total cumulative dose.

Metoclopramide therapy should be discontinued in patients who develop signs or symptoms of tardive dyskinesia. There is no known treatment for tardive dyskinesia. In some patients, symptoms may lessen or resolve after metoclopramide treatment is stopped.

Treatment with metoclopramide for longer than 12 weeks should be avoided in all but rare cases where therapeutic benefit is thought to outweigh the risk of developing tardive dyskinesia. See WARNINGS.

Figure 1-5. Black box warning for metoclopramide.

The Medication Administration Process

The medication process involves several steps:

1. The medication is ordered.
2. The medication order is interpreted (validating the accuracy and completion of the order) and transcribed as written.
3. The components of the Six Rights of Medication Administration are used to
   - prepare the ordered medication and
   - administer the medication to the patient.

THE MEDICATION ORDER

The administration of medications begins with the medication order. Technology has facilitated the process for prescribing medications and making the medication order more legible. It is important to remember that in the administration of medications, the medication order, whether it is electronically generated or handwritten, must contain the following basic components: patient identification information, drug name, ordered dose, route of administration, and frequency of administration (Fig. 1-6).

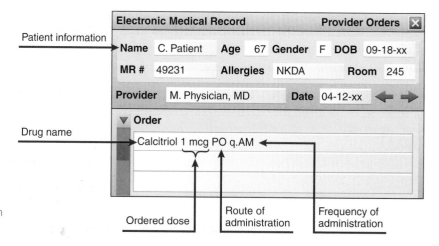

Figure 1-6. Medication order with medication administration components.

Safety considerations in reading the medication order begin by knowing the basic components that constitute the medication order and seeking clarification if any of the components are missing or are unclear.

INTERPRETATION AND TRANSCRIPTION OF THE MEDICATION ORDER

Once the medication order is written, the order needs to be interpreted and transcribed. The medication administration record (MAR) may be electronically generated by the pharmacist (Fig. 1-7), or the medication order may be interpreted and transcribed by the nurse into a MAR in paper format (Fig. 1-8). Regardless of the format, the MAR must

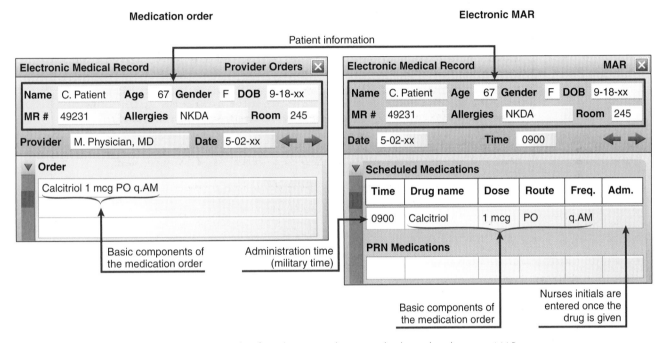

Figure 1-7. Example of medication order transcribed into the electronic MAR.

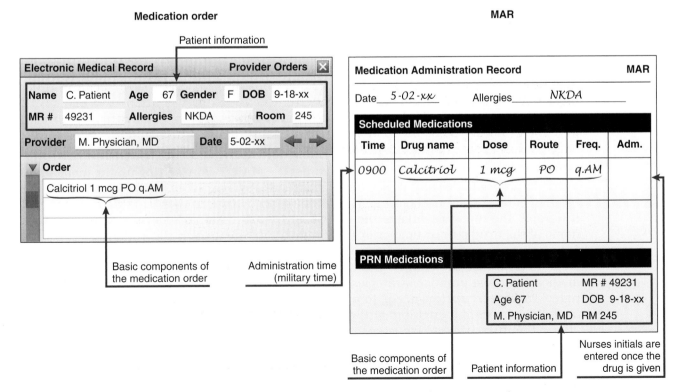

Figure 1-8. Example of medication order transcribed onto the MAR (paper format).

correctly identify the patient as well as identify all of the basic components of the ordered drug name, ordered dose, route, and frequency of administration ordered by the physician. Additional instructions for the safe administration of the drug may be ordered by the physician. The instructions guide the nurse in determining the safe administration of the drug based on the patient's clinical condition.

The actual time for the administration of the medication is based on the frequency ordered by the physician and the facility's standard times for the administration of medications. Notice how the basic components of the medication order appear on the electronic medication record and paper format of the MAR. After the drug has been given to the patient, the initials of the nurse are entered and recorded.

Military time is commonly used in clinical facilities. The benefits of using military time and instructions on reading and writing military time are discussed in Chapter 15, Calculating Infusion and Completion Time.

THE SIX RIGHTS OF MEDICATION ADMINISTRATION

The **Six Rights of Medication Administration** (Fig. 1-9) provide the guidelines for implementing safe medication administration practices. Each "right" provides the nurse the opportunity to question and clarify any misinterpretations in the administration of the drug that may lead to a medication error before administering the drug to the patient.

Patient safety is always an integral part of each "right" during the entire medication administration process. This includes the correlation of the medication with the patient's needs and the follow-up care of the patient after the administration of the drug. This requires the nurse to

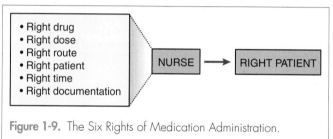

Figure 1-9. The Six Rights of Medication Administration.

■ know the drug's action

■ have an understanding of why the drug is ordered for the patient

■ carefully monitor the patient for the drug's therapeutic and side effects

 Safe practices in the medication administration process involve more than learning the skill of preparing and administering medications. Rather, safety in medication administration involves a deliberate collaborative approach to preventing medication errors.

The Preparation of the Medication

The first three "rights," **right drug, right dose,** and **right route,** are instituted during the preparation of the drug. Although the ordered medication is supplied by the pharmacist, the nurse is responsible for verifying that the MAR matches the physician's order (Fig. 1-10).

In preparing the right drug, the right dose, and the right route, the nurse begins by initially checking the name of the drug against the MAR. Before setting up the medication in the appropriate delivery device (medication cup, syringe, etc.), which is based on the route of administration, the nurse verifies the right drug against the MAR a second time. If needed, the nurse calculates the ordered dose at this time. The nurse will verify the name of the drug a third time prior to administering the drug to the patient.

Safety in the preparation of medications necessitates that the nurse implement steps to minimize the chance of a medication error in the preparation of the patient's medication. Best practice strategies include the preparation of medications in a designated **"no interruption area"** to allow the nurse to prepare the patient's medication in a distraction-free environment, employing a **"Medication Pass Time-Out,"** which allows the nurse time to focus specifically on checking medication orders, drug labels, MAR, and the like prior to preparing the medication, and wearing a "Do Not Disturb" vest as a visual signal to minimize interruptions during the medication preparation process.

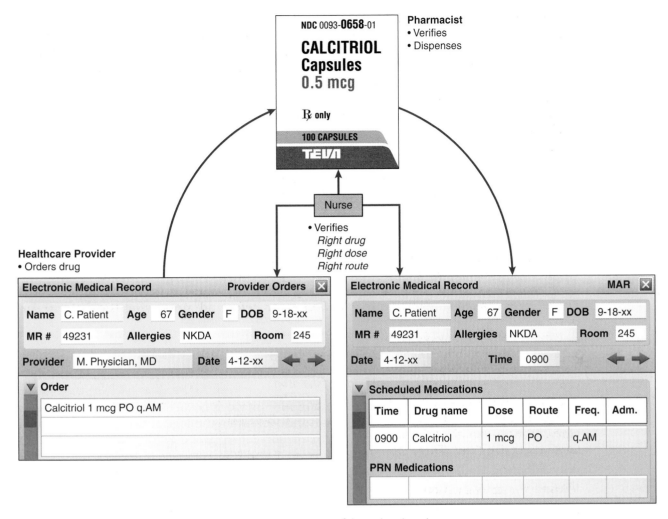

Figure 1-10. Preparation of the ordered medication.

The Right Time, the Right Patient, the Right Documentation

Administering the medication at the **right time,** to the **right patient,** and with the **right documentation** of the medication after it is administered completes the next three rights. To ensure medications are given at the right time, the nurse follows the medication administration times and guidelines set by the healthcare facility.

It is important to remember that the **right patient** is the focus of the Six Rights of Medication Administration. Misidentification of a patient has contributed to many medication errors. In 2003, The Joint Commission created the National Patient Safety Goals program to address areas of concern regarding patient safety. Its first national patient safety goal was to improve accuracy of patient identification when administering medications or providing treatments or procedures. Safe practice recommendations now require the healthcare worker to verify the patient using two patient identifiers (such as the patient's name and date of birth) and to incorporate newer methods such as bar coding for patient identification. At the patient's bedside, the nurse verifies the right patient using two patient identifiers (i.e., patient name, barcode patient identification), following the policies of the healthcare facility. After the administration of the medication, the nurse completes the last "right" by documenting all of the information that indicates that the patient has received the prescribed drug as ordered.

EBP *The institution of technology in the administration of medications has facilitated the use of best practices in minimizing potential errors by incorporating bar coding and scanning of drugs and patient identification. This type of best practice helps to verify the right drug, the right dose, the right time, and the right patient.*

Safety in Drug Dosage Calculations and Clinical Reasoning

In the calculation of the right dose, it is critical that the nurse use clinical reasoning as well as accurate math skills. It is important for the nurse to ask the question, "Does the answer make sense?" For example, the nurse uses clinical reasoning to question an answer that requires the administration of mutiple tablets or to seek guidance when a dose is greater than the usual dose identified in the drug reference.

Overall, clinical reasoning leads to decision making that is based on learned knowledge and experience. Clinical reasoning takes into account all the factors that may influence the clinical decision, such as the patient's age, disease process, and drug-drug interactions that may affect the administration of the drug. The authors recommend the use of a "Vigilant Process" or a systematic step-by-step approach for addressing the multiple factors associated with medication administration and use. The Vigilant Process is discussed in Chapter 22, Considerations for the Older Adult Population.

 CLINICAL REASONING 1-1
In the administration of medications it is important for the nurse to (select all that apply):

A. *inform the patient if the wrong drug or dose was administered.*
B. *decide on the appropriate route of administration.*
C. *use the physician's order to verify drug orders.*
D. *teach the patient the effects of a drug.*
E. *understand why the patient is taking the drug.*

In summary, the safe and accurate calculation of drug dosages requires the nurse to use a mathmatical method that is familiar and facilitates the logical setup and solving of the problem. Safety in medication administration involves the use of clinical reasoning and viewing the medication administration as a multidimensional process requiring not only adhering to the Six Rights of Medication Administration, but also seeking current drug information, monitoring the patient for the drug's effects, incorporating the individual needs of the patient, and making clinical decisions that promote patient safety.

Developing Competency

For questions 1 through 5, review the medication order shown and then select all statements that apply to the order.

1.
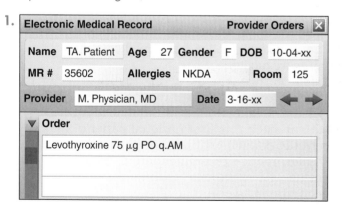

a. The medication order is written correctly.
b. The medication order has a dangerous symbol.
c. The ordered dose is 75 milligrams q.AM.

2.

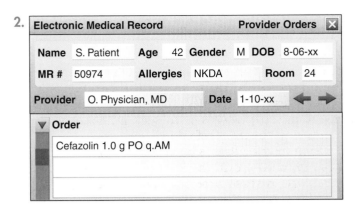

a. The medication order is written correctly.
b. The ordered dose has a trailing zero.
c. The nurse is correct to question the ordered dose.

3.

Electronic Medical Record   **Provider Orders** ☒

Name Y. Patient   **Age** 66 **Gender** M **DOB** 4-03-xx

MR # 23703   **Allergies** NKDA   **Room** 335

Provider D. Physician, MD   **Date** 4-30-xx ← →

▼ **Order**

Amoxicillin 250mg PO q.8h

a. The medication order is written incorrectly.
b. The ordered dose has a trailing zero.
c. "mg" should be spelled out to read "milligram."

4.

Electronic Medical Record   **Provider Orders** ☒

Name J. Patient   **Age** 58 **Gender** F **DOB** 6-05-xx

MR # 12560   **Allergies** NKDA   **Room** 115

Provider E. Physician, MD   **Date** 2-28-xx ← →

▼ **Order**

Penicillin G 1,200,000 u IM q.12h

a. The medication order is written correctly.
b. The dose should be written as 1.2 million.
c. Units (u) should not be abbreviated.

5.

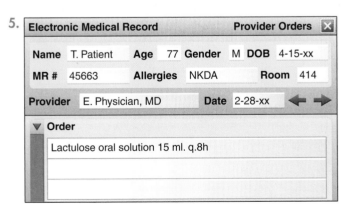

a. The medication order is written correctly.
b. "ml" should be written as "mL"
c. The period (.) after the ml is correct.

For questions 6 through 10, review the medication administration record shown and then choose the most appropriate clinical decision.

6.

Medication Administration Record					MAR

Date __10-2-xx__   Allergies __NKDA__

Scheduled Medications

Time	Drug name	Dose	Route	Freq.	Adm.
0800	Digoxin	.25 mg	PO	q.AM	

PRN Medications

S. Patient   MR # 51267
Age 52   DOB 6-08-xx
A. XXX M.D.   RM 134

The day shift nurse is reviewing the paper copy of a newly admitted patient's MAR. The most appropriate clinical decision for the nurse is to first
a. administer the 0800 dose as ordered.
b. check the M.D. order to verify dose.
c. ask another nurse to verify the dose.
d. question the dose with the pharmacist.

7.

Medication Administration Record					MAR

Date __8-14-xx__   Allergies __NKDA__

Scheduled Medications

Time	Drug name	Dose	Route	Freq.	Adm.
0900	Lasix	40 mg		q.AM	

PRN Medications

J. Patient   MR # 51267
Age 52   DOB 11-12-xx
H. XXX M.D.   RM 201

The nurse is reviewing the paper copy of a patient's MAR. The nurse has Lasix 40 mg tablets available. The most appropriate clinical decision for the nurse is to
a. not give the medication at 0900.
b. administer one 40 mg tablet of Lasix.
c. question the route with the pharmacist.
d. first check the M.D. order to verify the route.

8.

Medication Administration Record					MAR

Date __2-25-xx__   Allergies __NKDA__

Scheduled Medications

Time	Drug name	Dose	Route	Freq.	Adm.
2100	Benadryl	12.5 mg	PO	bed time	

PRN Medications

R. Patient   MR # 32012
Age 73   DOB 1-28-xx
G. XXX M.D.   RM 105

The nurse is reviewing the paper copy of a patient's MAR. For the 1500–2300 shift, the nurse is correct to
a. administer the Benadryl at 2100.
b. question the ordered dose with the pharmacist.
c. question the route with the pharmacist.
d. double-check the M.D. order.

9.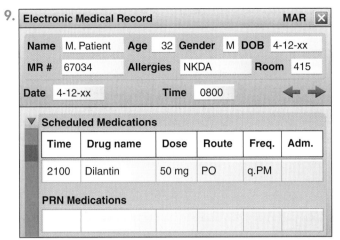

Electronic Medical Record   MAR ☒

| Name | M. Patient | Age | 32 | Gender | M | DOB | 4-12-xx |

| MR # | 67034 | | Allergies | NKDA | | Room | 415 |

| Date | 4-12-xx | | | Time | 0800 | | ← → |

▼ **Scheduled Medications**

Time	Drug name	Dose	Route	Freq.	Adm.
2100	Dilantin	50 mg	PO	q.PM	

PRN Medications

The nurse is reviewing the electronic MAR of the patient. For the 0700–1500 shift, the nurse is correct to
a. plan to administer the medication at 2100.
b. question the ordered dose with the pharmacist.
c. note no 0700–1500 medications ordered
d. double-check the MD order.

10.

Electronic Medical Record   MAR ☒

| Name | Q. Patient | Age | 45 | Gender | F | DOB | 7-04-xx |

| MR # | 22350 | | Allergies | NKDA | | Room | 125 |

| Date | 7-28-xx | | | Time | 0900 | | ← → |

▼ **Scheduled Medications**

Time	Drug name	Dose	Route	Freq.	Adm.
0900	Claritin	10 mg	PO	q.AM	SL

PRN Medications

The nurse is reviewing the electronic MAR of the patient. For the 1500–2300 shift, the nurse is correct to
a. interpret that the 0900 medication was given.
b. question the ordered dose with the pharmacist.
c. ask the patient whether the medication was given.
d. ask the day nurse whether the medication was given.

For questions 11 through 15, determine whether the statement is True or False.

11. High alert medications have an increased risk of causing significant patient harm. _____

12. Black box warnings are included in all prescription medications. _____

13. Safety in the use of medications includes the establishment of a partnership between the patient and the healthcare provider. _____

14. Promoting a culture of safety is the primary responsibility of physicians. _____

15. When a medication error occurs, the patient/family should be informed. _____

CHAPTER 2

The Drug Label

LEARNING OUTCOMES

Describe the information found on the drug label.

State how each component on the drug label is used in clinical practice.

The safe administration of medications includes an understanding of the information found on a drug label. The information on a drug label contains components used by the nurse to prepare medications and to apply several of the rights of medication administration. Table 2-1 identifies the important components found on a drug label. Although not all of the components are essential to the preparation of the medication, it is important to distinguish how each component may be used in clinical practice. Because the drug label design is unique to the drug manufacturer, the components on the drug label may be listed in different ways.

In the administration of medications, the nurse is guided by the Six Rights of Medication Administration. When preparing the medication for administration, the nurse will work with three of the rights of administration: the right drug, the right dose, and the right route.

Table 2-1. Components of a Drug Label

COMPONENTS OF A DRUG LABEL	
• Generic name	• Controlled substance
• Brand name	• Black box warning
• Dosage strength	• Storage information
• Route of administration	• Total amount in bottle
• Dosage and administration	• Lot number
• Instructions for mixing powdered medications	• Single-dose container versus multi-dose container
• Expiration date	• Manufacturer's name

The Right Drug

The drug label, along with the physician's order, provides the nurse with the initial step in verifying the right drug for administration. The physician orders the drug and the pharmacy sends the ordered drug. The nurse must then verify that the drug sent by the pharmacy is the same as the ordered drug. The name on the drug label may list the generic name of the drug or may list both the generic and brand names.

The Generic Name

The **generic name** is the universal chemical or pharmacological name of the drug. A drug has only one generic name. The generic name helps to identify drug groups by chemical structure or pharmacological properties. (For example, generic names ending in "-cillin" are part of the penicillin drug group.) When a drug label lists both the brand name and the generic name, such as in the Ceftin drug label in Figure 2-1, the generic name is usually listed under the brand name. The physician may order the drug using its generic name or its brand name.

THE GENERIC NAME AND THE UNITED STATES PHARMACOPEIA (USP)

The United States Pharmacopeia (USP) is an organization that sets pharmaceutical standards for the identity, quality, purity, and strength of prescription and over-the-counter drugs, as well as other healthcare products manufactured or sold in the United States. These standards are recognized in many countries and were developed with the primary interest of protecting the public health of people worldwide. The *United States Pharmacopeia and National Formulary* (USP-NF), the official book that contains a listing of drugs marketed in the United States, includes comprehensive information about each drug. The USP letters found after a generic drug name on the drug label indicate that the drug complies with the USP standards (see Fig. 2-2).

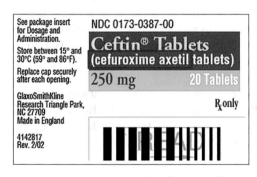

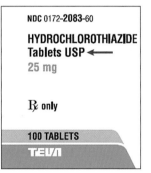

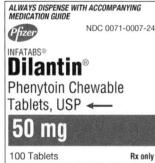

Figure 2-1. Generic name identified in red box.   **Figure 2-2.** USP letters on the drug label.

The Brand Name

The **brand name, trade name,** or **proprietary name** is the name given to the drug by a specific drug manufacturer. Every drug manufacturer that makes the same drug assigns a brand name to that drug. Therefore, the same drug can have several brand names. The brand name on the drug may have a combination of upper- and lowercase letters or may be written with just uppercase letters. Frequently the symbol ® is found on the right-hand corner of the brand name. This indicates that the drug name is registered and trademark protected. Thus, the production of the drug under the registered trademark name is restricted to the specific drug manufacturer. (See Fig. 2-3.)

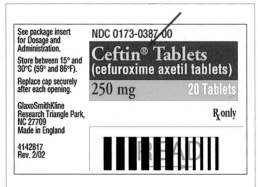

Figure 2-3. Drug label with registered trademark brand name.

The Drug Name and Tall Man Lettering

There are several drugs that have names that look alike and sound alike. The similarity of the drug names creates an environment that contributes to potential medication errors. To minimize the risk of medication errors, patient safety organizations such as the Institute for Safe Medication Practices (ISMP), the National Association of Boards of Pharmacy, and The Joint Commission have identified a list of look-alike drug names and instituted the use of tall man lettering to reduce the confusion between these drug names. ***Tall man lettering*** is the use of mixed case letters (lower- and uppercase) in a drug name with the specific purpose of highlighting a section of the drug name to help distinguish the name from other similar drug names. Table 2-2 provides an example of drug names that may be confused with other drug names and are now written using the tall man lettering format. A complete listing of additional drugs names written with tall man lettering can be found at http://www.ismp.org.

A drug name containing tall man lettering on the label provides an additional precautionary alert for all healthcare personnel who handle the drug. Tall man lettering may appear at the beginning, in the middle, or at the end of the drug name (Fig. 2-4). In adhering to the first right of medication administration (the right drug), the nurse is the final person that ensures that the right drug is given to the patient. It is imperative that the nurse question any discrepancies in the drug name prior to administering the drug to the patient.

Table 2-2. Drug Names Written Using the Tall Man Lettering Format

DRUG NAME	CONFUSED WITH
aceta**ZOLAMIDE**	aceto**HEXAMIDE**
chlorpro**MAZINE**	chlorpro**PAMIDE**
DAUNOrubicin	**DOXO**rubicin
dimenhy**DRINATE**	diphenhydr**AMINE**
DOPamine	**DOBUT**amine

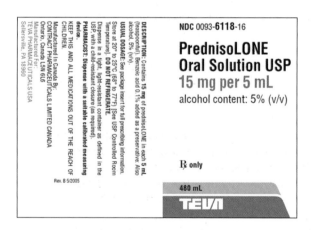
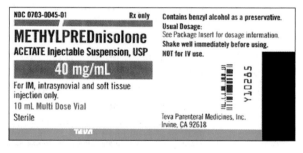

Figure 2-4. Drug names with tall man lettering.

APPLY LEARNED KNOWLEDGE 2-1

Circle "True" if the statement is correct. Circle "False" if the statement is incorrect.

1. The brand name refers to the chemical composition of the drug.   True   False

2. Tall man lettering is used for all drugs with generic names.   True   False

3. The generic name will always be listed on the drug label.   True   False

4. The brand name is assigned by the drug manufacturer.   True   False

5. The brand name is also known as the trade or proprietary name.   True   False

Table 2-3. Units of Measurement Commonly Seen on Drug Labels

UNIT OF MEASUREMENT AND ABBREVIATION	THE UNIT OF MEASUREMENT REPRESENTS	EXAMPLES		
			Strength of medication	Unit of measurement
gram (g)	Weight	Fortaz	1	g
milligram (mg)	Weight	Coreg	3.125	mg
microgram (mcg)	Weight	Lanoxin	125	mcg
milliequivalent (mEq)	The concentration of the electrolyte per liter of solution	Potassium chloride	20	mEq
unit	The potency of the drug	Heparin	5,000	units
		Regular insulin	10	units

The Strength of the Medication

The strength of the medication is another component found on every drug label. The strength of the medication signifies the strength of the active ingredient contained in one **dose** of the drug. The strength of the medication includes a number and a unit of measurement. The unit of measurement is listed after the strength of medication and represents the weight or potency of the drug. See Table 2-3 for units of measurement commonly seen on drug labels.

■ The gram, milligram, and the microgram are part of the metric system and refer to the weight of the drug. These units of measurement are written out completely or written with the approved abbreviation (g, mg, and mcg).

■ Electrolyte solutions are measured by **milliequivalents (mEq),** a unit of measurement that indicates the concentration of the electrolyte per liter of solution. Drugs with the mEq unit of measurement, such as potassium chloride, are ordered by the physician with this unit of measurement.

■ Some drugs are measured in units. Unlike units of measurement that represent the weight or quantity of a substance, a **unit** expresses the biological activity or potency of a substance that brings about a specific biological response in the body. Commonly used drugs such as heparin and insulin are measured in units. Because biological activity is unique to each drug, a unit of insulin is not the same as a unit of heparin. Drugs measured in units are ordered by the number of units to be administered. The Institute for Safe Medication Practices recommends that the word "unit" be used rather than the abbreviation "u" to avoid medication errors.

The Dosage Form

The form of the drug, called the dosage form, refers to the solid or liquid form that holds the strength of medication. The dosage form of the drug is available as

■ solid oral forms such as tablets **(scored, unscored, coated,** or **uncoated),** or capsules (spansules, caplets) (Fig. 2-5)

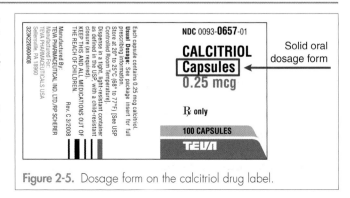

Figure 2-5. Dosage form on the calcitriol drug label.

- liquid preparations used for oral administration (**solutions, syrups,** and **suspensions**) (Fig. 2-6)
- **sterile** liquid preparations intended for parenteral administration (liquid medications and powders for injection) contained in a measured volume and expressed in mL (Fig. 2-7).

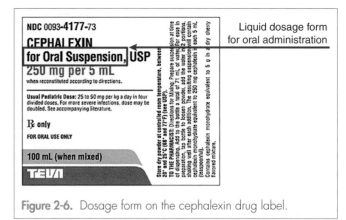

Figure 2-6. Dosage form on the cephalexin drug label.

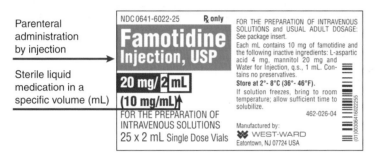

Figure 2-7. Dosage form on the famotidine drug label.

The Dosage Strength

The **dosage strength** is made up of two parts:

1. The strength of the medication with the unit of measurement
2. The dosage form, which includes the number of capsules, tablets, and so on (solid oral dosage form), or the specific volume of a liquid (oral or parenteral liquid dosage form) that contains the strength of the medication

The dosage strength for the solid oral dosage form (tablets, capsules, etc.) may be expressed in various formats on the drug label. On the side or front of the label, the nurse may find wording such as, "Each tablet contains . . .", or "Each capsule contains . . ." (Fig. 2-8) to indicate that the strength of the medication is in one tablet. The strength of the medication may be listed on the drug label without directly indicating the dosage strength (Fig. 2-9). It is implied that the strength of the drug is contained in one tablet.

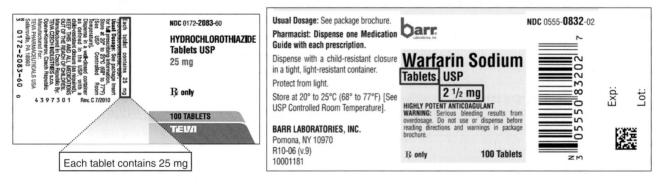

Figure 2-8. Dosage strength.

Figure 2-9. Dosage strength.

The dosage strength for liquid medications is usually expressed using a slash (/) between the strength of the medication and the dosage form. The slash " / " means "per" and when written as "/mL" is interpreted as meaning per 1 mL. For example, the dosage strength for the morphine drug label (15 mg/mL) can be written or expressed as 15 mg/mL, 15 mg per mL, or 15 mg/1 mL (Fig. 2-10).

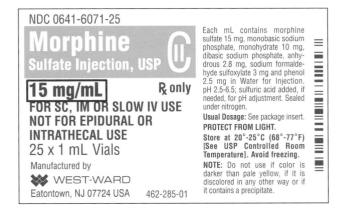

Figure 2-10. Morphine drug label identifying dosage strength.

A drug label may identify more than one dosage strength (Fig. 2-11). The nurse can choose any one of the dosage strengths from the drug label to solve for the ordered dose, as the dosage strengths listed are always equivalent.

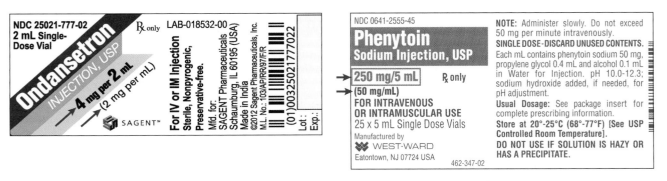

Figure 2-11. Drug labels identifying more than one dosage strength.

UNITS OF MEASUREMENT AND THE DOSAGE STRENGTH

There are also drug labels that identify the equivalent unit of measurement to help minimize errors in the calculation of drugs. The drug label in Figure 2-12, Lanoxin, identifies 62.5 mcg (0.0625 mg). The nurse can interpret this to indicate that 62.5 mcg is equivalent to 0.0625 mg. In working with the dosage strength, the nurse may use either 62.5 mcg/tablet or 0.0625 mg/tablet. Working with the metric units of measurement is found in Chapter 3, Systems of Measurement.

Figure 2-12. Equivalent units of measurement on a drug label.

FIXED DOSE COMBINATION DRUGS AND THE DOSAGE STRENGTH

There are drugs that contain two active ingredients and are manufactured in fixed dose combinations (Fig. 2-13). Although these drugs may be ordered separately, the fixed dose

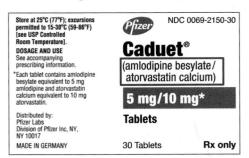

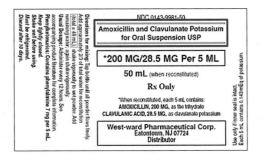

Figure 2-13. Examples of drug labels with fixed dose combinations.

combination may be more effective and convenient for certain patients. When the administration of a drug that is manufactured as a fixed dose combination is ordered, the physician's medication order will specifically indicate the drug names and the exact dosage of each of the active ingredients.

The dosage strength on the Caduet drug label can be read as 5 mg/10 mg per tablet. With fixed dose combination drug orders, the physician's order will include the number of tablets to administer, so a calculation will not be necessary (Fig. 2-14).

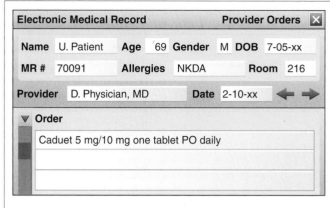

Figure 2-14. A physician's order for a fixed dose combination drug.

The Route of Administration

The route of administration provides the method of delivery by which a drug or other substance enters into the body. The ***absorption, distribution, metabolism,*** and ***excretion*** of a drug are influenced by the route of administration. In addition to administering the right drug, the nurse is responsible for administering the drug through the right route as ordered by the healthcare provider. It is important for the nurse to correctly administer drugs according to the approved route(s) identified on the drug label. Common routes of medication administration are listed in Table 2-4.

The route of administration is written in various places on the drug label. When looking at a drug label that contains the information for oral medications, such as tablets, capsules, and the like, the word "oral" as the route of administration is not written specifically on the drug label. It is understood that tablets, capsules, and so on are administered via the oral route. However, the route(s) of administration for sterile liquid dosage form (injections) and for oral liquid dosage form will be specifically written on the drug label (Fig. 2-15).

Table 2-4. Common Routes of Medication Administration

ROUTES OF ADMINISTRATION	DRUG ADMINISTRATION
Oral (PO)	By mouth/orally
Buccal (buc)	Between the gums and inner lining of the cheek
Sublingual (SL)	Under the tongue
Parenteral Injections	
• Intradermal (ID)	Into the top layers of the skin (dermis)
• Subcutaneous (subcut)	Into the subcutaneous tissue
• Intramuscular (IM)	Directly into a muscle
• Intravenous (IV)	Directly into a vein
Inhalation	Inhaled through the mouth or nose into the respiratory tract for absorption
Intranasal	Through the nasal mucosa
Intraauricular (otic)	Into the ear
Intravaginal	Into the vagina
Rectal (PR)	Into the rectum
Topical	Applied directly to the surfaces of the body or mucous membrane
Ophthalmic	Applied in the lower lid of the eye
Transdermal patches	Applied on the skin surface

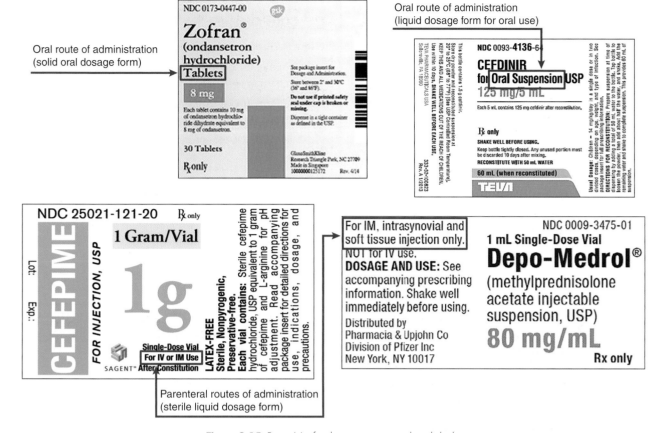

Figure 2-15. Route(s) of administration on drug labels.

APPLY LEARNED KNOWLEDGE 2-2

Review the drug label and answer the corresponding questions.

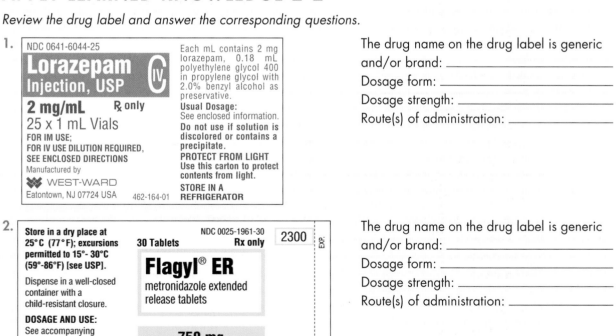

1.

The drug name on the drug label is generic and/or brand: _____

Dosage form: _____

Dosage strength: _____

Route(s) of administration: _____

2.

The drug name on the drug label is generic and/or brand: _____

Dosage form: _____

Dosage strength: _____

Route(s) of administration: _____

APPLY LEARNED KNOWLEDGE 2-2—cont'd

3.

Store at controlled room temperature 15°-30°C (59°-86°F).
Protect from light.

Dispense in a well-closed container as defined in the USP.

DOSAGE AND USE
See accompanying prescribing information.

*Each tablet contains quinapril HCl equivalent to 5 mg quinapril.

Distributed by:
Parke-Davis
Division of Pfizer Inc
NY, NY 10017

MADE IN IRELAND

Pfizer   NDC 0071-0527-23

Accupril®
(Quinapril HCl Tablets)

5 mg*

90 Tablets   **Rx only**

The drug name on the drug label is generic and/or brand: _____
Dosage form: _____
Dosage strength: _____
Route(s) of administration: _____

4.

Store at controlled room temperature 20° to 25°C (68° to 77°F) [see USP].
DOSAGE AND USE:
See accompanying prescribing information.

Each mL contains ibutilide fumarate, 0.1 mg. Also contains sodium chloride, 8.90 mg; sodium acetate trihydrate, 0.189 mg; water for injection. When necessary, pH was adjusted with sodium hydroxide and/or hydrochloric acid.

Distributed by Pharmacia & Upjohn Co
Division of Pfizer Inc, NY, NY 10017

NDC 0009-3794-01
10 mL Single-Dose Vial

Corvert®
(ibutilide fumarate injection)

1 mg/10 mL
(0.1 mg/mL)

For IV use only

Rx only

Pfizer Injectables

The drug name on the drug label is generic and/or brand: _____
Dosage form: _____
Dosage strength: _____
Route(s) of administration: _____

5.

NDC 24987-242-55   100 Tablets

LANOXIN®
(digoxin) Tablets, USP

125 mcg (0.125 mg)

Each scored tablet contains 125 mcg (0.125 mg).

Dist. by Covis Pharmaceuticals, Inc.
Cary, NC 27511
Mfd. by DSM Pharmaceuticals, Inc.
Greenville, NC 27834
Made in Germany   Rx only
100094   Rev. 6/13

See prescribing information for dosage information. Store at 25°C (77°F) in a dry place and protect from light (see insert). Dispense in tight, light-resistant container as defined in the USP. Keep out of reach of children. Do not use if printed safety seal under cap is broken or missing.

LOT/EXP AREA

011642

The drug name on the drug label is generic and/or brand: _____
Dosage form: _____
Dosage strength: _____
Route(s) of administration: _____

Dosage and Administration

The dosage and administration section on the drug label may be identified with wording such as "usual dosage," "dosage and use," "indication and use," or "dosage and administration" (Fig. 2-16). The usual dosage indicates the typical dosage or dose that is normally prescribed to treat a particular disorder or disease. The usual dosage of the drug may be listed on the label or contained in the package insert. Additional information regarding the safe and effective use of the drug is available in the package insert, drug reference book, or reliable electronic resources.

In the preparation and administration of drugs, nurses need to be knowledgeable regarding the usual dosage, drug dosages for specific populations, indication for use, drug precautions, and drug administration guidelines. For example, the dosage and administration information from the haloperidol package insert provides guidance in the administration of this intramuscular injection (Fig. 2-17). In addition to the injection site recommendation, the package insert includes extensive information for drug usage, side effects, reactions, contraindications, and other relevant information.

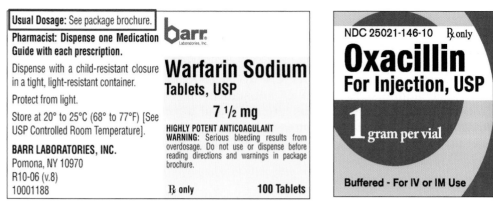

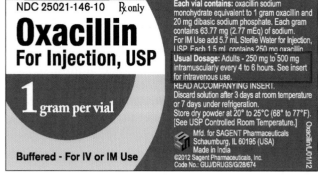

Figure 2-16. Dosage and administration information from the drug labels.

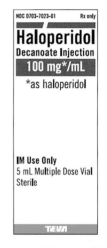

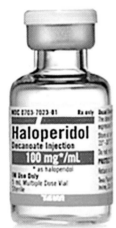

DOSAGE AND ADMINISTRATION

Haloperidol decanoate injection 50 mg/mL and haloperidol decanoate injection 100 mg/mL should be administered by <u>deep intramuscular injection</u>. A <u>21 gauge needle is recommended</u>. The maximum volume per injection site should not exceed 3 mL.

DO NOT ADMINISTER INTRAVENOUSLY.

Excerpt from **HALOPERIDOL DECANOATE-haloperidol decanoate injection Teva Parenteral Medicines, Inc. package insert 2012.**

Figure 2-17. Dosage and administration information from haloperidol package insert.

 *As patient advocates, nurses monitor the effects of drug therapy and question any drug order that is unclear or **exceeds the recommended guidelines** found on the drug label.*

Reconstitution of Powdered Drugs

Some drugs are not stable in liquid form and are manufactured in powdered form until ready for use. The powdered drug needs to be mixed, or **reconstituted,** into a liquid form before administering the drug through the oral or parenteral route. Reconstitution of powdered drugs is discussed in Chapter 12, Preparing Powdered Parenteral Medications.

The Expiration Date

The expiration date is not used in the calculation of the drug dosage but it is important information in the administration of the drug. The manufacturer's expiration date (month and year) is imprinted on the drug label and indicates the time frame in which the drug may be dispensed and used. The nurse should always check the expiration date of all drugs as part of preparation and administration of the drug to the patient. The expiration date can be located on the drug label or container.

Controlled Substances

Controlled substances are drugs or therapeutic agents that have the potential for abuse and addiction and may cause physical or mental harm. Controlled substances are regulated by state and federal laws and include narcotics, stimulants, depressants, hallucinogens, anabolic steroids, and chemicals used in the production of illegal substances. Controlled substances in the United States are regulated under the Controlled

Substances Act (CSA), Title II of the Comprehensive Drug Abuse Prevention and Control Act of 1970. Controlled substances are categorized under five schedules that are based on the drug's potential for abuse and the accepted medical use for it in the United States. (See Table 2-5.) The official list of controlled substances is updated and published annually in Title 21 Code of Federal Regulations (C.F.R.) §§ 1308.11 through 1308.15.

The nurse routinely administers controlled substances in the clinical area. The nurse can identify a controlled substance by the letter "C" and a roman numeral (I–V) found next to the drug name (Fig. 2-18). The letter "C" indicates that the drug is a controlled substance and the roman numeral signifies under which schedule the drug is categorized.

Table 2-5. Controlled Substance Schedules

Schedule I Controlled Substances (C I)

Substances in this schedule have no currently accepted medical use in the United States, a lack of accepted safety for use under medical supervision, and a high potential for abuse.

Examples of Schedule I

Heroin, lysergic acid diethylamide (LSD), marijuana a (cannabis), peyote, methaqualone, and 3, 4-methylenedioxymethamphetamine ("Ecstasy").

Schedule II Controlled Substances (C II)

Substances in this schedule have a high potential for abuse that may lead to severe psychological or physical dependence.

Examples of Schedule II

Narcotics: hydromorphone (Dilaudid), methadone (Dolophine), meperidine (Demerol), oxycodone (OxyContin, Percocet), and fentanyl (Sublimaze, Duragesic), morphine, opium, and codeine.

Stimulants: amphetamine (Dexedrine, Adderall), methamphetamine (Desoxyn), and methylphenidate (Ritalin).

Substances: amobarbital, glutethimide, and pentobarbital.

Schedule III Controlled Substances (C III)

Substances in this schedule have a potential for abuse less than substances in Schedules I or II and abuse may lead to moderate or low physical dependence or high psychological dependence.

Examples of Schedule III

Narcotics: combination products containing less than 15 milligrams of hydrocodone per dosage unit (Vicodin), products containing not more than 90 milligrams of codeine per dosage unit (Tylenol with Codeine), and buprenorphine (Suboxone).

Non-narcotics: benzphetamine (Didrex), phendimetrazine, ketamine, and anabolic steroids such as Depo-Testosterone.

Schedule IV Controlled Substances (C IV)

Substances in this schedule have a low potential for abuse relative to substances in Schedule III.

Examples of Schedule IV

Substances: alprazolam (Xanax), carisoprodol (Soma), clonazepam (Klonopin), clorazepate (Tranxene), diazepam (Valium), lorazepam (Ativan), midazolam (Versed), temazepam (Restoril), and triazolam (Halcion).

Schedule V Controlled Substances (C V)

Substances in this schedule have a low potential for abuse relative to substances listed in Schedule IV and consist primarily of preparations containing limited quantities of certain narcotics.

Examples of Schedule V

Substances: cough preparations containing not more than 200 milligrams of codeine per 100 milliliters or per 100 grams (Robitussin AC, Phenergan with Codeine), and ezogabine.

U.S. Department of Justice, Drug Enforcement Administration, Office of Diversion Control. *Controlled Substance Schedules.* http://www.deadiversion.usdoj.gov/schedules/index.html#define

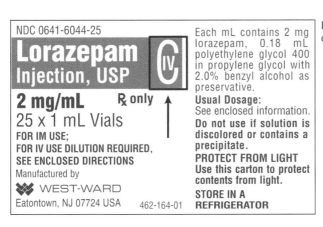

Lorazepam is a controlled substance categorized under Schedule IV.

Figure 2-18. Controlled substance identified on the drug label.

APPLY LEARNED KNOWLEDGE 2-3

Define the following words used in the administration of medication.

1. CII on a drug label: _____

2. Usual dosage: _____

3. Expiration date: _____

4. Reconstitution: _____

5. Dosage form: _____

Black Box Warning and the Role of the FDA

The United States Food and Drug Administration (FDA) is the government agency that is responsible for protecting the public health of consumers. One of the many functions of the FDA is to grant approval of drugs for human and animal use. FDA approval indicates that the FDA has determined that the benefits of the drug outweigh the risks of its intended medical use. The FDA regulates over-the-counter and prescription drug labeling and establishes drug manufacturing standards.

BLACK BOX WARNING

The FDA mandates that certain prescription drugs contain a black box warning. The black box warning is an indication that the drug carries significant **adverse effects** that may be life-threatening or may contribute to serious disability. Information about these adverse effects may be found in the package insert. The alert or warning is outlined with a black box on the drug label (Fig. 2-19). For example, on the Wellbutrin SR drug label, the black box warning refers to a Medication Guide that accompanies the drug and provides more information regarding the adverse effects of the drug.

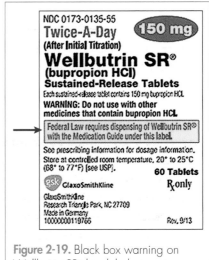

Figure 2-19. Black box warning on Wellbutrin SR drug label.

 For patient safety, the nurse must know why a drug has been ordered for the patient and must research the drug information for adverse effects. The nurse's ongoing contact with the patient provides an excellent opportunity for the nurse to monitor and assess the patient for adverse drug effects.

Single-Dose and Multi-Dose Containers

Parenteral medications used for injections or intravenous infusions are available in vials that may indicate "single-dose" or "multi-dose" use (see Figs. 2-20 and 2-21). Medications available in single dose vials are typically *preservative-free,* meaning that they do not contain *antimicrobial preservatives.* Antimicrobial preservatives help to minimize the growth of bacteria once a vial has been opened or needle-punctured. A vial labeled single-dose indicates that the vial is to be discarded after a dose of medication has been withdrawn, regardless of the volume of medication remaining in the vial. For example, if the physician ordered 2 mL of furosemide and there are 4 mL in the single-dose vial, the nurse would discard the vial after withdrawing the 2 mL dose.

Additional single dose containers include the prefilled syringe and ampule. The term "single-dose" is not specifically written on a prefilled syringe or an ampule. However, it is understood that a prefilled syringe is designated for one patient use and an ampule, once opened, cannot be resealed.

A multi-dose vial contains a preservative and may be used to administer multiple doses of the medication. It is recommended that an opened multi-dose vial be assigned to a single patient. To ensure the effectiveness of the drug, the United States Pharmacopeia recommends writing the date directly on the drug label to indicate when the multi-dose vial was opened or needle punctured. The opened multi-dose vial should be discarded within 28 days unless the manufacture indicates a different date (United States Pharmacopeia [USP] [2008, June 1]. Chapter 797: *Guidebook to pharmaceutical compounding— sterile preparations* [2nd ed.]).

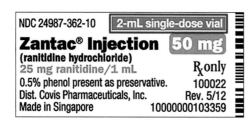

Figure 2-20. Single-dose vial drug label.

Figure 2-21. Multi-dose vial drug label.

Storage Information

All drug bottles have storage directions on the label. To maintain drug potency, drugs should be stored according to the manufacturer's guidelines. The drug label provides storage information such as "store at room temperature," "refrigerate after opening," and "protect from light." It is important to include storage directions when providing drug information to patients and families. Proper drug storage tips include the following:

■ Follow storage directions on the drug label (store drug at room temperature or in the refrigerator).

■ If refrigeration is required, make sure drugs do not freeze.

■ Store medications in a cool, dry area.

■ Maintain drugs in original drug containers.

■ Avoid prolong exposure of drugs to direct heat or sunlight.

■ Avoid storing drugs in the kitchen or bathroom because this exposes drugs to heat and humidity.

(U.S. Pharmacopeia, http://www.uspnf.com/uspnf/pub/index?usp=34&nf=29&s=1&officialOn=August 1, 2011. Accessed August 26, 2011.)

Total Amount in Bottle

The total amount identified on the drug label indicates the total number or quantity contained in a bottle or package. Although the total amount is not used in the calculations of drug doses, the nurse can assist patients and families to determine how many doses or number of days a drug will last or may provide advice as to when a prescription drug should be refilled. In healthcare facilities, the nurse is provided with a **unit dose** of a patient's ordered medication. The unit dose contains one dose of the medication. This eliminates the need for the storage of large quantities of medication bottles on the unit. (See Figs. 2-22 and 2-23.)

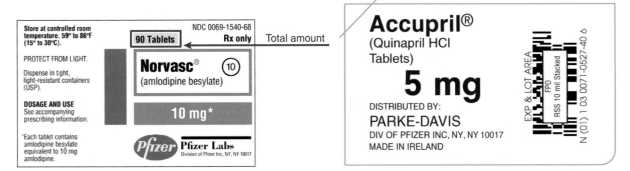

Figure 2-22. Total amount on drug label.   Figure 2-23. Unit dose.

 Safe medication administration is a collaborative process that includes the physician, the pharmacist, the nurse, and patient/family education.

Lot Number

Lot numbers are any unique combination of letters, numbers, or symbols that are assigned by the drug manufacturer to each group or batch of drug produced. The lot number is not used in the calculation of drugs but provides information so that in case of a drug recall, the batch of drug can be traced and the distribution identified.

Manufacturer's Name

The drug manufacturer's name will always appear on the drug label. It is important not to confuse the manufacturer's name with the name of the drug. Identifying information related to the drug name such as the registered trademark symbol, brand name, generic name, and tall man lettering will assist the nurse to differentiate the drug name from the manufacturer's name.

Working With Drug Labels

Knowing how to read a drug label prepares the nurse to recognize information critical to the calculation and administration of drugs. The nurse must use the drug label, along with the patient's medication record and the physician's order, to apply the first three rights of medication administration: the right drug, the right dose, and the right route (Fig. 2-24).

Because the nurse is central to the process of medication administration, it is important for the nurse to carefully review the information on the drug labels and question any discrepancies with the pharmacist and healthcare provider.

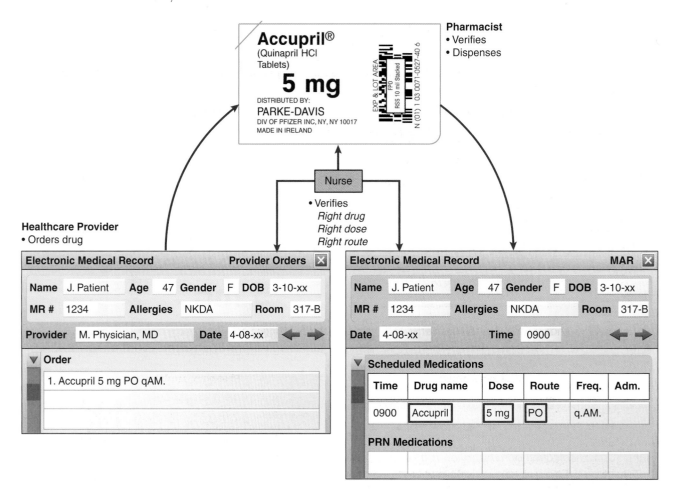

Figure 2-24. The first three rights of medication administration.

 CLINICAL REASONING 2-1

The nurse is making a home visit to a patient who is started on a new prescription for irbesartan and hydrochlorothiazide 300 mg/12.5 mg PO daily. The patient shows the nurse his previous prescription bottle because it has the same medication and asks whether he can continue taking this medication.

Patient's previous medication bottle.

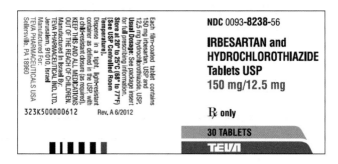

The nurse tells the patient that because the medication is the same, he can take two tablets daily from his previous medication until he gets the new medication. Has the nurse provided the correct information? Provide a rationale for your answer.

Developing Competency

Circle "Correct" or "Incorrect" for each of the following problems. For problems with incorrect answers, provide a rationale to support the answer.

1.

Physician's order:

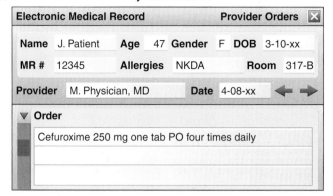

Pharmacy sends:

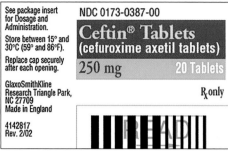

The physician has written the generic name of the drug. **Correct**   Incorrect

---

2.

Physician's order:

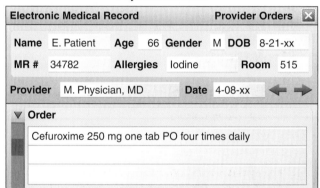

Pharmacy sends:

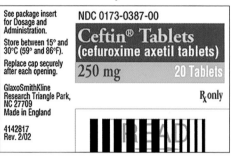

If cefuroxime is given four times a day, this medication will last 5 days. **Correct**   Incorrect

---

3.

The name of this drug is written using tall man lettering. **Correct**   Incorrect

4.

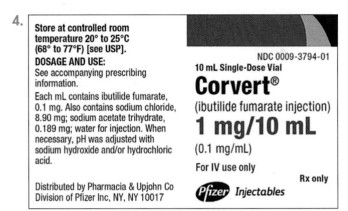

The nurse may administer multiple doses of this medication. **Correct**   Incorrect

---

5.

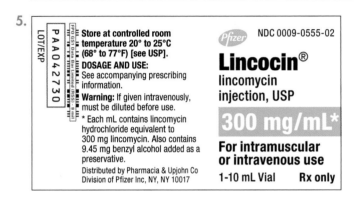

The dosage strength of this medication is 300 mg per 1 mL. **Correct**   Incorrect

---

6.

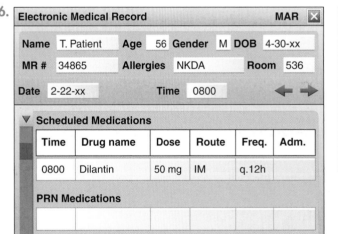

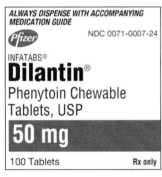

The nurse can administer the morning dose of this drug. **Correct**   Incorrect

---

7.

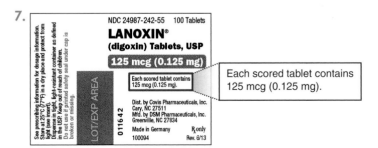

Each scored tablet contains 125 mcg (0.125 mg).

The nurse can administer half a tablet of Lanoxin if necessary. **Correct**   Incorrect

8.

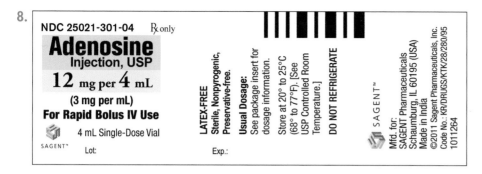

The dosage strength of this drug is 12 mg/4 mL or 3 mg/mL. **Correct**   Incorrect

9.

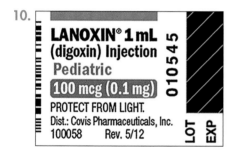

This drug is administered through the oral route. **Correct**   Incorrect

10.

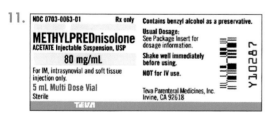

The dosage strength of this drug is 100 mcg/0.1 mg. **Correct**   Incorrect

For the following problems (11–15), choose the information that is listed on the drug label.

11.

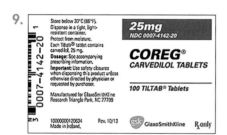

a. Black box warning
b. Multi-dose
c. IV route of administration

d. Total amount is 5 mL
e. Tall man lettering
f. Brand name

12.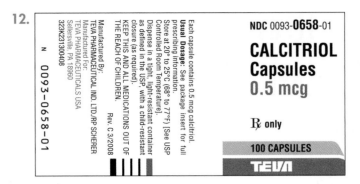

a. Unit dose
b. Dosage strength: 0.5 mcg in each capsule
c. Oral route of administration
d. Generic name
e. Tall man lettering
f. Brand name

13.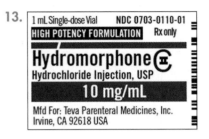

a. Multi-dose vial
b. Total amount: 1 mL
c. Brand name
d. Generic name
e. Tall man lettering
f. Controlled substance

14.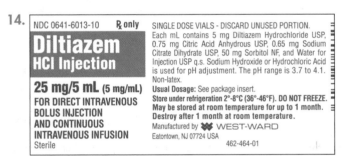

a. Dosage strength: 5 mg/mL
b. Dosage strength: 25 mg/5 mL
c. Brand name
d. Generic name
e. Storage information
f. Controlled substance

15.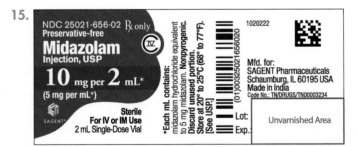

a. Multi-dose vial
b. Usual dosage
c. Brand name
d. Controlled substance
e. Tall man lettering
f. Storage information

Safety in Medication Administration

Unit Review—Evaluate for Clinical Decision Making

For questions 1 through 5, review the information provided and select all correct statement(s).

1. The nurse is preparing to administer 0900 medication to Mr. S. Patient. The nurse has a tablet of Digoxin 0.125 mg in the patient's medication drawer. In reviewing the 0900 medication order from the MAR. The nurse is most correct to first:
   a. Ask another nurse to review the order.
   b. Verify the route of administration.
   c. Check the dose against the drug label.
   d. Prepare to administer the drug orally.

Medication Administration Record					MAR

Date____10-2-xx____   Allergies____NKDA____

Scheduled Medications

Time	Drug name	Dose	Route	Freq.	Adm.
0900	Digoxin	0.125 mg		q.AM	

PRN Medications

S. Patient   MR # 64390
Age 64   DOB 2-25-xx
M. XXX M.D.   RM 413

2. Read the medication order and select the statement(s) that correspond to the order.
   a. The medication order is written correctly.
   b. The route of administration is ordered.
   c. The frequency of administration is missing.
   d. The ordered drug is administered directly into the muscle.

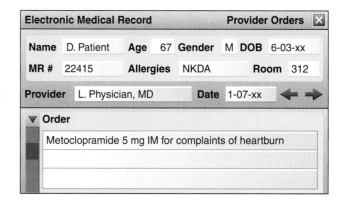

Electronic Medical Record		Provider Orders ☒

Name	D. Patient	**Age** 67 **Gender** M **DOB** 6-03-xx
MR # 22415	**Allergies** NKDA	**Room** 312

Provider L. Physician, MD   **Date** 1-07-xx ← →

▼ **Order**

Metoclopramide 5 mg IM for complaints of heartburn

3. Read the clindamycin drug label and select the statement(s) that correspond to the label.
   a. The generic name of the drug is on the label.
   b. This drug may be given orally.
   c. This drug is for parenteral use only.
   d. This drug is a controlled substance.

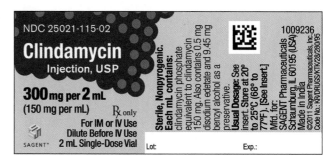

4. Read the Corvert drug label and select the statement(s) that correspond to the label.
   a. The generic name of the drug is on the drug label.
   b. The brand name of the drug is on the drug label.
   c. There are two equivalent dosage strengths.
   d. Corvert is a controlled substance.

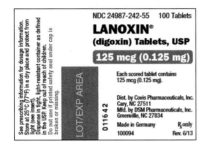

Store at controlled room temperature 20° to 25°C (68° to 77°F) [see USP].
DOSAGE AND USE:
See accompanying prescribing information.
Each mL contains ibutilide fumarate, 0.1 mg. Also contains sodium chloride, 8.90 mg; sodium acetate trihydrate, 0.189 mg; water for injection. When necessary, pH was adjusted with sodium hydroxide and/or hydrochloric acid.

Distributed by Pharmacia & Upjohn Co
Division of Pfizer Inc, NY, NY 10017

NDC 0009-3794-01
10 mL Single-Dose Vial
Corvert®
(ibutilide fumarate injection)
1 mg/10 mL
(0.1 mg/mL)
For IV use only
Rx only
Pfizer Injectables

5. Read the Lanoxin drug label and select the statement(s) that correspond to the label.
   a. The name of the drug contains tall man lettering.
   b. Digoxin is the generic name of the drug.
   c. The nurse may administer ½ tablet of Lanoxin if necessary.
   d. The drug label contains a black box warning.

NDC 24987-242-55   100 Tablets
LANOXIN®
(digoxin) Tablets, USP
125 mcg (0.125 mg)
Each scored tablet contains 125 mcg (0.125 mg).

Dist. by Covis Pharmaceuticals, Inc. Cary, NC 27511
Mfd. by DSM Pharmaceuticals, Inc. Greenville, NC 27834
Made in Germany   Rx only
100094   Rev. 6/13

Use the following MAR and drug label to answer questions 6 through 8.

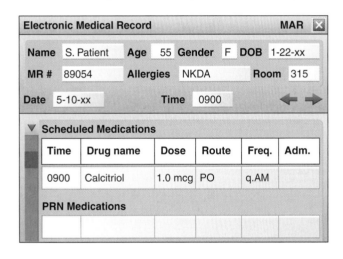

Electronic Medical Record   **MAR** ☒

| Name | S. Patient | Age | 55 | Gender | F | DOB | 1-22-xx |

| MR # | 89054 | Allergies | NKDA | Room | 315 |

| Date | 5-10-xx | Time | 0900 |

▼ Scheduled Medications

Time	Drug name	Dose	Route	Freq.	Adm.
0900	Calcitriol	1.0 mcg	PO	q.AM	

PRN Medications

NDC 0093-**0658**-01
CALCITRIOL
Capsules
0.5 mcg
Rx only
100 CAPSULES
TEVA

Manufactured By:
TEVA PHARMACEUTICAL IND. LTD./RP SCHERER
Manufactured For:
TEVA PHARMACEUTICALS USA
Sellersville, PA 18960   Rev. C 3/2008

Each capsule contains 0.5 mcg calcitriol.
Usual Dosage: See package insert for full prescribing information.
Store at 20° to 25°C (68° to 77°F) [See USP Controlled Room Temperature].
Dispense in a tight, light-resistant container as defined in the USP, with a child-resistant closure (as required).
KEEP THIS AND ALL MEDICATIONS OUT OF THE REACH OF CHILDREN.

N 0093-0658-01
323K23130O408

6. In reviewing the MAR, the nurse is correct to question the _____.

7. The unit of measurement on the drug label is _____.

8. The dosage strength of calcitriol is written as _____.

Use the following MAR and drug label to answer questions 9 and 10.

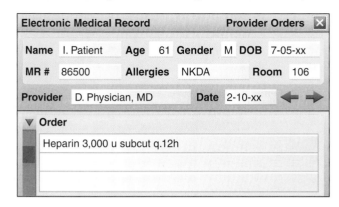

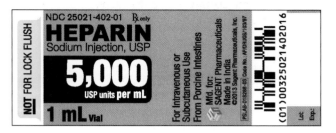

9. In reviewing the physician's order, the nurse is correct to question the _____.

10. The dosage strength of heparin is written as _____.

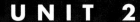

UNIT 2

Systems of Measurement

Safe practice in medication administration involves the calculation of drug dosages. This unit provides you with the foundation for working with both the metric system and the household system in the calculation of drug dosages. Understanding and working with the systems of measurement commonly used in health care is essential to safe nursing practice.

 APPLICATION TO NURSING PRACTICE

The nurse uses the metric and household systems to answer clinical questions, such as:

- *A drug contains 750 mcg of medication per tablet. How many mg does each tablet contain?*

- *The medication order is for 3 Tbs of a drug. How many mL will the nurse give?*

The nurse uses only standard rules when writing metric numbers, such as:

- *Always place a zero before a decimal fraction when there is no whole number.*

- *Omit trailing zeros.*

Finally, the nurse always thinks critically and evaluates the calculation of any dosage, asking questions such as:

- *Have I converted the metric units correctly?*

- *Have I used the correct metric to household equivalents?*

CHAPTER 3

The Metric System

LEARNING OUTCOMES

List the base units of metric measurement commonly used in clinical practice.

Identify the metric prefixes and symbols, and the numeric equivalents.

Write metric numbers using the standard rules for writing metric notations.

Convert between the metric units of measurement.

The metric system is a standard measuring system used throughout the world and is referred to as the International System of Units (SI Units). The base units of measurement used in clinical practice are the **meter,** the **gram,** and the **liter.** This system provides a systematic method for standardizing the conversion of numbers. The metric system is composed of prefixes and symbols that are used with the base units of measurement to identify larger and smaller quantities (Fig. 3-1).

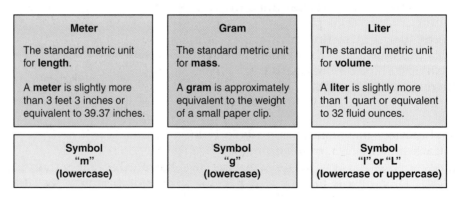

Meter	Gram	Liter
The standard metric unit for **length**.	The standard metric unit for **mass**.	The standard metric unit for **volume**.
A **meter** is slightly more than 3 feet 3 inches or equivalent to 39.37 inches.	A **gram** is approximately equivalent to the weight of a small paper clip.	A **liter** is slightly more than 1 quart or equivalent to 32 fluid ounces.
Symbol "m" (lowercase)	Symbol "g" (lowercase)	Symbol "l" or "L" (lowercase or uppercase)

Figure 3-1. Meter, gram, & liter.

The following are some examples of the application of the metric system in nursing practice:

- The patient walks 3 meters from the bed to the chair.
- The medication contains 1 gram of the drug in each tablet.
- The order is for the patient to receive 1 liter of intravenous fluid today.

The Decimal System

The key feature of the metric system is that it is based on the decimal system. Working with the metric system includes working with and understanding decimal numbers and decimal fractions.

The decimal system is based on the number 10, or powers of 10, so that multiplying or dividing by a multiple of ten (10, 100, 1000, etc.) will change the value of a number. For example, look at the number 1 in Table 3-1. Multiplying the number by a multiple of ten, such as 10, 100, or 1000, will increase the value of a number by ten, one hundred, or one thousand times.

Now look again at the number 1 in Table 3-2. Dividing the number by a multiple of ten, such as 10, 100, or 1000, will decrease the value of the number by one-tenth, one-hundredth, or one-thousandth. Note, a number that has a decimal point is referred to as a **decimal number.**

Table 3-1. Example of Multiplying a Number by 10

POWERS OF 10	MULTIPLY THE BASE NUMBER (1) BY 10	BASE NUMBER (1) × BY THE POWERS OF 10
10^1	One time	$1 \times 10 = \mathbf{10}$
10^2	Two times	$1 \times 10 \times 10 = \mathbf{100}$
10^3	Three times	$1 \times 10 \times 10 \times 10 = \mathbf{1,000}$

Table 3-2. Example of Dividing a Number by 10

POWERS OF 10	DIVIDE THE BASE NUMBER (1) BY A MULTIPLE OF 10	BASE NUMBER (1) DIVIDED BY THE POWERS OF 10 TO ARRIVE AT THE DECIMAL NUMBER
10^{-1}	$1 \div 10$	$1 \div 10 = \mathbf{0.1}$
10^{-2}	$1 \div 100$	$1 \div 100 = \mathbf{0.01}$
10^{-3}	$1 \div 1,000$	$1 \div 1,000 = \mathbf{0.001}$

The Decimal Point (.)

The decimal point is a symbol that identifies the separation of a whole number and a decimal fraction. The decimal point lies between the ones place (whole number placement) and the tenths place (fractional part of the decimal number). For example, using the number 2.5 (Fig. 3-2), the number to the left of the decimal point is the whole number (2) and the number to the right of the decimal point (.5) is the fractional part of the decimal number, or the decimal fraction.

A decimal number may consist of a whole number and a decimal fraction, as in 2.5, or may consist only of a decimal fraction, such as 0.5 or 0.75. A decimal fraction has a value of less than 1. In clinical practice, medication orders may be written as a whole number such as 2 tablets, or a number containing a decimal fraction such as 2.5 tablets or $2\frac{1}{2}$ tablets. The decimal fraction 0.5 and the fraction $\frac{1}{2}$ are equivalent.

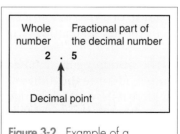

Figure 3-2. Example of a decimal number.

The decimal point is always placed to the right of a whole number. For example, using the whole number 6, the decimal point is placed to the right of the number (6 . 0 not 0 . 6).

The Use of a Zero and the Decimal Point

National organizations such as the Institute of Medicine, the Joint Commission on Accreditation of Healthcare Organizations, and the Institute for Safe Medication Practices recommend that a **leading zero** be placed before a decimal point for measurements less than 1. Notice how the leading zero is placed in the decimal fraction **0.**1 rather than just writing **.1**. Safety guidelines also state that a zero at the end of a decimal fraction, known as a **trailing zero** (e.g., **1.0**), should never be used in clinical practice because the decimal point may be overlooked and lead to the administration of an overdose.

The Decimal Fraction and Place Value

It is easy to understand the value or worth of a whole number. However, working with decimal fractions requires an understanding of how the placement of the decimal point determines the value of a number. For example, look at Figure 3-3. The decimal fraction 0.2 is in the tenths place. If the decimal point is moved from the tenths place to the hundredths place, the value of this decimal fraction becomes 0.02 or $\frac{2}{100}$. This is the same as dividing the decimal fraction by 10.

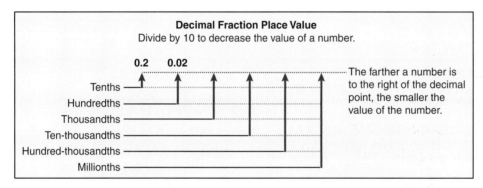

Figure 3-3. Change the value of a decimal fraction by dividing by 10.

The decimal fraction 0.02 can be divided by 10 to change value from the hundredths place to thousandths place, 0.002. Written in a fraction format, this would be $\frac{2}{1000}$.

Therefore, the value of a decimal fraction is 10 times smaller as it moves from the tenths place to the hundredths place, then from the hundredths place to the thousandths place and so on.

The value of the number can also be increased by 10 by simply multiplying the number by 10. For example, identify the millionth place in Figure 3-4. Multiply the decimal number 0.000005 (5 millionths) by 10 to change it to 0.00005 (5 hundred-thousandths). From the hundred-thousandths place, multiply 0.00005 by 10 to increase the decimal fraction to 0.0005 (5 ten-thousandths). Each time the decimal fraction is multiplied by 10, the number becomes larger.

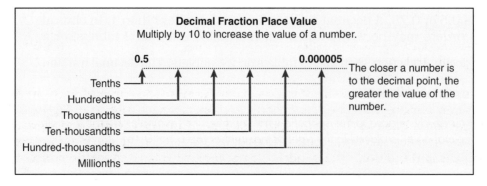

Figure 3-4. Change the value of a decimal fraction by multiplying by 10.

Did you know that each time you multiply or divide by 10 is the same as moving the decimal point one place? For example:

- *0.4 divided by 10 equals 0.04; this is the same as moving the decimal point one place from right to left: .0.4 = 0.04*
- *0.04 multiplied by 10 is the same as moving the decimal point one place from left to right: 0.04 = 0.4*

Understanding how the movement of the decimal point changes the value of a number is essential to safe practice in the administration of medications and other clinical nursing applications. For example:

■ One dose of a drug contains 0.6 grams of the medication. The physician orders 0.06 grams of the drug. In administering 0.06 grams, the nurse understands that a **smaller** dose of medication is being given to the patient.

■ One dose of a drug contains 0.003 grams of the medication. The physician orders 0.03 grams of the drug. In administering 0.03, the nurse understands that a **greater** dose of medication is being given to the patient.

APPLY LEARNED KNOWLEDGE 3-1

Circle "True" if the statement is correct. Circle "False" if the statement is incorrect.

1. 0.6 has a greater value than 0.75   True   ~~False~~

2. 0.08 has a lesser value than 0.00097   True   ~~False~~

3. 0.000003 has a lesser value that 0.001   ~~True~~   False

4. 0.638 has a greater value that 0.642   True   ~~False~~

5. 0.004 has a lesser value that 0.08   ~~True~~   False

The Metric System and the Standard Prefixes and Symbols

The metric system consists of base units of measurement and standard metric prefixes and symbols that represent the value of whole numbers and decimal fractions. For example, the whole number 1000 is represented by the prefix "kilo" and the symbol "k." The decimal fraction 0.1 is represented by the prefix "deci" and the symbol "d." The metric system contains prefixes that represent very large numbers. To effectively work with the metric system in clinical practice, it is necessary to identify the prefixes and symbols that are most commonly used for the calculation of drug dosages (Table 3-3).

Each prefix indicates a specific numeric value.

Table 3-3. Prefixes and Symbols Most Commonly Used in Drug Dosage Calculations

PREFIX	SYMBOL	NUMERIC VALUE
kilo	k	1000
centi	c	0.01
milli	m	0.001
micro	mc	0.000001

Setting up the prefixes in a line demonstrates the numeric value of each prefix and is helpful when working with the conversion of the units of measurement. Figure 3-5 shows the prefixes on a line starting with "kilo," the largest number (1000) and moving toward "micro," the smallest decimal fraction (0.000001). Note that the decimal fractions of ten-thousandths and hundred-thousandths do not have a designated metric prefix or symbol.

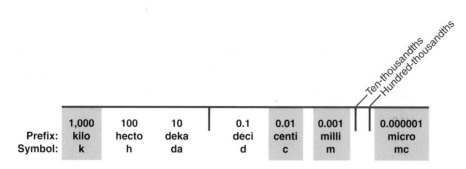

Figure 3-5. Commonly used metric prefixes and symbols in clinical practice.

Look at the line starting with the "kilo" prefix, notice how the numbers decrease in value ten times with each prefix. This is the same as dividing the numeric value of the prefix by 10. Likewise, the numbers increase in value ten times with each prefix going from right to left. This is the same as multiplying the numeric value of the prefix by 10.

APPLY LEARNED KNOWLEDGE 3-2

Circle "True" if the statement is correct. Circle "False" if the statement is incorrect.

1. The prefix "deci" represents a greater numeric value than "deka."   True   (False)

2. The prefix "centi" has a numeric value of 100.   True   (False)

3. The prefix "milli" has the same numeric value as the prefix "kilo."   True   False

4. The prefix "micro" represents the decimal fraction of 0.000001.   (True)   False

5. The prefix "hecto" has a greater value than the prefix "deka."   (True)   False

Using Metric Prefixes and Symbols

The metric prefix is always written before the base unit of measurement (liter, gram, meter). For example, the word "decigram" is formed by the metric prefix "deci" and the base unit of measurement "gram." The prefix represents a multiple of 10 and the base unit of measurement indicates the metric measurement related either to volume (liter), mass (gram), or length (meter). "Decigram" can be written as "dg" using the symbol "d" for "deci" and "g" for "gram."

Lowercase letters are used in writing the majority of the metric symbols. The exception to this is the symbol for liter. To avoid errors, the capital letter "L" is preferred because the lowercase letter "l" may be misread as the number one. Capital letters are not used in writing the metric symbols because the capital letter is a symbol for another measurement. For example, the symbol for meter is the lowercase "m." Using the capital letter "M" as the symbol for meter is not correct because this capital letter represents the prefix "mega." which means "million."

 *The lowercase letter "m" refers to both the base unit meter and the prefix "milli." To distinguish between them, remember that a prefix symbol is always placed before the base unit of measurement in defining a quantity (i.e., **mL**). If the "m" is by itself, then it represents the metric base unit for meter (i.e., 1 m).*

The Metric Line and the Base Units of Measurement

The base units of measurement are combined with the prefixes and symbols to create a line called the **metric line**. The base unit of measurement is placed on the metric line between the whole number deka and the decimal fraction deci (Fig 3-6). The metric line can be used by the nurse to convert metric units of measurement.

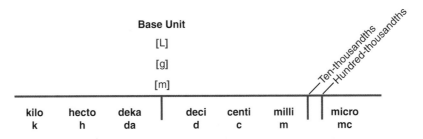

Figure 3-6. The metric line.

The Metric Line and Movement of the Decimal Point

The metric line provides a systematic way to convert between the metric units of measurement by moving the decimal point. Recall that the metric system is based on the decimal system, so that movement of the decimal point, from each unit of measurement on the metric line, changes the numeric value of the unit of measurement 10 times. Although the decimal fractions of ten-thousandths and hundred-thousandths do not have a designated metric symbol, the nurse must consider these decimal places in the movement of the decimal point.

For example, to use the metric line to convert from the **base unit** place to the **deci** (d) place requires identifying the symbols and then moving the decimal point in the correct direction. To convert:

■ First, identify the units of measurement on the metric line.

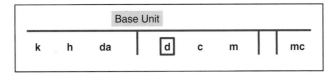

■ Second, recall that there is one decimal place between the base unit place and the deci place. Move the decimal point in the correct direction.

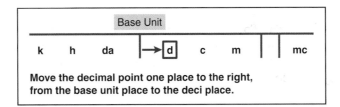

To convert from the **base unit** place to the **centi** place requires identifying the symbols on the metric line and, most important, recalling the correct number of decimal places between each prefix or symbol. To convert:

■ First, identify the units of measurement on the metric line.

■ Second, recall that there are two decimal places between the base unit place and the centi place. Move the decimal point in the correct direction.

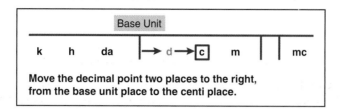

Move the decimal point two places to the right, from the base unit place to the centi place.

To convert from the **deka** place to the **kilo** place, begin by identifying the units of measurement on the metric line, recall the number of decimal places between each prefix or symbol, and then move the decimal point in the correct direction. To convert:

■ First, identify the units of measurement on the metric line.

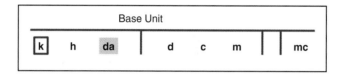

■ Second, recall that there are two decimal places between the deka place and the kilo place. Move the decimal point in the correct direction.

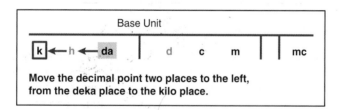

Move the decimal point two places to the left, from the deka place to the kilo place.

Memorizing the metric line with the prefix placement and the number of decimal places between each prefix allows the conversion from one unit of measurement to another on the metric line by the simple movement of the decimal point.

The decimal placements of ten-thousandths and hundred-thousandths are not identified by a metric prefix or symbol.
*To convert from the **milli** place to the **micro**, place move the decimal point three times.*

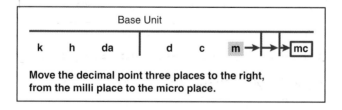

Move the decimal point three places to the right, from the milli place to the micro place.

*To convert from the **micro** place to the **milli**, place move the decimal point three times.*

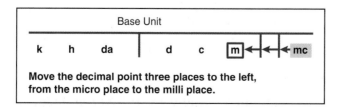

Move the decimal point three places to the left, from the micro place to the milli place.

Using the Metric Line to Solve Metric Problems

In clinical practice the nurse may need to convert between two metric units. Look at the following examples.

Example 1:

14 deciliters of water is equal to how many centiliters of water?

In this example, 14 is the quantity and deciliters and centiliters are the metric measurements. To solve the problem, use the metric line and apply the following steps:

Step 1: **Identify the starting place on the metric line.**

The starting place on the metric line identifies the quantity and the unit of measurement in the problem. In Example #1, the quantity is 14 and the base unit of measurement is the "liter." The prefix "deci" or the symbol "d" identifies the starting place. Look at the metric line and see how the number 14 is placed under the deci place and how liter is identified as the base unit.

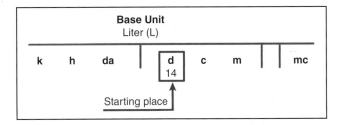

Step 2: **Identify the desired place on the metric line.**

The desired place on the metric line is the answer to the question. In Example #1, the desired unit of measurement is centiliters. How many decimal places will the decimal point need to be moved to convert from the starting place, deci, to the desired place, centi? Because working with the metric line involves the movement of the decimal point, it is important to look for the decimal point. If a number does not have a decimal point, remember to add a decimal point to the right of the whole number.

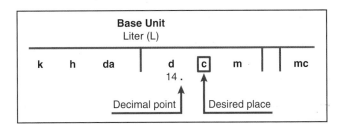

Step 3: **Convert to the desired place on the metric line by moving the decimal point.**

■ To move from the d (deci) place to the c (centi) place, move the decimal point one place (from left to right 14 **.0.**).
■ Add a zero as a placeholder.

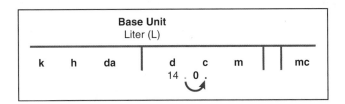

Therefore, 14 deciliters of water is equivalent to 140 centiliters of water.

In the administration of medications, the nurse may need to convert the dosage listed on a drug label. Consider this example:

Example 2:

The patient is given a medication bottle with the following drug label. What is the dose in grams (g)?

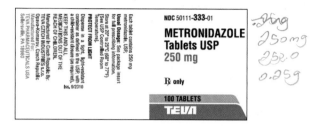

To solve, apply the following steps:

Step 1: **Identify the starting place on the metric line.**

In Example #2, the starting place on the metric line is milli (m) and 250 is the quantity. Look at the metric line and see how the number 250 is under the symbol "m." Gram is identified as the base unit.

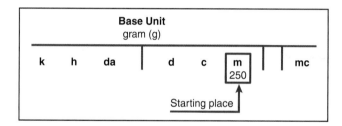

Step 2: **Identify the desired place on the metric line.**

The desired place on the metric line is the answer to the question. In Example #2, the desired unit of measurement is the base unit "g". How many places will the decimal point need to be moved to convert from the "m" place to the "g" place? Because this is a whole number, a decimal point must be added to the right of the number.

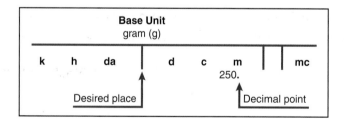

Step 3: **Convert to the desired place on the metric line by moving decimal point.**

To move from the m (milli) place to the g (gram) place, move the decimal point three places (from right to left). The first decimal point movement is from m (milli) to c (centi) 2 5 0., the second decimal place movement is from c (centi) to d (deci) 2. 5 0, and the third decimal place movement is from d (deci) to g (gram) .2 .5 0

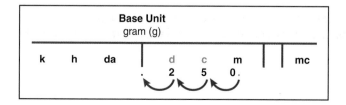

The answer 0.25 g is equivalent to a 250 mg dose of metronidazole.

Remember to always put a leading zero in front of a decimal fraction when there is no whole number.

APPLY LEARNED KNOWLEDGE 3-3

Use the metric line to convert the following problems.

Base Unit							
k	h	da		d	c	m		mc

1. 0.4 mg = ? mcg
   Starting place: ___mg___ Desired place: ___mcg___ Answer: 400mcg mcg

2. 1 m = ? km
   Starting place: ___m___ Desired place: ___km___ Answer: 0.001 Km

3. 0.3 kg = ? dag
   Starting place: ___kg___ Desired place: ___dag___ Answer: 30dag

4. 0.15 dL = ? mL
   Starting place: ___dL___ Desired place: ___ml___ Answer: 15ml

5. 550 mL = ? L
   Starting place: ___ml___ Desired place: ___L___ Answer: 0.55L

Standard Rules for Writing Metric Numbers

There are standard rules for writing metric numbers. Three of these standard rules (numbers 2, 5, and 6) are required by the Institute of Safe Medication Practices to be used by professional healthcare providers when communicating all medical information. It is important for healthcare providers to apply these standards in writing the metric notations.

1. Use arabic numbers, not roman numerals, with the metric symbols (e.g., 1 mg, 10 g, 3.5 L).
2. Always put a space between the arabic number and the metric symbol (e.g., 1 g).
3. Always place the arabic number before the metric symbol (e.g., 1 g or 2.5 mL).
4. Use decimal fractions (e.g., 0.5 mg or 0.75 cm), not fractional units (e.g., $\frac{1}{2}$ mg or $\frac{3}{4}$ cm).
5. For decimal fractions, always place a zero before the decimal point (e.g., 0.5 mL or 0.3 L).
6. Omit trailing zeros (e.g., 1 mL, not 1.0 mL).
7. Write the symbols in the singular form (e.g., 15 mL, not 15 mLs, or 100 kg, not 100 kgs).

 In clinical practice, the letters "mc" are used to represent the micro symbol. This safe practice helps healthcare providers avoid errors in interpreting and calculating drug dosages.

The Micro Symbol

The micro symbol (μ) is used in mathematics to identify the micro prefix. However, the Institute of Safe Medication Practices indicates that this symbol may be misinterpreted and may contribute to harmful medication errors. It is recommended that the micro symbol not be used by physicians or nurses to write drug orders or in communicating medical information. The symbol could be misinterpreted or confused for the metric symbol "m," which stands for the prefix "milli."

APPLY LEARNED KNOWLEDGE 3-4

Use the standard rules to evaluate the following metric numbers. For numbers that are stated incorrectly, use the standard metric rules to rewrite the metric number.

Metric Number	Correct	Incorrect		Metric Number	Correct	Incorrect
1. 0.3 mg	☒	☐		4. 250km	☒	☐ _250 km_
2. $\frac{3}{4}$ g	☐	☐ _0.75 g_		5. 60 mcgs	☐	☐ _60 mcg_
3. 1500 mL	☒	☐		6. XV L	☐	☐ _15 L_

CLINICAL REASONING 3-1

The home-care nurse is visiting a patient. The patient has two medication bottles with the same drug name, Drug A. The first medication bottle has printed on its label, "Drug A 500 mcg in each tablet." The second medication bottle has printed on its label, "Drug A 0.5 mg in each tablet." Is the nurse correct in informing the patient that the doses are equivalent? Provide a rationale for your answer.

In summary, the nurse uses the metric system in providing care to patients, especially in the administration of medications. Knowing how to work with the metric system to convert units of measurement will help the nurse to calculate and verify medications doses.

Developing Competency

Use the metric line to convert the following metric problems.

1. 0.002 kg×10= _?.02_ hg _0.02_
2. 25 dam÷10 = _?0.025_ m _250_
3. 5 dm×10= _? 50_ m _0.5_
4. 650 mL÷100= _?.65_ dL _6.5_
5. 700 mcg÷1000= _?0.07_ mg _0.7_
6. The nurse has a medication bottle with the following drug label. How many g will the patient take per tablet? _0.025g_

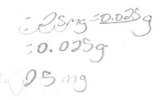

25mg=0.025g
=0.025g
25 mg

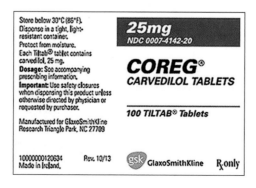

Store below 30°C (86°F). Dispense in a tight, light-resistant container. Protect from moisture. Each Tiltab® tablet contains carvedilol, 25 mg.
Dosage: See accompanying prescribing information.
Important: Use safety closures when dispensing this product unless otherwise directed by physician or requested by purchaser.

Manufactured for GlaxoSmithKline Research Triangle Park, NC 27709

25mg
NDC 0007-4142-20

COREG®
CARVEDILOL TABLETS

100 TILTAB® Tablets

10000000120634   Rev. 10/13   gsk GlaxoSmithKline   ℞ only

7. A drug is labeled 750 mcg of the active ingredient in each tablet. How many mg is this equivalent to? **0.75 mg**

8. The patient is to take 1.5 liters of water. How many mL will the patient take? **1500 ml**

9. The patient received 2000 mL of intravenous fluid. How many L of intravenous fluid did the patient receive? **2 L**

10. The patient is to take 0.1 L of water every hour. How many cL of water will the patient drink every hour? **10 cL**

11. The ordered dose is for 0.4 mcg. How many cg will the patient receive? **0.00004 cg**

12. The nurse will give 1 liter of intravenous fluid every 8 hours. How many mL will the patient receive every 8 hours? **1000 ml**

13. The patient is instructed to walk 100 meters every morning. How many km will the patient walk? **0.1 Km**

14. The nurse will give 1000 cL of a fluid to a patient. How many daL will the patient receive? **1 daL**

15. A drug contains 0.01 kilogram of a chemical substance. How many hg of the chemical does the drug contain? **0.1 hg**

Identify the metric notation error in following problems. Correct the problem by applying the metric notation rule.

		Metric Notation Error	Corrected Notation
16.	0.10 mL =	Trailing Zero	0.1 ml
17.	$\frac{1}{2}$ mg =	Fraction	0.5 mg
18.	15 mls =	"s" Added mL	15 ml
19.	5cm =	no space	5 cm
20.	m 3 =	"m" on left Side	3 m

CHAPTER 4

The Household System

LEARNING OUTCOMES

Identify the common household units of measurement used in clinical practice.

Write the household units of measurement using the correct abbreviations.

Identify the equivalent measurements for the household and metric units.

Use metric equivalent measurements to convert common household measurements.

Solve drug dosage problems using household units.

The household system consists of units of measurement used for measuring liquid volume, weight, and distance. Common household utensils used for measuring liquid volume vary in size and are only an approximation of the quantity. To assist patients, especially in the home-care setting, the nurse must be familiar with equivalencies between common household utensils and more accurate measuring devices. Many pharmacies provide measuring devices with liquid medications for use in the home. See Table 4-1 for common household measurements and abbreviations.

Table 4-1. Common Household Measurements and Abbreviations

HOUSEHOLD UNIT OF MEASUREMENT	STANDARD ABBREVIATION	OTHER COMMON ABBREVIATIONS
tablespoon	Tbs	Tbsp, tbsp, tbs (T)
teaspoon	tsp	Tsp (t)
ounce	oz	
drops	gtt	
glass	(none)	
cup	(none)	
pound	lb	
inch	in	

The use of "T" for tablespoon and "t" for teaspoon may be misinterpreted, increasing the risk of a medication error. For safe practice, it is best to use the full standard abbreviation (such as Tbs or tsp).

Because the household system is not a precise system of measurement, standard household measurements are converted to metric equivalent measurements to identify precise quantities (Table 4-2).

Table 4-2. Household and Metric Equivalents

HOUSEHOLD UNIT OF MEASUREMENT	STANDARD ABBREVIATION	HOUSEHOLD APPROXIMATIONS	METRIC EQUIVALENT
tablespoon	Tbs	3 tsp	15 mL
teaspoon	tsp	(none)	5 mL
ounce	oz	6 tsp, 2 Tbs	30 mL
drops	gtt	(none)	none
glass	(none)	6 oz	180 mL
		8 oz	240 mL
cup	(none)	6 oz	180 mL
		8 oz	240 mL
pound	lb	2.2 lb	1 kg
inch	in	1 in	2.54 cm

Household System Notations

There are few specific guidelines for writing household notations. However, as with the metric system, it is recommended that the singular form be used when writing standard household abbreviations.

For example, the singular form "oz" is used for both ounce and ounces.

■ Give **1 oz** of a liquid medication.
■ Give **6 oz** of a liquid medication.

The same applies when using the abbreviations for teaspoons and tablespoons.

■ Give **3 tsp** of a liquid medication.
■ Administer **1 tsp** of the ordered drug.
■ Give **2 Tbs** of a liquid medication.
■ Administer **1 Tbs** of the ordered drug.

Because nurses continuously work with medication orders, the nurse can take the lead in promoting the use of standard abbreviations by all healthcare professionals who write medication orders using the household system.

Converting Within the Household Units of Measurement

To convert from one household unit of measurement to another household unit of measurement requires simple memorization of a few measurements. Knowing these equivalent measurements is helpful in solving simple problems.

HOUSEHOLD UNITS OF MEASUREMENT		HOUSEHOLD EQUIVALENT MEASUREMENTS
For 1 ounce (oz)	memorize	2 (Tbs, 6 tsp)
For 1 tablespoon	memorize	3 tsp

Example:

The medication order is for 2 Tbs of a drug. How many oz will the nurse give?

To solve this problem, simply recall the equivalent measurement: 2 Tbs is equal to 1 oz.

APPLY LEARNED KNOWLEDGE 4-1

Fill in the standard abbreviation and the equivalent measurements, as appropriate, for the household and metric systems.

	Standard Abbreviation(s)	Household Equivalent Measurement	Metric Equivalent Measurement
1. ounce =	_____	_____	_____
2. drops =	_____	_____	_____
3. tablespoon =	_____	_____	_____
4. teaspoon =	_____	_____	_____
5. glass (8 oz) =	_____	_____	_____
6. cup (6 oz) =	_____	_____	_____

Using the Household and Metric Systems

The most frequently used household units of measurement in clinical practice are the tablespoon, the teaspoon, the ounce, the glass, and the cup. In the following example, the physician's order identifies the amount of guaifenesin in mL. To determine the household equivalent measurement, the nurse recalls that 5 mL is equal to 1 tsp.

Example of Physician's Order:

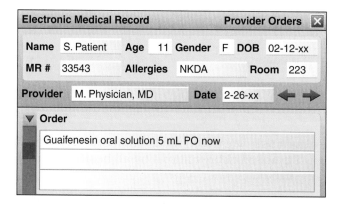

Electronic Medical Record	Provider Orders ☒

Name S. Patient   **Age** 11 **Gender** F **DOB** 02-12-xx

MR # 33543   **Allergies** NKDA   **Room** 223

Provider M. Physician, MD   **Date** 2-26-xx ⬅ ➡

▼ **Order**

Guaifenesin oral solution 5 mL PO now

It is important to remember that the household system is not precise and the measurement of liquid medications will vary with the use of common household utensils such as the teaspoon, the tablespoon, and household glasses and cups. Patients and families need to be taught to use standard measuring equipment to ensure accurate measurement of liquid medications.

CLINICAL REASONING 4-1

The doctor orders 2 tsp of a liquid antibiotic for the patient every 12 hours. The nurse instructs the patient to take 1 oz of the medication at 9 a.m. and the other ounce at 9 p.m. Has the nurse provided the patient with the correct instructions? Provide a rationale for your answer.

Developing Competency

Read the problem, and then select the correct household to metric equivalent measurement(s) to recall for solving the problem.

1. The medication order is for 3 Tbs of a drug. How many mL will the nurse give?
   a. 2 Tbs equals 30 mL
   b. 6 tsp equals 30 mL
   c. 1 Tbs equals 15 mL
   d. 1 oz equals 30 mL

2. The patient says that he routinely takes 2 tsp of a drug. How many mL does the patient take?
   a. 1 Tbs equals 3 tsp
   b. 6 tsp equals 30 mL
   c. 1 tsp equals 5 mL
   d. 1 oz equals 6 tsp

3. The nurse gives 0.5 oz of a medication. How many mL does the patient receive?
   a. 1 Tbs equals 3 tsp
   b. 15 mL equals 1 Tbs
   c. 1 oz equals 30 mL
   d. 1 oz equals 6 tsp

4. The patient is instructed to drink one 8 oz glass of water with the medication. How many mL will the patient drink?
   a. 2 Tbs equals 1 oz
   b. 1 oz equals 30 mL
   c. 3 tsp equals 15 mL
   d. 1 oz equals 6 tsp

5. The nurse records that the patient took 675 mL of fluid during the morning. How many ounces did the patient drink?
   a. 2 Tbs equals 1 oz
   b. 1 oz equals 30 mL
   c. 3 tsp equals 15 mL
   d. 1 oz equals 6 tsp

6. The order is to give the patient 20 mL of a drug. How many tsp does the patient receive?
   a. 5 mL equals 1 tsp
   b. 15 mL equals 3 tsp
   c. 1 oz equals 30 mL
   d. 2 Tbs equals 6 tsp

7. The nurse is preparing to mix 2 Tbs of a drug into a glass of water. How many mL will the nurse add to the water?
   a. 1 Tbs equals 3 tsp
   b. 15 mL equals 1 Tbs
   c. 1 Tbs equals 15 mL
   d. 1 oz equals 6 tsp

8. The order is to give the patient 30 mL of a drug. How many Tbs will the nurse instruct the patient to take?
   a. 15 mL equals 1 Tbs
   b. 3 tsp equals 15 mL
   c. 2 Tbs equals 6 tsp
   d. 1 oz equals 30 mL

9. The patient receives 6 Tbs of a drug. How many ounces will the patient take?
   a. 3 tsp equals 15 mL
   b. 1 oz equals 6 tsp
   c. 1 Tbs equals 15 mL
   d. 1 oz equals 2 Tbs

10. The medication order is to give the patient 12 ounces of juice. How many mL will the patient drink?
    a. 1 oz equals 30 mL
    b. 1 oz equals 6 tsp
    c. 15 mL equals 3 tsp
    d. 1 Tbs equals 3 tsp

Systems of Measurement
Unit Review—Evaluate for Clinical Decision Making

*For each question, use your clinical judgment to determine whether the nurse's decision is **Correct** or **Incorrect**. For incorrect problems, write the correct answer.*

1. To convert from the kilo placement to the hecto placement, move the decimal point one place, from left to right.

Correct	Incorrect	Answer: _____

2. The doctor's order is for 100 mcg of a tablet. The nurse is planning to administer a tablet labeled 1 mg.

Correct	Incorrect	Answer: _____

3. The following is the medication order: Give 1.0 mg of Drug A. The nurse is most correct to ask the doctor to clarify the order.

Correct	Incorrect	Answer: _____

4. The patient drank 2.5 L of fluid for the shift. The nurse reports that the patient drank 250 mL.

Correct	Incorrect	Answer: _____

5. The nurse is preparing to administer 375 mg of a drug. The nurse calculates that 0.0375 g will need to be administered.

Correct	Incorrect	Answer: _____

6. The nurse is asked to administer 0.5 mg. The nurse calculates that 50 mcg is the equivalent dose of the drug.

Correct	Incorrect	Answer: _____

7. The following is the medication order: Give 3 μg of Drug D. The nurse is most correct to give one tablet labeled Drug D 3 mg.

Correct	Incorrect	Answer: _____

8. The medication order is for 3 Tbs of a drug. The nurse prepares 1.5 ounces of the drug.

Correct	Incorrect	Answer: _____

9. The patient says that he routinely takes 2 tsp of the prescribed liquid drug. The nurse prepares 30 mL of the drug.

Correct	Incorrect	Answer: _____

10. The order is to give 0.5 oz of a medication. The nurse prepares 15 mL of the drug.

Correct	Incorrect	Answer: _____

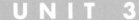

UNIT 3

Methods of Calculation

dministration of medications involves validating the correct dosage. This may require the nurse to do a mathematical calculation using the metric and household units of measurement. This unit discusses four of the main methods used in clinical calculations. For safe practice, choose the method that is best for you, and continue to use it with all of your dosage calculations.

⚠ APPLICATION TO NURSING PRACTICE

The nurse has an order to administer glycopyrrolate 150 mcg IV this morning. The pharmacy sends a vial of glycopyrrolate, and the nurse prepares to administer the drug to the patient.

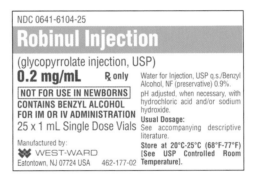

To accurately calculate the dosage for this medication, the nurse uses clinical reasoning to determine the following:

- *What is the dosage strength of this drug?*
- *How will I convert between mg and mcg?*
- *Does the answer make sense?*

CHAPTER 5

Linear Ratio and Proportion

LEARNING OUTCOMES

Define ratio *and* proportion.

Discuss how dosage strength is used in ratio and proportion.

Set up a ratio and proportion using the linear format.

Solve drug dosage calculation problems using the linear ratio and proportion method.

The medication administration process involves many members of the healthcare team: the physician prescribes the medication, the pharmacist dispenses the medication, and the nurse gives the medication to the patient. As the healthcare professional who administers the medication to the patient, the nurse has the responsibility to verify the ordered dose.

Safe medication administration requires that before giving any medication, the nurse must validate the **dosage.** Sometimes a calculation is required to determine how much of the medication to give. One method of solving a dosage calculation is the ratio and proportion method. This is a very useful method for nurses, as it can be used to solve all dosage and clinical math calculations.

Ratios

A **ratio** is a comparison of two numbers that have a relationship to each other. In nursing practice, there are many numbers that are related to each other. For example:

- A patient weighs 185 lb on admission and 182 lb after taking a diuretic medication.
- 10 milligrams of medication is contained in each capsule.
- The patient's pulse at 7:00 a.m. is 86 beats per minute. At noon, the patient's pulse is 78 beats per minute.

Numbers that are related can be written in a **linear** mathematical format.

LINEAR FORMAT

A ratio set up in a linear format uses a colon (**:**) to show the relationship between two numbers.

Two numbers expressed in a ratio look like this:

> 185 lb : 182 lb
>
> 10 mg : 1 capsule
>
> 86 beats per minute : 78 beats per minute

The linear format is read:

> 185 lb **is to** 182 lb
>
> 10 mg **is to** 1 capsule
>
> 86 beats per minute **is to** 78 beats per minute

 Did you know that the colon (:) used in the linear format, together with the line (—) used when writing a ratio as a fraction, are both derived from the symbol for division (÷)?

Proportions

A ratio by itself does not help the nurse calculate a drug dosage. To solve a dosage problem, the nurse needs to use a **proportion.** In math, a proportion is a statement that two ratios are equal. Stated another way, a proportion is an equation of two ratios. Like a ratio, a proportion can be written using a linear format.

LINEAR FORMAT

A proportion in a linear format uses a double colon (::) to show the relationship between the two ratios. Here are two examples:

> 1 : 2 :: 2 : 4
>
> 10 mg : 1 capsule :: 20 mg : 2 capsules

In each of these examples, it is easy to see that the two linear ratios are equal.

The linear proportion is read:

> 1 is to 2 **as** 2 is to 4
>
> 10 mg is to 1 capsule **as** 20 mg is to 2 capsules

When using a linear proportion to calculate a drug dosage, only three of the four numbers are known. Setting up a proportion is an easy way to solve for the fourth number.

THE MEANS AND THE EXTREMES

With a linear proportion, each of the numbers has a name. The numbers on the ends of the proportion are called the **extremes.** The numbers in the middle are called the **means.**

Look at the means and the extremes in the proportion 1 : 2 :: 2 : 4.

It is easy to remember the names: "e" for ends or extremes, and "m" stands for middle or means.

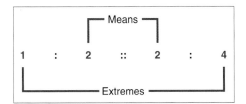

Information Needed to Set Up a Linear Proportion

To calculate a drug dosage using a linear proportion, the nurse uses two sources of information:

■ The ordered dose of medication from the physician's order

■ The dosage strength from the drug label

Each is used in setting up one ratio in the proportion used to solve a dosage calculation.

THE ORDERED DOSE

The physician who prescribes the medication specifies the drug name, dose, route, and frequency or time of administration. The ordered **dose** contains the **strength** of the medication (a number) with a **unit of measurement.**

Here is an example of a physician's order for a medication on the electronic medical record:

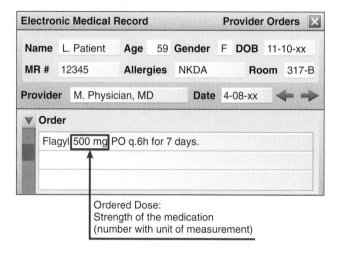

THE DOSAGE STRENGTH FROM THE DRUG LABEL

The pharmacy supplies the medication and the nurse identifies specific information from the drug label needed to set up the dosage calculation. In reviewing the drug label, the nurse will identify the following:

■ The strength of the medication

■ The dosage form in which the medication is available

Look at each part of the medication label in Figure 5-1.

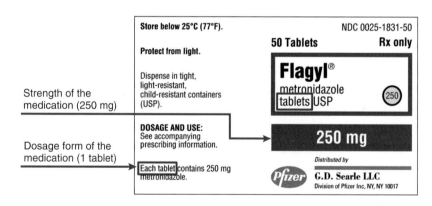

Figure 5-1. Information on the drug label: the dosage strength.

Notice that the strength of a medication is made up of a number and a unit of measurement.

The dosage form of a medication is made up of the number of capsules, tablets, and so on (solid oral dosage form) or the specific volume of liquid (oral or parenteral liquid dosage form) that contains the strength of the medication.

The strength and the dosage form of the medication are a ratio—250 mg : 1 tablet. Together, they are called the **dosage strength** of the medication. Refer to Chapter 2, The Drug Label, for more information on the dosage strength of a medication.

The dosage strength can be written in several ways on a drug label. Here are some examples. Notice where the dosage strength is found on each drug label and how it is written as a linear ratio:

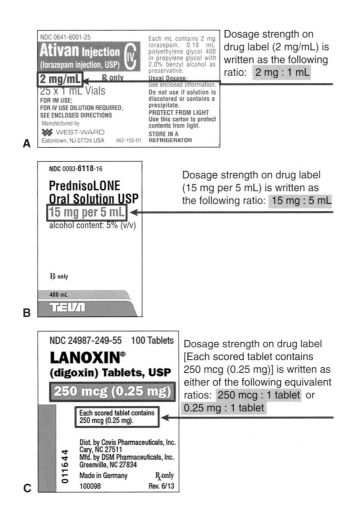

Dosage strength on drug label (2 mg/mL) is written as the following ratio: 2 mg : 1 mL

Dosage strength on drug label (15 mg per 5 mL) is written as the following ratio: 15 mg : 5 mL

Dosage strength on drug label [Each scored tablet contains 250 mcg (0.25 mg)] is written as either of the following equivalent ratios: 250 mcg : 1 tablet or 0.25 mg : 1 tablet

APPLY LEARNED KNOWLEDGE 5-1

Write the linear ratio that expresses the correct dosage strength for the medications below.

1.

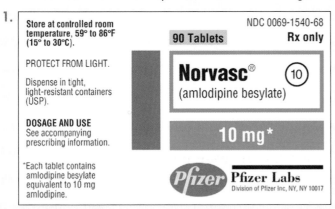

APPLY LEARNED KNOWLEDGE 5-1—cont'd

2.
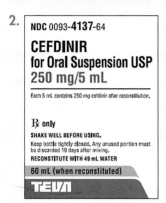

3.
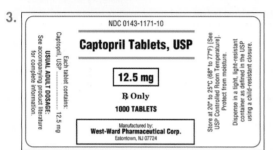

4.

NDC 24987-362-10   2-mL single-dose vial
Zantac® Injection   50 mg
(ranitidine hydrochloride)
25 mg ranitidine/1 mL   R̶x only
0.5% phenol present as preservative.   100022
Dist. Covis Pharmaceuticals, Inc.   Rev. 5/12
Made in Singapore   10000000103359

5.
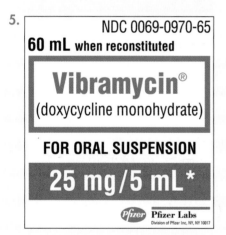

Solving Dosage Calculations With a Linear Proportion

A linear proportion can be used to solve any drug dosage calculation. A proportion contains two equal ratios, and if three of the four numbers in a proportion are known, it is easy to find the value of the unknown fourth number (or "x").

With most dosage calculations, the dosage strength of the medication is used as the first ratio.

■ This first ratio is called the **known ratio,** as its two parts are always known from the drug label (the strength of medication and the dosage form in which the medication is available).

■ The second ratio in the proportion is called the **unknown ratio,** as it contains the ordered dose and the unknown quantity. In setting up the ratio with an unknown, "x" represents the unknown quantity.

See Figure 5-2 for an example of how the dosage strength on the drug label (the known ratio) and the ordered dose (part of the unknown ratio) are used in setting up a proportion.

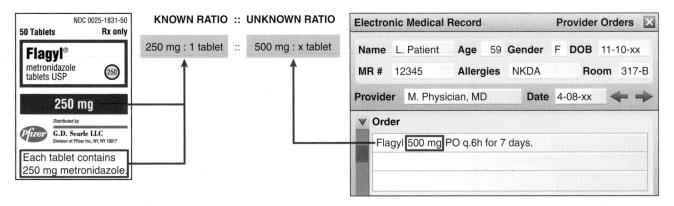

Figure 5-2. Setting up the known and the unknown ratios.

In the example in Figure 5-2, the nurse has an order to give 500 mg of Flagyl. The medication is available in 250 mg tablets. The nurse needs to know how many tablets to administer to the patient.

STEPS FOR SETTING UP AND SOLVING A LINEAR PROPORTION

Here are the steps to set up and solve a linear proportion using the known and unknown ratios:

- **First,** write the known ratio: the dosage strength from the drug label. Notice that the units of measurement are included as well as the numbers.

> **KNOWN RATIO   ::**
>
> 250 mg : 1 tablet ::

- **Second,** write the unknown ratio: the ordered dose and the unknown amount to administer, which is written as "*x*."

The proportion using the known and unknown ratios is now set up.

> **KNOWN RATIO   ::   UNKNOWN RATIO**
>
> 250 mg : 1 tablet :: 500 mg : *x* tablet

- **Third,** check the units of measurement. Both ratios must contain the same two units in the same order.

Each ratio in the proportion has the same two units, mg and tablets. The unit of measurement of the first

> **KNOWN RATIO   ::   UNKNOWN RATIO**
>
> 250 mg : 1 tablet :: 500 mg : *x* tablet

number of both ratios (mg) is the same, and the unit of measurement of the second number of both ratios (tablet) is the same.

If the ratios and the units are not set up in the correct order, the answer will not be correct. If the units are not the same, a conversion must be done. Conversions are discussed at the end of this chapter.

- **Fourth,** Solve for *x* by multiplying the means and the extremes.
  - Multiply the means and the extremes (work only with the numbers, not the units of measurement).
  - Clear the *x* by dividing both sides of the equation by the number in front of the *x*.
  - Solve for *x*.
  - Put the answer back in the original equation to find the correct unit of measurement.
  - Think critically: Does the answer make sense?

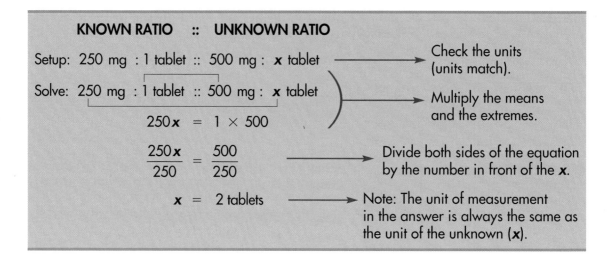

KNOWN RATIO   ::   UNKNOWN RATIO

Setup: 250 mg : 1 tablet :: 500 mg : **x** tablet   ⟶ Check the units (units match).

Solve: 250 mg : 1 tablet :: 500 mg : **x** tablet

$$250x = 1 \times 500$$

⟶ Multiply the means and the extremes.

$$\frac{250x}{250} = \frac{500}{250}$$

⟶ Divide both sides of the equation by the number in front of the **x**.

$$x = 2 \text{ tablets}$$

⟶ Note: The unit of measurement in the answer is always the same as the unit of the unknown (**x**).

*The important rule to remember in working with linear proportions is that the **product** of the means is equal to the product of the extremes. Or, the answer of the multiplication of the means equals the answer of the multiplication of the extremes. This provides a convenient way to double check that the answer is correct: if the answer is put back into the setup, then the products of the means and the extremes should be equal. For example, in the above calculation: $250 \times 2 = 1 \times 500$. The calculation is correct.*

Here is another example of how to set up and solve a dosage calculation using a linear proportion. Note that the question asks for the number of mg per dose, rather than the number of mL to administer.

Example:

The patient tells the home health nurse that she takes 8 mL of Vibramycin syrup twice a day. How many mg of Vibramycin does the patient receive in each dose?

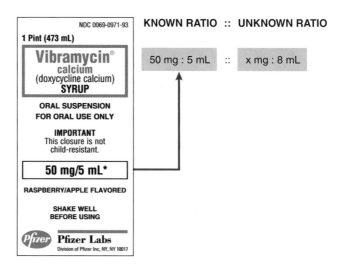

KNOWN RATIO :: UNKNOWN RATIO

50 mg : 5 mL :: x mg : 8 mL

Depending on the setup, the unknown (*x*) may be the first or second number of the unknown ratio. It is most important for the nurse to ensure that units of measurement are set up in the same order in each of the ratios.

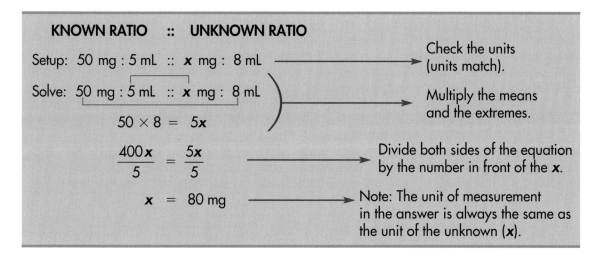

APPLY LEARNED KNOWLEDGE 5-2

Determine which proportion is set up correctly. Calculate the answer.

1. The order is for 16 mg of a medication. The dosage strength of the medication is 4 mg in one drop. How many drops will the nurse administer?
   a. 16 mg : 1 drop :: 4 mg : **x** drop
   b. 4 mg : 1 drop :: 16 mg : **x** drop

2. The patient is to receive 500 grams of a drug daily. The drug bottle is labeled 650 grams in 1 mL. How many mL should the nurse administer?
   a. 500 gram : **x** mL :: 1 mL : 650 gram
   b. 650 gram : 1 mL :: 500 gram : **x** mL

3. The pharmacy sends a drug labeled 20 mg per tablet. The nurse administers 0.5 tablet. How many mg did the nurse administer?
   a. 20 mg : 1 tablet :: **x** mg : 0.5 tablet
   b. 1 tablet : 20 mg :: 0.5 mg : **x** tablet

4. The patient is to receive 5 mg of Drug Z now. The pharmacy sends a dose of Drug Z labeled 2.5 mg in 0.5 mL. How many mL should the nurse administer?
   a. 2.5 mg : **x** mL :: 5 mg : 0.5 mL
   b. 2.5 mg : 0.5 mL :: 5 mg : **x** mL

5. The patient takes 6 doses of a medication each day. The medication contains 4 mg in each dose. The nurse needs to know how many mg the patient takes each day.
   a. 4 mg : 1 dose :: **x** mg : 6 doses
   b. 4 mg : 6 dose :: **x** mg : 1 dose

Setting Up the Proportion When the Units of Measurement Are Not the Same

In each of the examples presented, the units of measurement in the ratios have been the same. But in many dosage calculations, the medication order is in one unit of measurement, and the pharmacy provides the drug with a different unit of measurement. To solve a dosage calculation when there are different units of measurement, a **conversion** is needed.

WORKING WITH CONVERSIONS WITHIN THE METRIC SYSTEM

If a unit of measurement from the metric system needs to be converted to another unit of measurement within the metric system, the metric line is used to **convert** to the equivalent unit of measurement. To promote safety in medication administration, it is recommended that the units of measurement be converted toward the unit on the drug label. That way, the answer has the same unit of measurement as the drug that the nurse has available from the pharmacy.

Example 1:

The physician orders Enalaprilat 625 mcg IV stat. The nurse has the following vial of Enalaprilat. How many mL will the nurse administer to the patient? (See Fig. 5-3.)

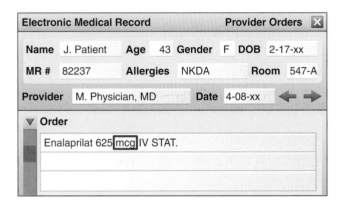
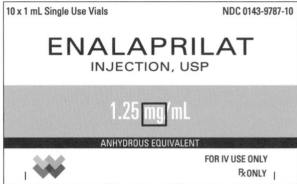

Figure 5-3. Physician's order for Enalaprilat injection.

To solve this problem, begin by setting up the known and the unknown ratios.

■ Known ratio: 1.25 mg : 1 mL
■ Unknown ratio: 625 mcg : x mL

The units do not match. A conversion is required.

In this example, mcg is the unit of measurement from the physician's order and mg is the unit of measurement from the drug label. To convert from mcg (the starting place) to mg (the desired place), move the decimal point three places to the left.

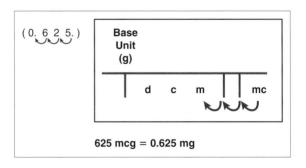

The units are now the same and the problem can be solved.

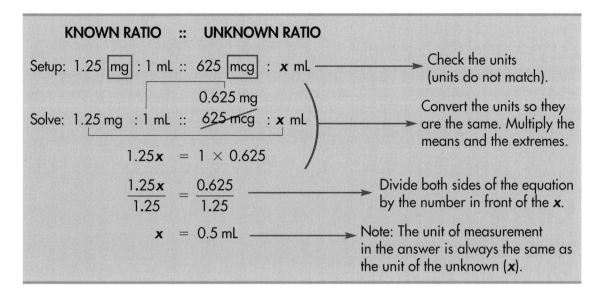

Example 2:

The physician orders Cleocin 0.375 g IM q.12h. The nurse has the following vial of Cleocin. How many mL will the nurse administer to the patient? (See Fig. 5-4.)

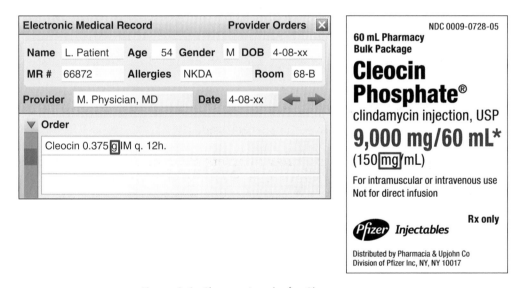

Figure 5-4. Physician's order for Cleocin injection.

To solve this problem, begin by setting up the known and the unknown ratios. There are two equivalent dosage strengths listed on the drug label. For simplicity, use the smaller number.

■ Known ratio: 150 mg : 1 mL

■ Unknown ratio: 0.375 g : x mL

The units do not match. A conversion is required.

In this example, g is the unit of measurement from the physician's order and mg is the unit of measurement from the drug label. To convert from g (the starting place) to mg (the desired place), move the decimal point three places to the right.

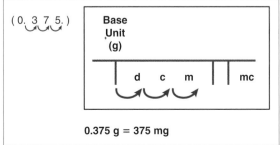

The units are now the same and the problem can be solved.

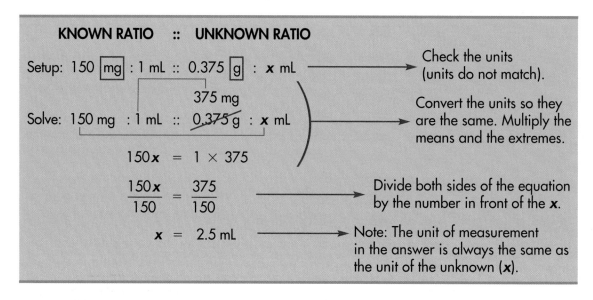

APPLY LEARNED KNOWLEDGE 5-3

*Convert the metric units and solve for **x** in the proportions below.*

1. 500 mg : 1 pill :: 0.25 g : **x** pill _____

2. 0.25 mg : 1 mL :: 62.5 mcg : **x** mL _____

3. 32 mcg : 1 capsule :: 0.096 mg : **x** capsule _____

4. 0.2 g : 1 tsp :: 500 mg : **x** tsp _____

5. 2.5 g : 1 ounce :: 4000 mg : **x** ounce _____

Working With Conversions Between the Metric and the Household Systems

Sometimes, the nurse needs to convert between metric and household units of measurement before the problem can be solved. The metric line and the household equivalent measurements are used to convert the units so that they are the same.

Example 1:

The physician orders 125 mg of cefdinir oral suspension p.o. two times a day for the patient who is to be discharged home. The pharmacy dispenses the medication with a dosing spoon that measures in teaspoons (tsp). How many tsp should the nurse instruct the patient to take with each dose? (See Fig. 5-5.)

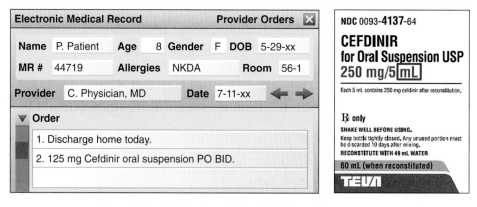

Figure 5-5. Physician's order for Cefdinir oral suspension.

To solve this problem, begin by setting up the known and the unknown ratios.

■ Known ratio: 250 mg : 5 mL

■ Unknown ratio: 125 mg : x tsp

The metric units match. But the mL and tsp units do not match. A conversion is required.

To convert mL to the household measurement tsp, use the equivalent measurement 1 tsp = 5 mL.

The units are now the same and the problem can be solved.

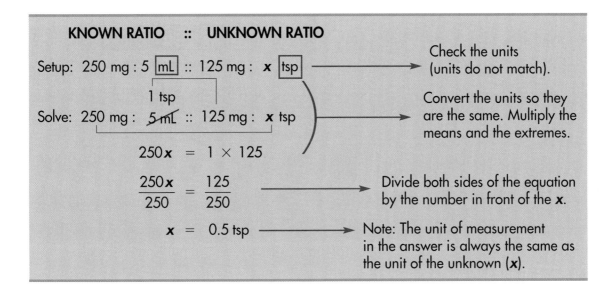

Working With the Conversion of Multiple Units of Measurement

In some calculations, the nurse will need to convert multiple units of measurement before solving the problem. When multiple conversions are required, the nurse systematically does one conversion at a time. The order of the conversions does not matter.

Example 1:

The physician orders Vibramycin 0.125 g p.o. twice daily for a patient who is going home from the hospital. The pharmacy sends the following bottle of Vibramycin. How many teaspoons will the nurse instruct the patient to take? (See Fig. 5-6.)

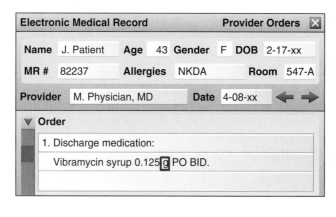

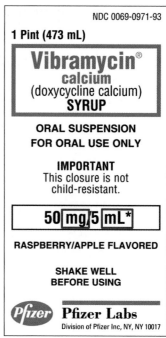

Figure 5-6. Physician's order for Vibramycin syrup.

To solve this problem, begin by setting up the known and the unknown ratios.

■ Known ratio: 50 mg : 5 mL

■ Unknown ratio: 0.125 g : x tsp

The metric units do not match and the mL and tsp units do not match. Two conversions are needed.

Conversion # 1: In the example, g is the unit of measurement from the physician's order and mg is the unit of measurement from the drug label. To convert from g (the starting place) to mg (the desired place), move the decimal point three places to the right.

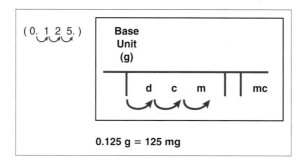

After this first conversion, the metric units are the same (mg).

Conversion # 2: The question, "How many teaspoons will the nurse instruct the patient to take?" requires the answer in the household measurement unit of tsp. To convert mL in the known ratio to tsp, use the household equivalent measurement of 1 tsp = 5 mL.

The units in the proportion now match and the problem can be solved.

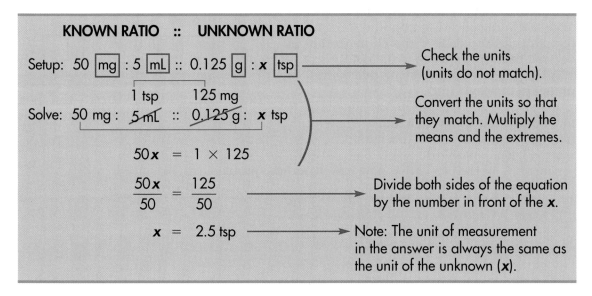

Example 2:

The physician orders Vibramycin oral suspension 0.075 g p.o. twice daily. The pharmacy sends the following bottle of Vibramycin oral suspension and a measuring spoon that measures in teaspoons and tablespoons (Tbs). How many tsp will the nurse instruct the patient to take per dose? How many Tbs per dose? (See Fig. 5-7.)

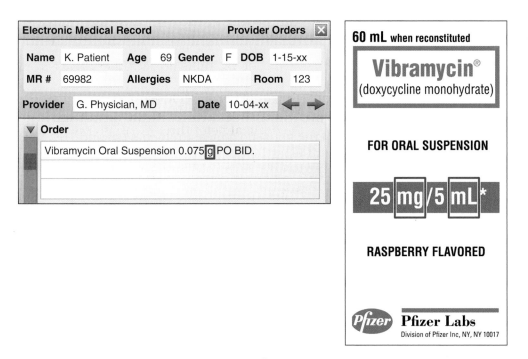

Figure 5-7. Physician's order for Vibramycin oral suspension.

To solve this problem, begin by setting up the known and the unknown ratios.

■ Known ratio: 25 mg : 5 mL

■ Unknown ratio: 0.075 g : x tsp

The metric units do not match and the mL and tsp units do not match. To answer the first question in the problem, "How many tsp will the nurse instruct the patient to take per dose?", two conversions are needed.

Conversion 1: In the example, g is the unit of measurement from the physician's order and mg is the unit of measurement from the drug label. To convert from g (the starting place) to mg (the desired place), move the decimal point three places to the right.

After this first conversion, the metric units are the same (mg).

Conversion 2: A conversion table is used to identify the equivalent measurement between mL and tsp in the first ratio: 5 mL = 1 tsp.

The units in the proportion now match and the problem can be solved.

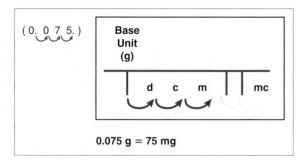

0.075 g = 75 mg

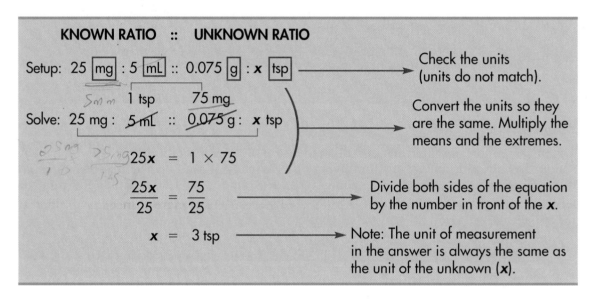

The nurse will instruct the patient to take 3 tsp of Vibramycin oral suspension with each dose. To answer the question "How many Tbs per dose?" an additional conversion is needed.

Conversion 3: To convert between the household measurements tsp and Tbs, the nurse recalls the equivalent measurement 3 tsp = 1 Tbs.

The nurse can instruct the patient to take 1 Tbs of Vibramycin oral suspension with each dose.

WORKING WITH CONVERSIONS FOR OTHER CLINICAL CALCULATIONS

In addition to drug dosage calculations, the linear ratio and proportion method can be used to solve a variety of other clinical calculations. These types of problems usually include the following:

■ The conversion of units within the household system such as teaspoons to tablespoons and tablespoons to ounces

■ The conversion of household to metric equivalent measurements such as pound to kilogram, mL to ounce, and inch to centimeter

In these types of problems, there is no dosage strength to be read from a drug label to set up the known ratio. Instead, the nurse uses the household and metric equivalency as the known ratio in the setup.

CONVERSIONS WITHIN THE HOUSEHOLD SYSTEM FOR OTHER CLINICAL CALCULATIONS

If a unit of measurement from the household system needs to be converted to another household unit, a conversion table is used to identify the equivalent measurements.

Example 1:

The patient measures 1¹/₂ tsp of medication in an oral dosing spoon. How many Tbs of medication has the patient measured?

This example requires a conversion between two household units, tsp and Tbs. The known equivalent measurement of 3 tsp = 1 Tbs is used as the known ratio in the setup.

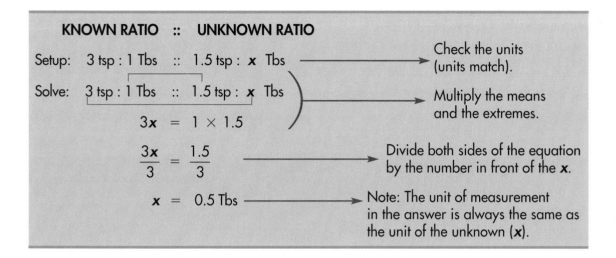

Example 2:

A patient takes 6 tablespoons of nutritional supplement. How many ounces (oz) does the patient receive?

This example requires a conversion between two household units, Tbs and oz. The known equivalent measurement of 2 Tbs = 1 oz is used as the known ratio in the setup.

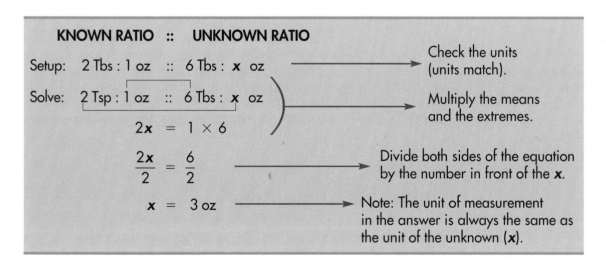

CONVERSIONS BETWEEN THE HOUSEHOLD AND METRIC SYSTEMS FOR OTHER CLINICAL CALCULATIONS

The next example involves a conversion between a household and a metric unit of measurement for a clinical application other than a dosage calculation.

Example 1:

A patient weighs 143 lb. How many kg does the patient weigh?

This example requires a conversion between a household unit of measurement (lb) and a metric unit of measurement (kg). To convert from lb to kg, the equivalent measurement 1 kg = 2.2 lb is used as the known ratio in the setup.

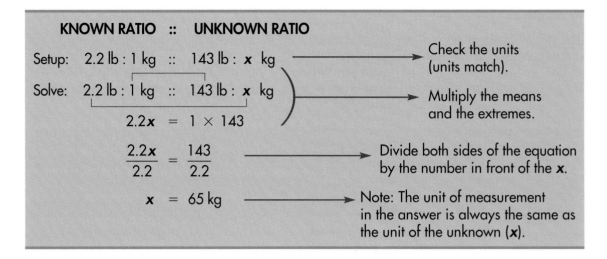

KNOWN RATIO :: UNKNOWN RATIO

Setup: 2.2 lb : 1 kg :: 143 lb : **x** kg → Check the units (units match).

Solve: 2.2 lb : 1 kg :: 143 lb : **x** kg → Multiply the means and the extremes.

$$2.2x = 1 \times 143$$

$$\frac{2.2x}{2.2} = \frac{143}{2.2}$$ → Divide both sides of the equation by the number in front of the **x**.

$$x = 65 \text{ kg}$$ → Note: The unit of measurement in the answer is always the same as the unit of the unknown (**x**).

CLINICAL REASONING 5-1
The patient tells the home care nurse that he is taking 1 Tbs of Griseofulvin Oral Suspension every morning. Is the patient taking the correct amount of medication? Provide a rationale for your answer.

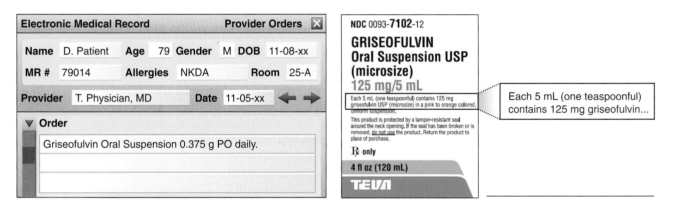

Electronic Medical Record		Provider Orders	✕
Name D. Patient	**Age** 79 **Gender** M **DOB** 11-08-xx		
MR # 79014	**Allergies** NKDA	**Room** 25-A	
Provider T. Physician, MD	**Date** 11-05-xx ← →		
▼ **Order**			
Griseofulvin Oral Suspension 0.375 g PO daily.			

NDC 0093-**7102**-12

GRISEOFULVIN
Oral Suspension USP
(microsize)
125 mg/5 mL

Each 5 mL (one teaspoonful) contains 125 mg
griseofulvin USP (microsize) in a pink to orange colored,
uniform suspension.

This product is protected by a tamper-resistant seal
around the neck opening. If the seal has been broken or is
removed, <u>do not use</u> the product. Return the product to
place of purchase.

℞ only

4 fl oz (120 mL)

TEVA

Each 5 mL (one teaspoonful) contains 125 mg griseofulvin...

In summary, the nurse can use linear ratio and proportion to solve all math problems encountered in the clinical area. The dosage strength of the medication is the known ratio when setting up the proportion for a dosage calculation. The same steps are used in solving all proportions: checking the units of measurement, converting the units of measurement so that they are the same, and multiplying the means and the extremes to solve for *x*, the unknown.

Developing Competency

Write the dosage strength of the medication as a linear ratio.

1.

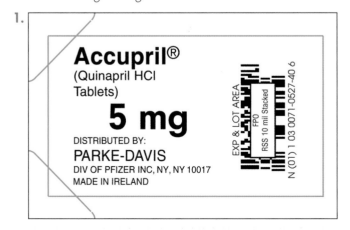

Accupril®
(Quinapril HCl
Tablets)

5 mg

DISTRIBUTED BY:
PARKE-DAVIS
DIV OF PFIZER INC, NY, NY 10017
MADE IN IRELAND

N (01) 1 03 0071-0527-40 6
RSS 10 mil Stacked
FPO
EXP & LOT AREA

2.

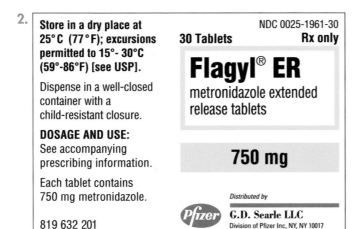

Store in a dry place at
25°C (77°F); excursions
permitted to 15°- 30°C
(59°-86°F) [see USP].

Dispense in a well-closed
container with a
child-resistant closure.

DOSAGE AND USE:
See accompanying
prescribing information.

Each tablet contains
750 mg metronidazole.

819 632 201

NDC 0025-1961-30
30 Tablets   **Rx only**

Flagyl® ER
metronidazole extended
release tablets

750 mg

Distributed by
Pfizer **G.D. Searle LLC**
Division of Pfizer Inc, NY, NY 10017

3.

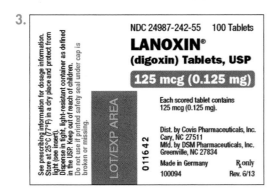

See prescribing information for dosage information.
Store at 25°C (77°F) in a dry place and protect from
light (see insert).
Dispense in tight, light-resistant container as defined
in the USP. Keep out of reach of children.
Do not use if printed safety seal under cap is
broken or missing.

LOT/EXP AREA

011642

NDC 24987-242-55   100 Tablets
LANOXIN®
(digoxin) Tablets, USP
125 mcg (0.125 mg)

Each scored tablet contains
125 mcg (0.125 mg).

Dist. by Covis Pharmaceuticals, Inc.
Cary, NC 27511
Mfd. by DSM Pharmaceuticals, Inc.
Greenville, NC 27834
Made in Germany   R̥only
100094   Rev. 6/13

Review the information provided and determine whether the nurse has set up the problem correctly.

4. A drug is labeled 0.1 mg per 10 mL. The doctor has ordered 0.25 mg of the drug. The nurse sets up the following proportion to calculate the dose:

10 mL : 0.1 mg :: x mL : 0.25 mg

Has the nurse set up the problem correctly?   _____

5. A medication has 350 grams in each tablet. The doctor has ordered 700 grams p.o. daily. The nurse sets up the following proportion to calculate the dose:

700 g : 1 tablet :: 350 g : x tablet

Has the nurse set up the problem correctly?   _____

Set up a linear proportion and solve the problem.

6. The label on the medication container states 0.25 gram tablets. The patient is to receive 0.125 gram each morning. How many tablets will the patient receive?   _____

7. The patient is to receive 8.75 mg of a medication. The pharmacy sends the medication to the nurse in a container labeled 2.5 mg/mL. How many mL will the patient receive?   _____

8. The medication is available in 0.05 mg scored pills. The order is for 0.125 mg. How many pills will the patient receive?   _____

Use the information in each question to solve the problem.

9. The patient tells the nurse that he takes 12 mL of Ceftin four times daily. How many mg does the patient receive per dose?

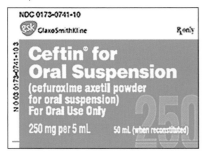

NDC 0173-0741-10
gsk GlaxoSmithKline   R̥only

Ceftin® for
Oral Suspension
(cefuroxime axetil powder
for oral suspension)
For Oral Use Only

250 mg per 5 mL   50 mL (when reconstituted)

10. The pharmacy sends the nurse the following bottle of PrednisoLONE Oral Solution. The order is to administer 0.03g PO daily. How many tsp will the patient receive?

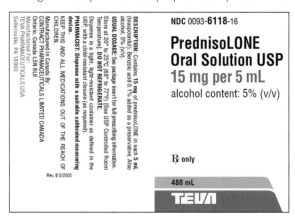

_____

11. The patient is to receive 6 mg of IV morphine q.4h as needed for severe pain. How many mL will the nurse give per dose?

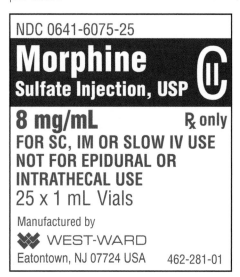

_____

12. The doctor orders granisetron 450 mcg IV 30 minutes prior to chemotherapy. The nurse has the following vials of granisetron. How many mL will the nurse give to the patient?

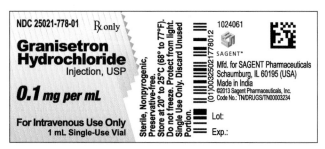

_____

13. The patient is to receive 350 mg of a medication. The medication is labeled 250 mg in 15 mL. How many ounces will the nurse administer?   _____

14. The physician's order is for 0.01 g p.o. each morning. How many tablets will the nurse instruct the patient to take?

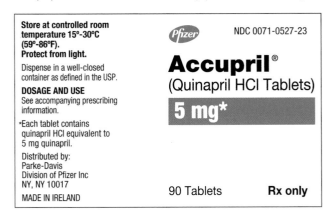

15. The patient is to drink 2000 mL of water daily. Bottled water is available in a 400 mL size. How many bottles will the patient need to drink daily? _____

16. The pharmacy sends the nurse the following medication. How many capsules will the nurse give to the patient if the physician's order is for calcitriol 1.5 mcg p.o. daily?

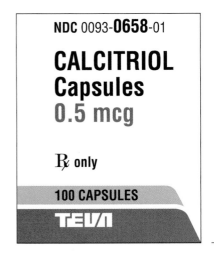

17. The nurse is to give 6.25 mg of carvedilol p.o. twice a day. How many tablets of carvedilol will the patient receive each day?

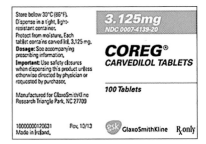

18. The nurse practitioner orders 60 mg of Fluoxetine Oral Solution p.o. daily for the patient. The pharmacy sends the following bottle of Fluoxetine. How many tsp will the patient receive?

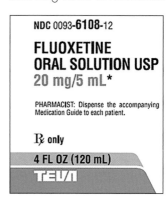

NDC 0093-**6108**-12

FLUOXETINE ORAL SOLUTION USP
20 mg/5 mL*

PHARMACIST: Dispense the accompanying Medication Guide to each patient.

℞ only

4 FL OZ (120 mL)

TEVA

---

19. The order is for METHYLPREDnisolone Acetate 30 mg IM now. The pharmacy sends the following vial of METHYLPREDnisolone Acetate. How many mL will the nurse administer?

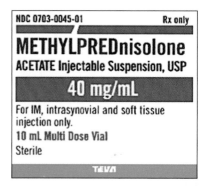

NDC 0703-0045-01   Rx only

METHYLPREDnisolone
ACETATE Injectable Suspension, USP

40 mg/mL

For IM, intrasynovial and soft tissue injection only.
10 mL Multi Dose Vial
Sterile

TEVA

---

20. The following is the medication order: Give 0.75 g of Cephalexin Oral Suspension p.o. q.12h. The following bottle of Cephalexin is available. How many oz will the nurse administer to the patient with each dose?

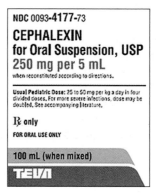

NDC 0093-**4177**-73

CEPHALEXIN for Oral Suspension, USP
250 mg per 5 mL
when reconstituted according to directions.

Usual Pediatric Dose: 25 to 50 mg per kg a day in four divided doses. For more severe infections, dose may be doubled. See accompanying literature.

℞ only
FOR ORAL USE ONLY

100 mL (when mixed)

TEVA

CHAPTER 6

Fractional Ratio and Proportion

LEARNING OUTCOMES

Define ratio and proportion.

Discuss how dosage strength is used in ratio and proportion.

Set up a ratio and proportion using the fractional format.

Solve drug dosage calculation problems using the fractional ratio and proportion method.

The medication administration process involves many members of the healthcare team: the physician prescribes the medication, the pharmacist dispenses the medication, and the nurse gives the medication to the patient. As the healthcare professional who administers the medication to the patient, the nurse has the responsibility to verify the ordered dose.

Safe medication administration requires that before giving any medication, the nurse must validate the ***dosage.*** Sometimes a calculation is required to determine how much of the medication to give. One method of solving a dosage calculation is the ratio and proportion method. This is a very useful method for nurses, as it can be used to solve all dosage and clinical math calculations.

Ratios

A ***ratio*** is a comparison of two numbers that have a relationship to each other. In nursing practice, there are many numbers that are related to each other. For example:

- A patient weighs 185 lb on admission and 182 lb after taking a diuretic medication.
- 10 milligrams of medication is contained in each capsule.
- The patient's pulse at 7:00 a.m. is 86 beats per minute. At 12 noon, the patient's pulse is 78 beats per minute.

Numbers that are related can be written in a ***fractional*** mathematical format.

FRACTIONAL FORMAT

A ratio set up in a fractional format uses a line (—) to show the relationship between two numbers.

Two numbers expressed in a ratio look like this:

$$\frac{185 \text{ lb}}{182 \text{ lb}} \qquad \frac{10 \text{ mg}}{1 \text{ capsule}} \qquad \frac{86 \text{ beats/minute}}{78 \text{ beats/minute}}$$

The fractional format is read:

- 185 lb **divided by** 182 lb

- 10 mg **divided by** 1 capsule

- 86 beats per minute **divided by** 78 beats per minute

Proportions

A ratio by itself does not help the nurse calculate a drug dosage. To solve a dosage problem, the nurse needs to use a **proportion.** In math, a proportion is a statement that two ratios are equal. Another way to say this is that a proportion is an equation of two ratios. Like a ratio, a proportion can be written using a fractional format.

FRACTIONAL FORMAT

A proportion in a fractional format uses an equal sign (=) to show the relationship between the two ratios. Here are two examples:

$$\frac{1}{2} = \frac{2}{4} \qquad \frac{10 \text{ mg}}{1 \text{ capsule}} = \frac{20 \text{ mg}}{2 \text{ capsules}}$$

In each of these examples, it is easy to see that the two fractional ratios are equal. The fractional proportion is read:

1 divided by 2 **equals** 2 divided by 4

10 mg divided by 1 capsule **equals** 20 mg divided by 2 capsules

When using a fractional proportion to calculate a drug dosage, only three of the four numbers are known. Setting up a proportion is an easy way to solve for the fourth number.

Information Needed to Set Up a Fractional Proportion

To calculate a drug dosage using a fractional proportion, the nurse uses two sources of information:

■ The ordered dose of medication from the physician's order

■ The dosage strength from the drug label

Each is used in setting up one ratio in the proportion used to solve a dosage calculation.

THE ORDERED DOSE

The physician who prescribes the medication specifies the drug name, dose, route, and frequency or time of administration. The ordered **dose** contains the **strength** of the medication (a number) with a **unit of measurement.**

To the right is an example of a physician's order for a medication on the electronic medical record.

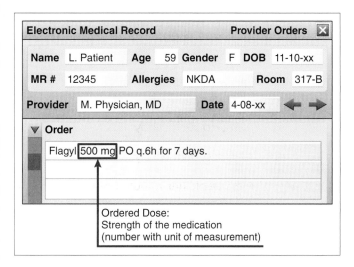

THE DOSAGE STRENGTH FROM THE DRUG LABEL

The pharmacy supplies the medication and the nurse identifies specific information from the drug label needed to set up the dosage calculation. In reviewing the drug label, the nurse will identify the following:

■ The strength of the medication

■ The dosage form in which the medication is available

Look at each part of the medication label in Figure 6-1.

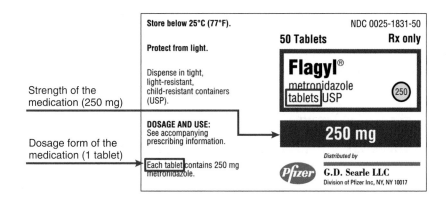

Figure 6-1. Information on the drug label: the dosage strength.

Notice that the strength of a medication is made up of a number and a unit of measurement.

The dosage form of a medication is made up of the number of capsules, tablets, and so on (solid oral dosage form) or the specific volume of liquid (oral or parenteral liquid dosage form) that contains the strength of the medication.

The strength and the dosage form of the medication are a ratio $\dfrac{250 \text{ mg}}{1 \text{ tablet}}$.

Together they are called the **dosage strength** of the medication. Refer to Chapter 2, The Drug Label, for more information on the dosage strength of a medication.

The dosage strength can be written in several ways on a drug label. Here are some examples. Notice where the dosage strength is found on each drug label and how it is written as a fractional ratio:

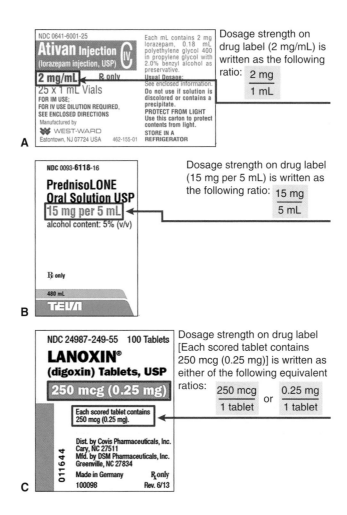

Dosage strength on drug label (2 mg/mL) is written as the following ratio: $\dfrac{2\ mg}{1\ mL}$

Dosage strength on drug label (15 mg per 5 mL) is written as the following ratio: $\dfrac{15\ mg}{5\ mL}$

Dosage strength on drug label [Each scored tablet contains 250 mcg (0.25 mg)] is written as either of the following equivalent ratios: $\dfrac{250\ mcg}{1\ tablet}$ or $\dfrac{0.25\ mg}{1\ tablet}$

APPLY LEARNED KNOWLEDGE 6-1

Write the fractional ratio that expresses the correct dosage strength for the medications below.

1.
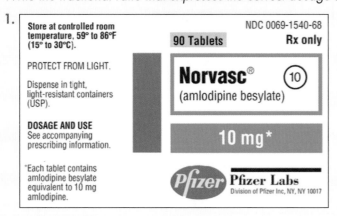

_____

APPLY LEARNED KNOWLEDGE 6-1—cont'd

2.

NDC 0093-**4137**-64

CEFDINIR
for Oral Suspension USP
250 mg/5 mL

Each 5 mL contains 250 mg cefdinir after reconstitution.

℞ only

SHAKE WELL BEFORE USING.
Keep bottle tightly closed. Any unused portion must
be discarded 10 days after mixing.
RECONSTITUTE WITH 49 mL WATER

60 mL (when reconstituted)

TEVA

_____

3.

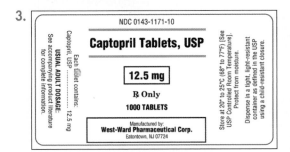

NDC 0143-1171-10

Captopril Tablets, USP

12.5 mg

℞ Only
1000 TABLETS

Each Tablet contains:
Captopril, USP
USUAL ADULT DOSAGE:
See accompanying product literature
for complete information.
Captopril, USP .... 12.5 mg

Store at 20° to 25°C (68° to 77°F) [See
USP Controlled Room Temperature].
Protect from moisture.
Dispense in a tight, light-resistant
container as defined in the USP
using a child-resistant closure.

Manufactured by:
West-Ward Pharmaceutical Corp.
Eatontown, NJ 07724

_____

4.

NDC 24987-362-10 | **2-mL single-dose vial**

Zantac® Injection | **50 mg**
(ranitidine hydrochloride)
25 mg ranitidine/1 mL   ℞ only
0.5% phenol present as preservative.   100022
Dist. Covis Pharmaceuticals, Inc.   Rev. 5/12
Made in Singapore   10000000103359

_____

5.

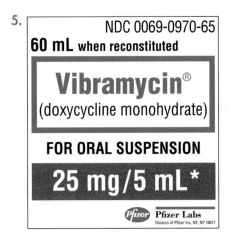

NDC 0069-0970-65

60 mL when reconstituted

Vibramycin®
(doxycycline monohydrate)

FOR ORAL SUSPENSION

25 mg/5 mL*

Pfizer   **Pfizer Labs**
Division of Pfizer Inc, NY, NY 10017

_____

Solving Dosage Calculations With a Fractional Proportion

A fractional proportion can be used to solve any drug dosage calculation. A proportion contains two equal ratios, and if three of the four numbers in a proportion are known, it is easy to find the value of the unknown fourth number (or "x").

With most dosage calculations, the dosage strength of the medication is used as the first ratio.

■ This first ratio is called the **known ratio,** as its two parts are always known from the drug label (the strength of medication and the dosage form in which the medication is available).

■ The second ratio in the proportion is called the **unknown ratio,** as it contains the ordered dose and the unknown quantity. In setting up the ratio with an unknown, **"x"** represents the unknown quantity.

See Figure 6-2 for an example of how the dosage strength on the drug label (the known ratio) and the ordered dose (part of the unknown ratio) are used in setting up a proportion.

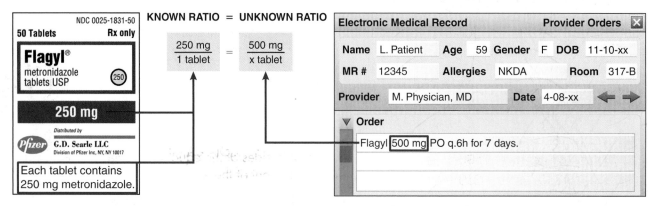

Figure 6-2. Setting up the known and the unknown ratios.

In the example in Figure 6-2, the nurse has an order to give 500 mg of Flagyl. The medication is available in 250 mg tablets. The nurse needs to know how many tablets to administer to the patient.

STEPS FOR SETTING UP AND SOLVING A FRACTIONAL PROPORTION

Here are the steps to set up and solve a fractional proportion using the known and unknown ratios:

■ **First,** write the known ratio: the dosage strength from the drug label. Notice that the units of measurement are included as well as the numbers.

■ **Second,** write the unknown ratio: the ordered dose and the unknown amount to administer, which is written as "x."

The proportion using the known and unknown ratios is now set up.

■ **Third,** check the units of measurement. Both ratios must contain the same two units in the same order.

Each ratio in the proportion has the same two units, mg and tablets. The units of measurement in the

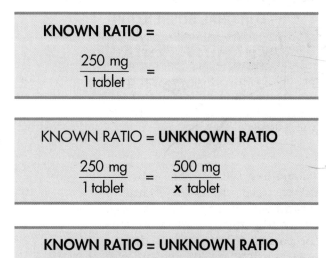

numerators (mg) are the same, and the units of measurement in the denominators (tablet) are the same.

If the ratios and the units are not set up in the correct order, the answer will not be correct. If the units are not the same, a conversion must be done. Conversions are discussed at the end of this chapter.

■ **Fourth**, Solve for **x** by **cross multiplication.**
- Multiply the numerator of one fraction by the denominator of the other fraction, and vice versa (work only with the numbers, not the units of measurement).
- Clear the x by dividing both sides of the equation by the number in front of the x.
- Solve for x.
- Put the answer back in the original equation to find the correct unit of measurement.
- Think critically: Does the answer make sense?

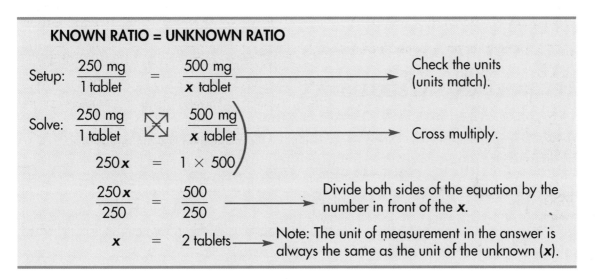

 The important rule to remember in working with fractional proportions is that the **products** of cross multiplication are always equal. This provides a convenient way to double-check that the answer is correct: if the answer is put back into the setup, then the products of cross multiplication of the two ratios should be equal. For example, in the above calculation, $250 \times 2 = 1 \times 500$. The calculation is correct.

Here is another example of how to set up and solve a dosage calculation using a fractional proportion. Note that the question asks for the number of mg per dose, rather than the number of mL to administer.

Example:

The patient tells the home-health nurse that she takes 8 mL of Vibramycin syrup twice a day. How many mg of Vibramycin does the patient receive in each dose?

Depending on the setup, the unknown (x) may be in the numerator or the denominator of the

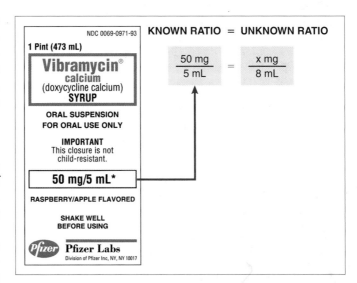

unknown ratio. It is most important for the nurse to ensure that units of measurement are set up in the same order in each of the ratios.

KNOWN RATIO = UNKNOWN RATIO

Setup: $\dfrac{50 \text{ mg}}{5 \text{ mL}} = \dfrac{x \text{ mg}}{8 \text{ mL}}$ ⟶ Check the units (units match).

Solve: $\dfrac{50 \text{ mg}}{5 \text{ mL}} \diagdown\!\!\!\!\diagup \dfrac{x \text{ mg}}{8 \text{ mL}}$ ⟶ Cross multiply.

$50 \times 8 = 5x$

$\dfrac{400}{5} = \dfrac{5x}{5}$ ⟶ Divide both sides of the equation by the number in front of the x.

$x = 80 \text{ mg}$ ⟶ Note: The unit of measurement in the answer is always the same as the unit of the unknown (x).

APPLY LEARNED KNOWLEDGE 6-2

Determine which proportion is set up correctly. Calculate the answer.

1. The order is for 16 mg of a medication. The dosage strength of the medication is 4 mg in one drop. How many drops will the nurse administer?

   A. $\dfrac{16 \text{ mg}}{1 \text{ drop}} = \dfrac{4 \text{ mg}}{x \text{ drop}}$ B. $\dfrac{4 \text{ mg}}{1 \text{ drop}} = \dfrac{16 \text{ mg}}{x \text{ drop}}$

2. The patient is to receive 500 grams of a drug daily. The drug bottle is labeled 650 grams in 1 mL. How many mL should the nurse administer?

   A. $\dfrac{500 \text{ gram}}{x \text{ mL}} = \dfrac{1 \text{ mL}}{650 \text{ gram}}$ B. $\dfrac{650 \text{ gram}}{1 \text{ mL}} = \dfrac{500 \text{ gram}}{x \text{ mL}}$

3. The pharmacy sends a drug labeled 20 mg per tablet. The nurse administers 0.5 tablet. How many mg did the nurse administer?

   A. $\dfrac{20 \text{ mg}}{1 \text{ tablet}} = \dfrac{x \text{ mg}}{0.5 \text{ tablet}}$ B. $\dfrac{1 \text{ tablet}}{20 \text{ mg}} = \dfrac{0.5 \text{ mg}}{x \text{ tablet}}$

4. The patient is to receive 5 mg of Drug Z now. The pharmacy sends a dose of Drug Z labeled 2.5 mg in 0.5 mL. How many mL should the nurse administer?

   A. $\dfrac{2.5 \text{ mg}}{x \text{ mL}} = \dfrac{5 \text{ mg}}{0.5 \text{ mL}}$ B. $\dfrac{2.5 \text{ mg}}{0.5 \text{ mL}} = \dfrac{5 \text{ mg}}{x \text{ mL}}$

5. The patient takes 6 doses of a medication each day. The medication contains 4 mg in each dose. The nurse needs to know how many mg the patient takes each day.

   A. $\dfrac{4 \text{ mg}}{1 \text{ dose}} = \dfrac{x \text{ mg}}{6 \text{ dose}}$ B. $\dfrac{4 \text{ mg}}{6 \text{ dose}} = \dfrac{x \text{ mg}}{1 \text{ dose}}$

SETTING UP THE PROPORTION WHEN THE UNITS OF MEASUREMENT ARE NOT THE SAME

In each of the examples presented, the units of measurement in the ratios have been the same. But in many dosage calculations, the medication order is in one unit of measurement, and the pharmacy provides the drug with a different unit of measurement. To solve a dosage calculation when there are different units of measurement, a **conversion** is needed.

WORKING WITH CONVERSIONS WITHIN THE METRIC SYSTEM

If a unit of measurement from the metric system needs to be converted to another unit of measurement within the metric system, the metric line is used to **convert** to the equivalent unit of measurement. To promote safety in medication administration, it is recommended that the units of measurement be converted toward the unit on the drug label. That way, the answer has the same unit of measurement as the drug that the nurse has available from the pharmacy.

Example 1:

The physician orders Enalaprilat 625 mcg IV stat. The nurse has the following vial of Enalaprilat. How many mL will the nurse administer to the patient? (See Fig. 6-3.)

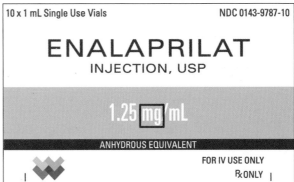

Figure 6-3. Physician's order for Enalaprilat Injection.

To solve this problem, begin by setting up the known and the unknown ratios.

■ Known ratio: $\dfrac{1.25 \text{ mg}}{1 \text{ mL}}$

■ Unknown ratio: $\dfrac{625 \text{ mcg}}{x \text{ mL}}$

The units do not match. A conversion is required.

In this example, mcg is the unit of measurement from the physician's order and mg is the unit of measurement from the drug label. To convert from mcg (the starting place) to mg (the desired place), move the decimal point three places to the left.

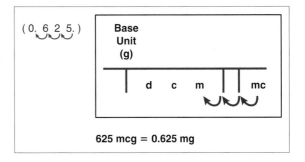

The units are now the same and the problem can be solved.

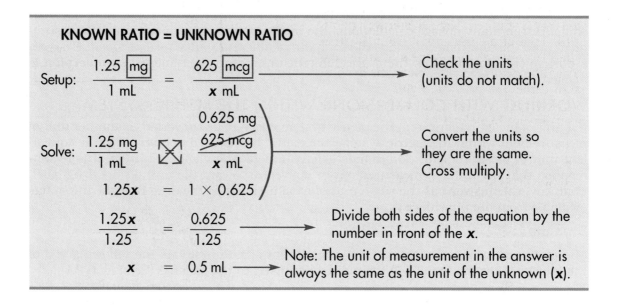

KNOWN RATIO = UNKNOWN RATIO

Setup: $\dfrac{1.25 \boxed{\text{mg}}}{1 \text{ mL}} = \dfrac{625 \boxed{\text{mcg}}}{x \text{ mL}}$ ⟶ Check the units (units do not match).

Solve: $\dfrac{1.25 \text{ mg}}{1 \text{ mL}}$ ⤬ $\dfrac{\overset{0.625 \text{ mg}}{\cancel{625 \text{ mcg}}}}{x \text{ mL}}$ ⟶ Convert the units so they are the same. Cross multiply.

$1.25x = 1 \times 0.625$

$\dfrac{1.25x}{1.25} = \dfrac{0.625}{1.25}$ ⟶ Divide both sides of the equation by the number in front of the **x**.

$x = 0.5 \text{ mL}$ ⟶ Note: The unit of measurement in the answer is always the same as the unit of the unknown (**x**).

Example 2:

The physician orders Cleocin 0.375 g IM q.12h. The nurse has the following vial of Cleocin. How many mL will the nurse administer to the patient? (See Fig. 6-4.)

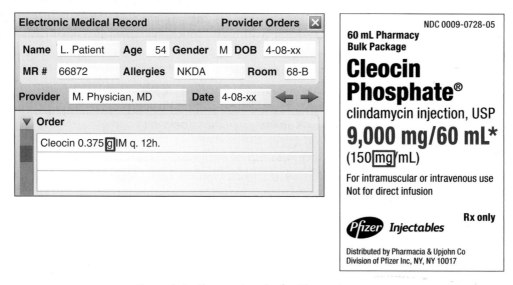

Figure 6-4. Physician's order for Cleocin Injection.

To solve this problem, begin by setting up the known and the unknown ratios. There are two equivalent dosage strengths listed on the drug label. For simplicity, use the smaller numbers.

■ Known ratio: $\dfrac{150 \text{ mg}}{1 \text{ mL}}$

■ Unknown ratio: $\dfrac{0.375 \text{ g}}{x \text{ mL}}$

The units do not match. A conversion is required.

In this example, g is the unit of measurement from the physician's order and mg is the unit of measurement from the drug label. To convert from g (the starting place) to mg (the desired place), move the decimal point three places to the right.

The units are now the same and the problem can be solved.

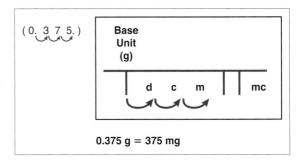

$0.375 \text{ g} = 375 \text{ mg}$

KNOWN RATIO = UNKNOWN RATIO

Setup: $\dfrac{150 \; \boxed{\text{mg}}}{1 \text{ mL}} = \dfrac{0.375 \; \boxed{\text{g}}}{x \text{ mL}}$ ⟶ Check the units (units do not match).

Solve: $\dfrac{150 \text{ mg}}{1 \text{ mL}} \; \bowtie \; \dfrac{\overset{375 \text{ mg}}{\cancel{0.375 \text{ g}}}}{x \text{ mL}}$ ⟶ Convert the units so they are the same. Cross multiply.

$150x = 1 \times 375$

$\dfrac{150x}{150} = \dfrac{375}{150}$ ⟶ Divide both sides of the equation by the number in front of the x.

$x = 2.5 \text{ mL}$ ⟶ Note: The unit of measurement in the answer is always the same as the unit of the unknown (x).

APPLY LEARNED KNOWLEDGE 6-3

Convert the metric units and solve for x in the proportions below.

1. $\dfrac{500 \text{ mg}}{1 \text{ pill}} = \dfrac{0.25 \text{ g}}{x \text{ pill}}$ _____

2. $\dfrac{0.25 \text{ mg}}{1 \text{ mL}} = \dfrac{62.5 \text{ mcg}}{x \text{ mL}}$ _____

3. $\dfrac{32 \text{ mcg}}{1 \text{ capsule}} = \dfrac{0.096 \text{ mg}}{x \text{ capsule}}$ _____

4. $\dfrac{0.2 \text{ g}}{1 \text{ tsp}} = \dfrac{500 \text{ mg}}{x \text{ tsp}}$ _____

5. $\dfrac{2.5 \text{ g}}{1 \text{ ounce}} = \dfrac{4000 \text{ mg}}{x \text{ ounce}}$ _____

WORKING WITH CONVERSIONS BETWEEN THE METRIC AND THE HOUSEHOLD SYSTEMS

Sometimes the nurse needs to convert between metric and household units of measurement before the problem can be solved. The metric line and the household equivalent measurements are used to convert the units so that they are the same.

Example 1:

The physician orders 125 mg of Cefdinir oral suspension PO two times a day for the patient who is to be discharged home. The pharmacy dispenses the medication with a dosing spoon that measures in tsp. How many tsp should the nurse instruct the patient to take with each dose? (See Fig. 6-5.)

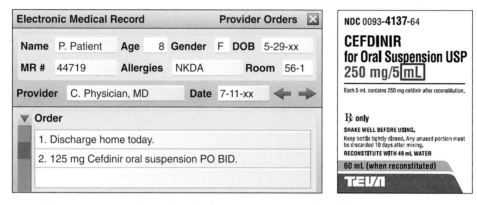

Figure 6-5. Physician's order for Cefdinir oral suspension.

To solve this problem, begin by setting up the known and the unknown ratios.

■ Known ratio: $\dfrac{250 \text{ mg}}{5 \text{ mL}}$

■ Unknown ratio: $\dfrac{125 \text{ mg}}{x \text{ tsp}}$

The metric units match. But the mL and tsp units do not match. A conversion is required.

To convert mL to the household measurement tsp, use the equivalent measurement of 1 tsp = 5 mL.

The units are now the same and the problem can be solved.

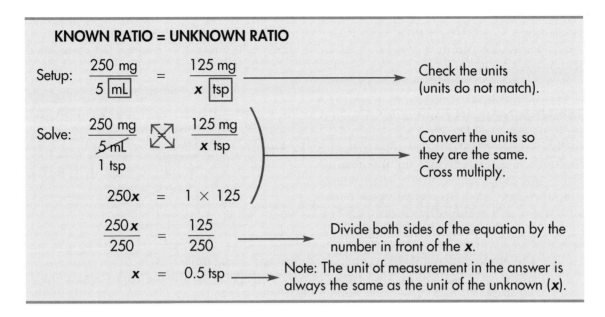

WORKING WITH THE CONVERSION OF MULTIPLE UNITS OF MEASUREMENT

In some calculations, the nurse will need to convert multiple units of measurement before solving the problem. When multiple conversions are required, the nurse systematically does one conversion at a time. The order of the conversions does not matter.

Example 1:

The physician orders Vibramycin syrup 0.125 g PO twice daily for a patient who is going home from the hospital. The pharmacy sends the following bottle of Vibramycin. How many teaspoons will the nurse instruct the patient to take? (See Fig. 6-6.)

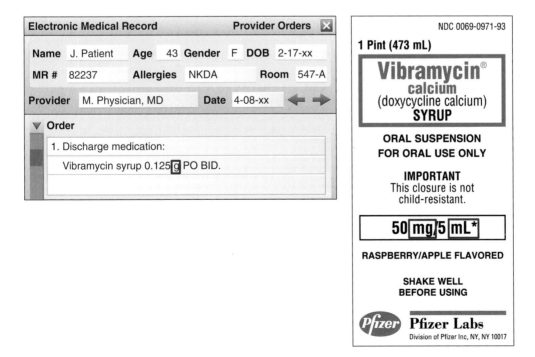

Figure 6-6. Physician's order for Vibramycin syrup.

To solve this problem, begin by setting up the known and the unknown ratios.

■ Known ratio: $\dfrac{50 \text{ mg}}{5 \text{ mL}}$

■ Unknown ratio: $\dfrac{0.125 \text{ g}}{x \text{ tsp}}$

The metric units do not match and the mL and tsp units do not match. Two conversions are needed.

Conversion 1: In the example, g is the unit of measurement from the physician's order and mg is the unit of measurement from the drug label. To convert from g (the starting place) to mg (the desired place), move the decimal point three places to the right.

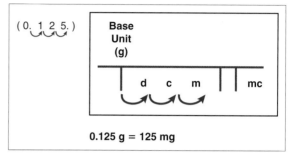

0.125 g = 125 mg

After this first conversion, the metric units are the same (mg).

Conversion 2: The question "How many teaspoons will the nurse instruct the patient to take?" requires the answer in the household measurement tsp. To convert mL in the known ratio to tsp, use the household equivalent measurement of 1 tsp = 5 mL.

The units in the proportion now match and the problem can be solved.

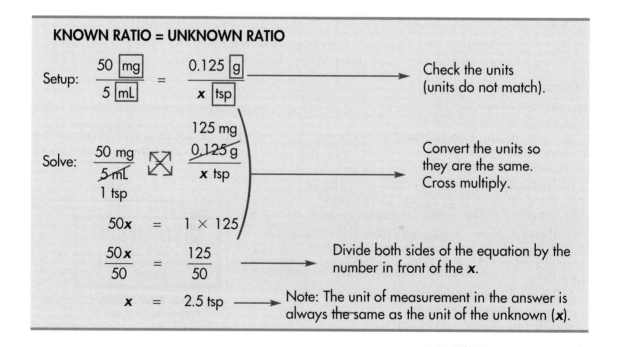

KNOWN RATIO = UNKNOWN RATIO

Setup: $\dfrac{50\ \boxed{mg}}{5\ \boxed{mL}} = \dfrac{0.125\ \boxed{g}}{x\ \boxed{tsp}}$ ⟶ Check the units (units do not match).

Solve: $\dfrac{\underset{1\text{ tsp}}{\dfrac{50 \text{ mg}}{\cancel{5\text{ mL}}}}}{} \boxtimes \dfrac{\overset{125\text{ mg}}{\cancel{0.125\text{ g}}}}{x \text{ tsp}}$ ⟶ Convert the units so they are the same. Cross multiply.

$50x\ =\ 1 \times 125$

$\dfrac{50x}{50}\ =\ \dfrac{125}{50}$ ⟶ Divide both sides of the equation by the number in front of the **x**.

$x\ =\ 2.5 \text{ tsp}$ ⟶ Note: The unit of measurement in the answer is always the same as the unit of the unknown (**x**).

Example 2:

The physician orders Vibramycin oral suspension 0.075 g PO twice daily. The pharmacy sends the following bottle of Vibramycin oral suspension and a measuring spoon that measures in teaspoons and tablespoons. How many tsp will the nurse instruct the patient to take per dose? How many Tbs per dose? (See Fig. 6-7.)

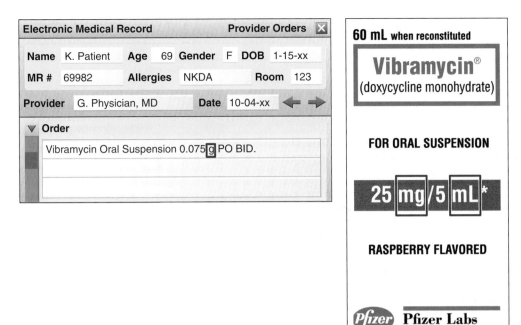

Figure 6-7. Physician's order for Vibramycin oral suspension.

To solve this problem, begin by setting up the known and the unknown ratios.

■ Known ratio: $\dfrac{25 \text{ mg}}{5 \text{ mL}}$

■ Unknown ratio: $\dfrac{0.075 \text{ g}}{x \text{ tsp}}$

The metric units do not match and the mL and tsp units do not match. To answer the first question in the problem—"How many tsp will the nurse instruct the patient to take per dose?"—two conversions are needed.

Conversion 1: In the example, g is the unit of measurement from the physician's order and mg is the unit of measurement from the drug label. To convert from g (the starting place) to mg (the desired place), move the decimal point three places to the right.

After this first conversion, the metric units are the same (mg).

Conversion 2: A conversion table is used to identify the equivalent measurement between mL and tsp in the first ratio:

5 mL = 1 tsp.

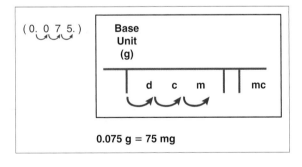

The units in the proportion now match and the problem can be solved.

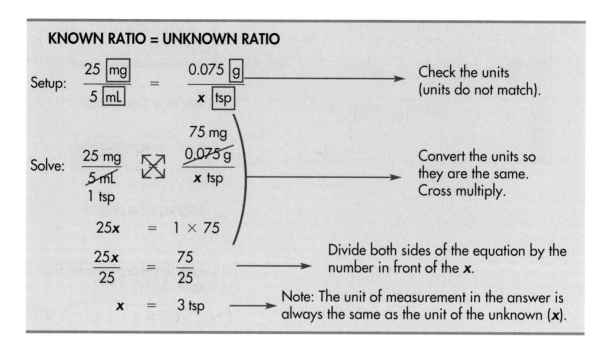

KNOWN RATIO = UNKNOWN RATIO

Setup: $\dfrac{25\ \boxed{mg}}{5\ \boxed{mL}} = \dfrac{0.075\ \boxed{g}}{x\ \boxed{tsp}}$ → Check the units (units do not match).

Solve: $\dfrac{25\ mg}{\overset{5\ mL}{\underset{1\ tsp}{}}} \quad \dfrac{\overset{75\ mg}{0.075\ g}}{x\ tsp}$ → Convert the units so they are the same. Cross multiply.

$25x = 1 \times 75$

$\dfrac{25x}{25} = \dfrac{75}{25}$ → Divide both sides of the equation by the number in front of the **x**.

$x = 3\ tsp$ → Note: The unit of measurement in the answer is always the same as the unit of the unknown (**x**).

The nurse will instruct the patient to take 3 tsp of Vibramycin oral suspension with each dose. To answer the question "How many Tbs per dose?" an additional conversion is needed.

Conversion 3: To convert between the household measurements tsp and Tbs, the nurse recalls the equivalent measurement of 3 tsp = 1 Tbs.

The nurse can instruct the patient to take 1 Tbs of Vibramycin oral suspension with each dose.

Working With Conversions for Other Clinical Calculations

In addition to drug dosage calculations, the fractional ratio and proportion method can be used to solve a variety of other clinical calculations. These types of problems usually include:

■ the conversion of units within the household system such as teaspoons to tablespoons and tablespoons to ounces

■ the conversion of household to metric equivalent measurements such as pound to kilogram, mL to ounce, and inch to centimeter

In these types of problems, there is no dosage strength from a drug label to set up the known ratio. Instead, the nurse uses the household and metric equivalency as the known ratio in the setup.

CONVERSIONS WITHIN THE HOUSEHOLD SYSTEM FOR OTHER CLINICAL CALCULATIONS

If a unit of measurement from the household system needs to be converted to another household unit, a conversion table is used to identify the equivalent measurements.

Example 1:

The patient measures 1½ tsp of medication in an oral dosing spoon. How many Tbs of medication has the patient measured?

This example requires a conversion between two household units, tsp and Tbs. The known equivalent measurement of 3 tsp = 1 Tbs is used as the known ratio in the setup.

KNOWN RATIO = UNKNOWN RATIO

Setup: $\dfrac{3 \text{ tsp}}{1 \text{ Tbs}} = \dfrac{1.5 \text{ tsp}}{x \text{ Tbs}}$ ⟶ Check the units (units match).

Solve: $\dfrac{3 \text{ tsp}}{1 \text{ Tbs}} \diagup\hspace{-1em}\diagdown \dfrac{1.5 \text{ tsp}}{x \text{ Tbs}}$ ⟶ Cross multiply.

$3x = 1 \times 1.5$

$\dfrac{3x}{3} = \dfrac{1.5}{3}$ ⟶ Divide both sides of the equation by the number in front of the **x**.

$x = 0.5 \text{ Tbs}$ ⟶ Note: The unit of measurement in the answer is always the same as the unit of the unknown (**x**).

Example 2:

A patient takes 6 Tbs of nutritional supplement. How many oz does the patient receive?

This example requires a conversion between two household units, Tbs and oz. The known equivalent measurement of 2 Tbs = 1 oz is used as the known ratio in the setup.

KNOWN RATIO = UNKNOWN RATIO

Setup: $\dfrac{2 \text{ Tbs}}{1 \text{ oz}} = \dfrac{6 \text{ Tbs}}{x \text{ oz}}$ ⟶ Check the units (units match).

Solve: $\dfrac{2 \text{ Tbs}}{1 \text{ oz}} \diagup\hspace{-1em}\diagdown \dfrac{6 \text{ Tbs}}{x \text{ oz}}$ ⟶ Cross multiply.

$2x = 1 \times 6$

$\dfrac{2x}{2} = \dfrac{6}{2}$ ⟶ Divide both sides of the equation by the number in front of the **x**.

$x = 3 \text{ oz}$ ⟶ Note: The unit of measurement in the answer is always the same as the unit of the unknown (**x**).

CONVERSIONS BETWEEN THE HOUSEHOLD AND METRIC SYSTEMS FOR OTHER CLINICAL CALCULATIONS

The next example involves a conversion between a household and a metric unit of measurement for a clinical application other than a dosage calculation.

Example 1:

A patient weighs 143 lb. How many kg does the patient weigh?

This example requires a conversion between the household unit of measurement (lb) and the metric unit of measurement (kg). To convert from lb to kg, the equivalent measurement of 1 kg = 2.2 lb is used as the known ratio in the setup.

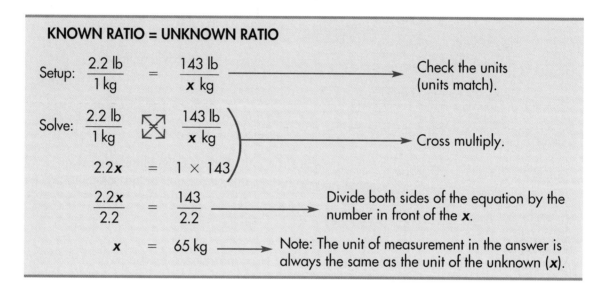

KNOWN RATIO = UNKNOWN RATIO

Setup: $\dfrac{2.2 \text{ lb}}{1 \text{ kg}} = \dfrac{143 \text{ lb}}{x \text{ kg}}$ → Check the units (units match).

Solve: $\dfrac{2.2 \text{ lb}}{1 \text{ kg}} \bowtie \dfrac{143 \text{ lb}}{x \text{ kg}}$ → Cross multiply.

$2.2x = 1 \times 143$

$\dfrac{2.2x}{2.2} = \dfrac{143}{2.2}$ → Divide both sides of the equation by the number in front of the x.

$x = 65 \text{ kg}$ → Note: The unit of measurement in the answer is always the same as the unit of the unknown (x).

 CLINICAL REASONING 6-1

The patient tells the home care nurse that he is taking 1 Tbs of Griseofulvin Oral Suspension every morning. Is the patient taking the correct amount of medication? Provide a rationale for your answer.

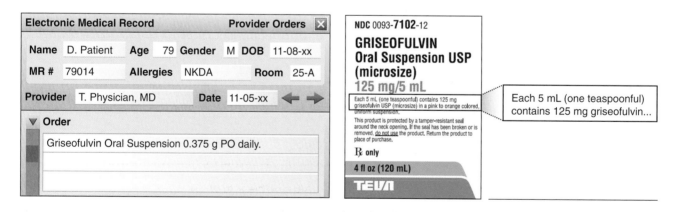

Electronic Medical Record		Provider Orders	☒
Name D. Patient	**Age** 79 **Gender** M **DOB** 11-08-xx		
MR # 79014	**Allergies** NKDA	**Room** 25-A	
Provider T. Physician, MD	**Date** 11-05-xx ⬅ ➡		
▼ **Order**			
Griseofulvin Oral Suspension 0.375 g PO daily.			

NDC 0093-**7102**-12

GRISEOFULVIN
Oral Suspension USP
(microsize)
125 mg/5 mL

Each 5 mL (one teaspoonful) contains 125 mg griseofulvin USP (microsize) in a pink to orange colored, uniform suspension.

This product is protected by a tamper-resistant seal around the neck opening. If the seal has been broken or is removed, <u>do not use</u> the product. Return the product to place of purchase.

℞ only

4 fl oz (120 mL)

TEVA

Each 5 mL (one teaspoonful) contains 125 mg griseofulvin...

In summary, the nurse can use fractional ratio and proportion to solve all math problems encountered in the clinical area. The dosage strength of the medication is the known ratio when setting up the proportion for a dosage calculation. The same steps are used in solving all proportions: checking the units of measurement, converting the units of measurement so they are the same, and cross multiplying the fractions to solve for x, the unknown.

Developing Competency

Write the dosage strength of the medications as a fractional ratio.

1.

Accupril®
(Quinapril HCl
Tablets)

5 mg

DISTRIBUTED BY:
PARKE-DAVIS
DIV OF PFIZER INC, NY, NY 10017
MADE IN IRELAND

_____

2.

Store in a dry place at
25°C (77°F); excursions
permitted to 15°- 30°C
(59°-86°F) [see USP].

Dispense in a well-closed
container with a
child-resistant closure.

DOSAGE AND USE:
See accompanying
prescribing information.

Each tablet contains
750 mg metronidazole.

819 632 201

NDC 0025-1961-30
30 Tablets   **Rx only**

Flagyl® ER
metronidazole extended
release tablets

750 mg

Distributed by
Pfizer **G.D. Searle LLC**
Division of Pfizer Inc, NY, NY 10017

_____

3.

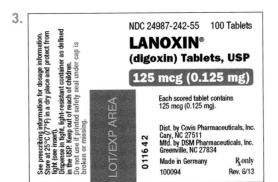

NDC 24987-242-55   100 Tablets
LANOXIN®
(digoxin) Tablets, USP
125 mcg (0.125 mg)

Each scored tablet contains
125 mcg (0.125 mg).

Dist. by Covis Pharmaceuticals, Inc.
Cary, NC 27511
Mfd. by DSM Pharmaceuticals, Inc.
Greenville, NC 27834
Made in Germany   R only
100094   Rev. 6/13

_____

Review the information provided and determine if the nurse set up the problem correctly.

4. A drug is labeled 0.1 mg per 10 mL. The doctor has ordered 0.25 mg of the drug. The nurse sets up the following proportion to calculate the dose: $\dfrac{10 \text{ mL}}{0.1 \text{ mg}} = \dfrac{x \text{ mL}}{0.25 \text{ mg}}$

Has the nurse set up the problem correctly? _____

5. A medication has 350 grams in each tablet. The doctor has ordered 700 grams PO daily. The nurse sets up the following proportion to calculate the dose: $\dfrac{700 \text{ g}}{1 \text{ tablet}} = \dfrac{350 \text{ g}}{x \text{ tablet}}$

Has the nurse set up the problem correctly? _____

Set up a fractional proportion and solve each problem.

6. The label on the medication container states 0.25 g tablets. The patient is to receive 0.125 g each morning. How many tablets will the patient receive? _____

7. The patient is to receive 8.75 mg of a medication. The pharmacy sends the medication to the nurse in a container labeled 2.5 mg/mL. How many mL will the patient receive? _____

8. The medication is available in 0.05 mg scored pills. The order is for 0.125 mg. How many pills will the patient receive? _____

Review the information and solve each problem.

9. The patient tells the nurse that he takes 12 mL of Ceftin four times daily. How many mg does the patient receive per dose?

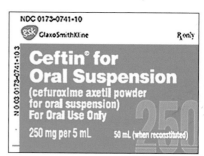

10. The pharmacy sends the nurse the following bottle of PrednisoLONE Oral Solution. The order is to administer 0.03g PO daily. How many tsp will the patient receive?

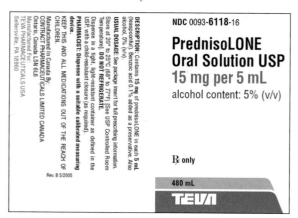

11. The patient is to receive 6 mg of IV morphine q.4h as needed for severe pain. How many mL will the nurse give per dose?

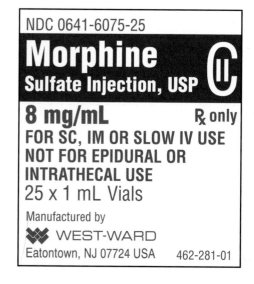

12. The doctor orders granisetron 450 mcg IV 30 minutes prior to chemotherapy. The nurse has the following vials of granisetron. How many mL will the nurse give to the patient?

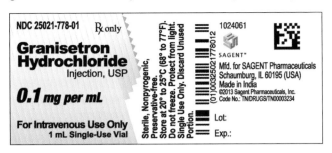

13. The patient is to receive 350 mg of a medication. The medication is labeled 250 mg in 15 mL. How many ounces will the nurse administer? _____

14. The physician's order is for 0.01 g PO each morning. How many tablets will the nurse instruct the patient to take?

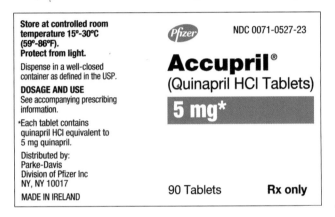

15. The patient is to drink 2,000 mL of water daily. Bottled water is available in 400 mL size. How many bottles will the patient need to drink daily? _____

16. The pharmacy sends the nurse the following medication. How many capsules will the nurse give to the patient if the physician's order is for calcitriol 1.5 mcg PO daily?

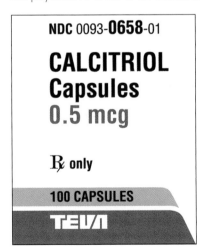

17. The nurse is to give 6.25 mg of carvedilol PO twice a day. How many tablets of carvedilol will the patient receive each day?

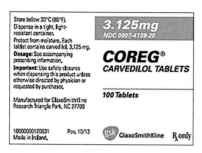

_____

18. The nurse practitioner orders 60 mg of Fluoxetine Oral Solution PO daily for the patient. The pharmacy sends the following bottle of Fluoxetine. How many tsp will the patient receive?

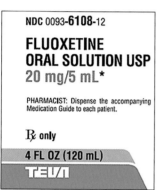

_____

19. The order is for METHYLPREDnisolone Acetate 30 mg IM now. The pharmacy sends the following vial of METHYLPREDnisolone Acetate. How many mL will the nurse administer?

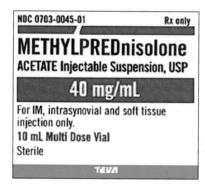

_____

20. The medication order reads as follows: Give 0.75 g of Cephalexin Oral Suspension PO q.12h. The following bottle of Cephalexin is available. How many oz will the nurse administer to the patient?

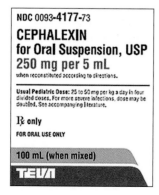

_____

Dimensional Analysis

Define conversion factor.

Discuss dosage strength as a conversion factor.

Set up a dimensional analysis problem using appropriate conversion factors.

Solve drug dosage calculation problems using dimensional analysis.

The medication administration process involves many members of the healthcare team: the physician prescribes the medication, the pharmacist dispenses the medication, and the nurse gives the medication to the patient. As the healthcare professional who administers the medication to the patient, the nurse has the responsibility to verify the ordered dose.

Safe medication administration requires that before giving any medication, the nurse must validate the **dosage.** Sometimes a calculation is required to determine how much of the medication to give. One method of solving a dosage calculation is to use the dimensional analysis method. This is a very useful method for nurses, as it can be used to solve all dosage and clinical math calculations. Dimensional analysis allows the nurse to set up one equation to solve the problem, even if multiple conversions are required.

The Dimensional Analysis Method

Dimensional analysis is a method of calculation that uses a series of equivalent measurements to change one unit of measurement to another to solve a problem. The equivalent measurements are set up as a series of fractions, called **conversion factors,** used to cancel unnecessary units of measurement, leaving only the unit desired for the answer.

Conversion Factors

A conversion factor contains two equivalent measurements written as a fraction in which the numerator is equivalent to the denominator. For example, the metric to household equivalent 2.54 cm = 1 inch can be written as a conversion factor: $\frac{2.54 \text{ cm}}{1 \text{ in}}$.

To work with conversion factors in dimensional analysis, the equivalent measurement must be set up so that the unnecessary units of measurement in the problem cancel. Equivalent measurements can therefore be placed as the numerator or as the denominator.

For example, the problem is "The patient has a cut that is 2 inches in length. How many cm is the cut?" Therefore, the answer must be in "cm," so the equivalent measurement (conversion factor) must be set up to cancel the unit, inches, leaving the unit desired for the answer (cm).

Setting up the equivalent measurement correctly is critical to solving the problem.

Standard equivalent measurements can be memorized or found in a **conversion table** (Table 7-1).

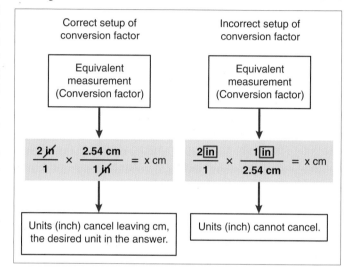

Table 7-1. Conversion Tables of Commonly Used Metric and Household Equivalents

METRIC EQUIVALENT MEASUREMENTS

1 g = 1,000 mg
1 mg = 1,000 mcg
1 mcg = 0.001 mg
1 kg = 1000 g
1 L = 1,000 mL
1 mm = 0.001 m

HOUSEHOLD UNIT OF MEASUREMENT	HOUSEHOLD EQUIVALENT	METRIC EQUIVALENT
1 tablespoon	3 tsp	15 mL
1 teaspoon	—	5 mL
1 ounce	6 tsp, 2 Tbs	30 mL
1 glass	6 oz	180 mL
	8 oz	240 mL
1 cup	6 oz	180 mL
	8 oz	240 mL
—	2.2 lb	1 kg
—	1 in	2.54 cm

Drug Dosage Calculations

In working with drug dosage calculation problems, the nurse may use several conversion factors to solve for the answer. A key conversion factor in drug dosage calculations is the **dosage strength** of the medication found on the drug label. The dosage strength and the ordered dose of medication start the setup of the drug dosage calculation problem.

Information Needed to Set Up a Drug Dosage Dimensional Analysis Problem

To set up a drug dosage problem, the nurse uses two sources of information:

- the ordered dose of medication from the physician's order
- the dosage strength from drug label

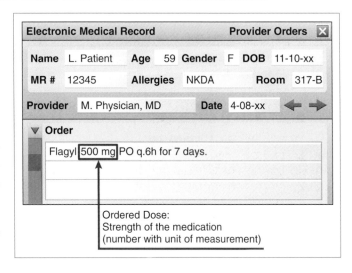

THE ORDERED DOSE

The physician who prescribes the medication specifies the drug name, dose, route, and frequency or time of administration. The ordered **dose** contains the **strength** of the medication (a number) and a **unit of measurement.** An example of a physician's order for a medication on an electronic medical record is shown to the right.

THE DOSAGE STRENGTH FROM THE DRUG LABEL

The pharmacy supplies the medication and the nurse identifies specific information from the drug label to set up the dosage calculation. In reviewing the drug label, the nurse will identify the following:

- The strength of the medication
- The **dosage form** in which the medication is available

Look at each part of the Flagyl medication label (Fig. 7-1).

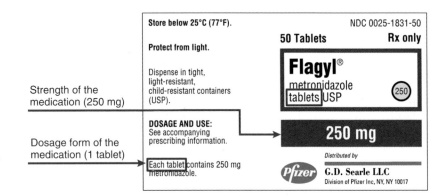

Figure 7-1. Information on the drug label: the dosage strength.

Notice that the strength of a medication is made up of a number and a unit of measurement.

The dosage form of a medication is made up of the number of capsules, tablets, and so on (solid oral dosage form) or the specific volume of liquid (oral or parenteral liquid dosage form) that contains the strength of the medication.

Together, the strength and the dosage form of the medication are called the **dosage strength.** Refer to Chapter 2, The Drug Label, for more information on the dosage strength of a medication.

STEPS FOR SETTING UP AND SOLVING A DIMENSIONAL ANALYSIS PROBLEM

To begin the setup of a drug dosage calculation problem, the nurse needs the following information:

- the ordered dose
- the dosage strength
- the unit of measurement for the answer

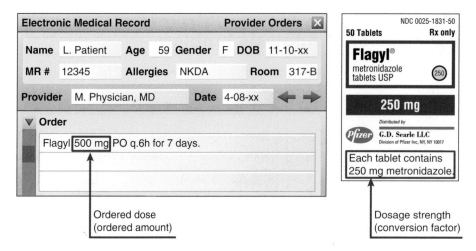

Figure 7-2. Physician's order for Flagyl and Flagyl drug label.

In Figure 7-2, the nurse has an order to give 500 mg of Flagyl. The medication is available in 250 mg tablets. How many tablets will the nurse administer to the patient?

STEPS FOR SETTING UP AND SOLVING IN DIMENSIONAL ANALYSIS

To set up and solve a dimensional analysis problem, five steps are necessary.
   Steps for setting up and solving this problem:

■ **First,** write in the ordered dose as a fraction, called the **ordered amount.**

$$\frac{\text{Ordered}}{\text{Amount}} \times$$

$$\frac{500\ \text{mg}}{1} \times$$

■ **Second,** write in the amount to be given to the patient, called the **desired amount.** The desired amount contains the unknown quantity (represented by the symbol "x") with the unit of measurement. This is the answer to the problem.

$$\frac{\text{Ordered}}{\text{Amount}} \times \quad = \frac{\textbf{Desired}}{\textbf{Amount}}$$

$$\frac{500\ \text{mg}}{1} \times \quad = \boldsymbol{x}\ \text{tablet}$$

■ **Third,** add the conversion factor(s).

   The dosage strength from the drug label is the first conversion factor, placed after the ordered amount. The dosage strength is written as a fraction and is set up so that the unit of measurement in the numerator is the same as (or related to) the unit of measurement in the desired amount.

$$\frac{\text{Ordered}}{\text{Amount}} \times \frac{\textbf{Dosage}}{\textbf{Strength}} = \frac{\text{Desired}}{\text{Amount}}$$

$$\frac{500\ \text{mg}}{1} \times \frac{1\ \text{tablet}}{250\ \text{mg}} = \boldsymbol{x}\ \text{tablet}$$

■ **Fourth,** cancel the units.

   Notice how the two mg units of measurement in the setup cancel, leaving only the unit that is in the desired amount, tablet.

$$\frac{\textbf{Ordered}}{\textbf{Amount}} \times \frac{\textbf{Dosage}}{\textbf{Strength}} = \frac{\textbf{Desired}}{\textbf{Amount}}$$

$$\frac{500\ \cancel{\text{mg}}}{1} \times \frac{1\ \text{tablet}}{250\ \cancel{\text{mg}}} = \boldsymbol{x}\ \text{tablet}$$

■ **Fifth,** solve for x.
   • Multiply the numerators. Multiply the denominators.
   • Solve for x.
   • Think critically: Does the answer make sense?

$$\frac{\text{Ordered}}{\text{Amount}} \times \frac{\text{Dosage}}{\text{Strength}} = \frac{\text{Desired}}{\text{Amount}}$$

Setup: $\dfrac{500 \text{ mg}}{1} \times \dfrac{1 \text{ tablet}}{250 \text{ mg}} = x \text{ tablet}$ ⟶ Set up the equation. Determine the setup of the conversion factor.

Solve: $\dfrac{500 \text{ mg}}{1} \times \dfrac{1 \text{ tablet}}{250 \text{ mg}} = x \text{ tablet}$ ⟶ Cancel the units of measurement. Check the remaining units.

$\dfrac{500 \times 1}{1 \times 250} = x \text{ tablet}$

$\dfrac{500}{250} = 2 \text{ tablets}$ ⟶ Solve for x.

Here is another example of how to set up and solve a dosage calculation using dimensional analysis. Notice how the five steps are used to solve the problem in this example:

The order is to give Vibramycin oral suspension 80 mg PO twice daily. How many mL of Vibramycin will the nurse administer with each dose?

Steps to set up and solve the drug dosage problem:

■ **First,** write in the ordered amount.

The ordered amount is placed first in the setup.

■ **Second,** write in the desired amount.

The desired amount contains the unknown quantity (represented by the symbol "x").

■ **Third,** add the conversion factors.

The dosage strength is set up so that the unit in the numerator is the same as (or is related to) the unit in the desired amount.

■ **Fourth,** cancel the units.

■ **Fifth,** solve for x.

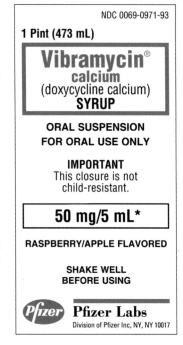

NDC 0069-0971-93

1 Pint (473 mL)

Vibramycin®
calcium
(doxycycline calcium)
SYRUP

ORAL SUSPENSION
FOR ORAL USE ONLY

IMPORTANT
This closure is not
child-resistant.

50 mg/5 mL*

RASPBERRY/APPLE FLAVORED

SHAKE WELL
BEFORE USING

Pfizer **Pfizer Labs**
Division of Pfizer Inc, NY, NY 10017

$$\frac{\text{Ordered}}{\text{Amount}} \times \frac{\text{Dosage}}{\text{Strength}} = \frac{\text{Desired}}{\text{Amount}}$$

Setup: $\dfrac{80 \text{ mg}}{1} \times \dfrac{5 \text{ mL}}{50 \text{ mg}} = x \text{ mL}$ ⟶ Set up the equation. Determine the setup of the conversion factor.

Solve: $\dfrac{80 \text{ mg}}{1} \times \dfrac{5 \text{ mL}}{50 \text{ mg}} = x \text{ mL}$ ⟶ Cancel the units of measurement. Check the remaining units.

$\dfrac{80 \times 5}{1 \times 50} = x \text{ mL}$

$\dfrac{400}{50} = 8 \text{ mL}$ ⟶ Solve for x.

APPLY LEARNED KNOWLEDGE 7-1

Write the dosage strength as a conversion factor for the problems below, and then solve the problem.

1. The MD orders 5 mg of Norvasc PO daily. How many tablets will the nurse administer?

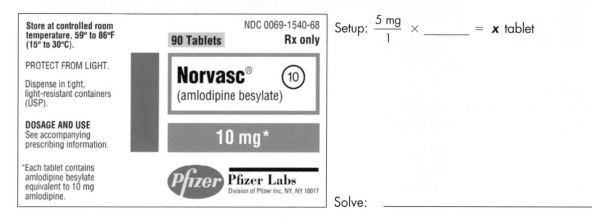

Setup: $\dfrac{5 \text{ mg}}{1} \times$ _____ = **x** tablet

Solve: _____

2. The order is for 300 mg of Cefdinir oral suspension PO q.12h. How many mL will the nurse administer with each dose?

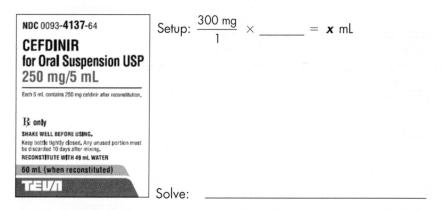

Setup: $\dfrac{300 \text{ mg}}{1} \times$ _____ = **x** mL

Solve: _____

3. The patient is to receive 25 mg Captopril PO BID. How many tablets will the nurse instruct the patient to take with each dose?

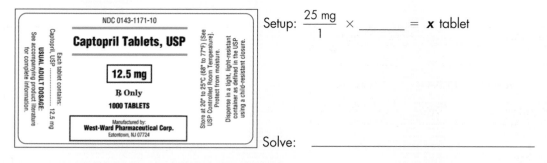

Setup: $\dfrac{25 \text{ mg}}{1} \times$ _____ = **x** tablet

Solve: _____

4. The order is for Zantac 40 mg IV q.8h. How many mL will the nurse administer with each dose?

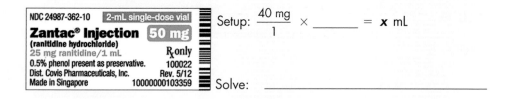

Setup: $\dfrac{40 \text{ mg}}{1} \times$ _____ = **x** mL

Solve: _____

APPLY LEARNED KNOWLEDGE 7-1—cont'd

5. The MD orders Vibramycin oral suspension 200 mg PO daily. How many mL will the nurse administer?

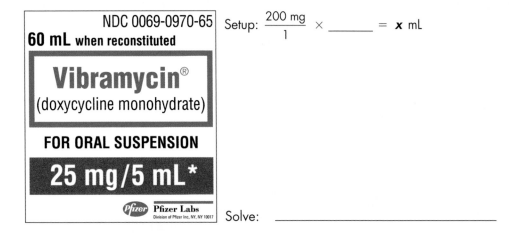

Setup: $\dfrac{200\ mg}{1} \times$ _____ = **x** mL

Solve: _____

Using More Than One Conversion Factor

In each of the examples presented, the units of measurement in the problem have been the same. But in many dosage calculations, the medication order is in one unit of measurement, and the pharmacy provides the drug with a different unit of measurement. To solve a dosage calculation when there are different units, additional conversion factors are used to change the unit of measurement in the ordered amount to that in the desired amount.

WORKING WITH CONVERSIONS WITHIN THE METRIC SYSTEM

If the units of measurement are all in the metric system, a metric equivalent measurement can be used as a conversion factor in the problem. See the following two examples:

Example 1:

The physician orders Enalaprilat 625 mcg IV STAT. The nurse has the following vial of Enalaprilat. How many mL will the nurse administer to the patient? (See Fig. 7-3.)

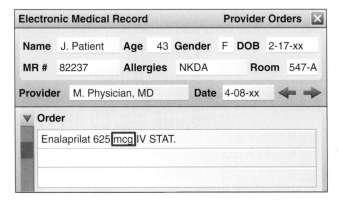
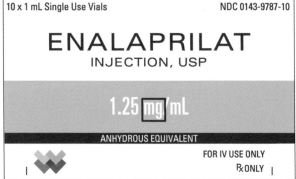

Figure 7-3. Physician's order for Enalaprilat injection.

To solve this problem, begin by applying the first three steps:

■ **First,** write in the ordered amount.
■ **Second,** write in the desired amount,
■ **Third,** set up the dosage strength as the first conversion factor.

$$\frac{\text{Ordered}}{\text{Amount}} \times \frac{\text{Dosage}}{\text{Strength}} = \frac{\text{Desired}}{\text{Amount}}$$

$$\frac{625 \boxed{\text{mcg}}}{1} \times \frac{1 \text{ mL}}{1.25 \boxed{\text{mg}}} = \textbf{x} \text{ mL}$$

The mcg unit in the ordered amount is not the same as the mg unit of the dosage strength. An extra conversion factor is required. The equivalent measurement 1 mg = 1,000 mcg is used as a conversion factor.

Now apply the final steps: cancel the units and solve for *x.*

$$\frac{\text{Ordered}}{\text{Amount}} \times \frac{\text{Dosage}}{\text{Strength}} \times \frac{\text{Conversion}}{\text{Factor}} = \frac{\text{Desired}}{\text{Amount}}$$

Setup: $\dfrac{625 \text{ mcg}}{1} \times \dfrac{1 \text{ mL}}{1.25 \text{ mg}} \times \dfrac{1 \text{ mg}}{1000 \text{ mcg}} = \textbf{x} \text{ mL}$ ⟶ Set up the equation. Determine the setup of the conversion factors.

Solve: $\dfrac{625 \text{ mcg}}{1} \times \dfrac{1 \text{ mL}}{1.25 \text{ mg}} \times \dfrac{1 \text{ mg}}{1000 \text{ mcg}} = \textbf{x} \text{ mL}$ ⟶ Cancel the units of measurement. Check the remaining units.

$$\frac{625 \times 1 \times 1}{1 \times 1.25 \times 1000} = \textbf{x} \text{ mL}$$

$$\frac{625}{1250} = 0.5 \text{ mL}$$

⟶ Solve for **x.**

Example 2:

The physician orders Cleocin 0.375 g IM q.12h. The nurse has the following vial of Cleocin. How many mL will the nurse administer to the patient? (See Fig. 7-4.)

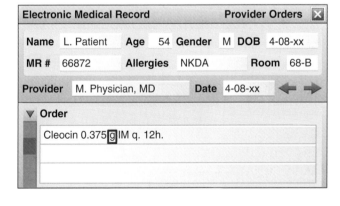
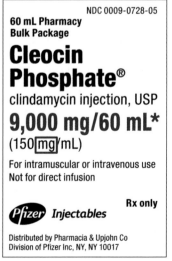

Figure 7-4. Physician's order for Cleocin injection.

To solve this problem, begin by applying the first three steps:

■ **First,** write in the ordered amount.
■ **Second,** write in the desired amount.
■ **Third,** set up the dosage strength as the first conversion factor.

$$\frac{\text{Ordered}}{\text{Amount}} \times \frac{\text{Dosage}}{\text{Strength}} = \frac{\text{Desired}}{\text{Amount}}$$

$$\frac{0.375 \boxed{\text{g}}}{1} \times \frac{1 \text{ mL}}{150 \boxed{\text{mg}}} = \textbf{x} \text{ mL}$$

There are two equivalent dosage strengths listed on the drug label. For simplicity, use the smaller numbers.

The g unit in the ordered amount does not match the mg unit of the dosage strength. An extra conversion factor is required. The equivalent measurement 1 g = 1,000 mg is used as a conversion factor.

Now apply the final steps: cancel the units and solve for x.

$$\frac{\text{Ordered}}{\text{Amount}} \times \frac{\text{Conversion}}{\text{Strength}} \times \frac{\text{Conversion}}{\text{Factor}} = \frac{\text{Desired}}{\text{Amount}}$$

Setup: $\dfrac{0.375 \text{ g}}{1} \times \dfrac{1 \text{ mL}}{150 \text{ mg}} \times \dfrac{1000 \text{ mg}}{1 \text{ g}} = \textbf{x} \text{ mL}$ → Set up the equation. Determine the setup of the conversion factors.

Solve: $\dfrac{0.375 \cancel{\text{g}}}{1} \times \dfrac{1 \text{ mL}}{150 \cancel{\text{mg}}} \times \dfrac{1000 \cancel{\text{mg}}}{1 \cancel{\text{g}}} = \textbf{x} \text{ mL}$ → Cancel the units of measurement. Check the remaining units.

$$\frac{0.375 \times 1 \times 1000}{1 \times 150 \times 1} = \textbf{x} \text{ mL}$$

$$\frac{375}{150} = 2.5 \text{ mL}$$

→ Solve for **x.**

APPLY LEARNED KNOWLEDGE 7-2

Fill in the correct conversion factor for the dimensional analysis problems below. Solve for x.

1. $\dfrac{0.25 \text{ g}}{1} \times \dfrac{1 \text{ pill}}{500 \text{ mg}} \times \boxed{} = \textbf{x} \text{ pill}$ _____

2. $\dfrac{0.625 \text{ g}}{1} \times \dfrac{1 \text{ mL}}{25 \text{ mg}} \times \boxed{} = \textbf{x} \text{ mL}$ _____

3. $\dfrac{0.096 \text{ mg}}{1} \times \dfrac{1 \text{ capsule}}{32 \text{ mcg}} \times \boxed{} = \textbf{x} \text{ capsule}$ _____

Continued

APPLY LEARNED KNOWLEDGE 7-2—cont'd

4. $\dfrac{500 \text{ mg}}{1} \times \dfrac{1 \text{ tsp}}{0.2 \text{ g}} \times \boxed{} = \mathbf{x} \text{ tsp}$ _____

5. $\dfrac{4000 \text{ mg}}{1} \times \dfrac{1 \text{ oz}}{2.5 \text{ g}} \times \boxed{} = \mathbf{x} \text{ oz}$ _____

WORKING WITH CONVERSIONS BETWEEN THE METRIC AND THE HOUSEHOLD SYSTEMS

Sometimes the nurse needs to convert between metric and household units of measurement. In this case, the metric and household equivalent measurements (see Table 7-1) are used as conversion factors.

Example:

The physician orders 125 mg of Cefdinir oral suspension PO two times a day for the patient who is to be discharged home. The pharmacy dispenses the medication with a dosing spoon that measures in tsp. How many tsp should the nurse instruct the patient to take with each dose? (See Fig. 7-5.)

Electronic Medical Record		Provider Orders ☒
Name P. Patient	Age 8 Gender F DOB 5-29-xx	
MR # 44719	Allergies NKDA	Room 56-1
Provider C. Physician, MD	Date 7-11-xx ← →	

▼ Order

1. Discharge home today.
2. 125 mg Cefdinir oral suspension PO BID.

NDC 0093-**4137**-64

CEFDINIR
for Oral Suspension USP
250 mg/5 [mL]

Each 5 mL contains 250 mg cefdinir after reconstitution.

℞ only

SHAKE WELL BEFORE USING.
Keep bottle tightly closed. Any unused portion must be discarded 10 days after mixing.
RECONSTITUTE WITH 49 mL WATER
60 mL (when reconstituted)

TEVA

Figure 7-5. Physician's order for Cefdinir oral suspension.

To solve this problem, begin by applying the first three steps:

- **First,** write in the ordered amount.
- **Second,** write in the desired amount.
- **Third,** set up the dosage strength as the first conversion factor.

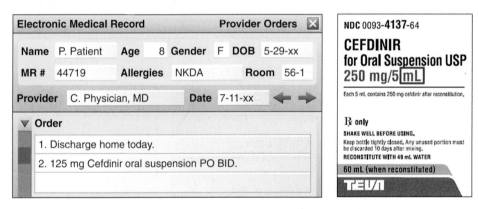

$$\dfrac{\text{Ordered}}{\text{Amount}} \times \dfrac{\text{Dosage}}{\text{Strength}} = \dfrac{\text{Desired}}{\text{Amount}}$$

$$\dfrac{125 \text{ mg}}{1} \times \dfrac{5 \boxed{\text{mL}}}{250 \text{ mg}} = \mathbf{x} \boxed{\text{tsp}}$$

Notice that the mL unit in the dosage strength is not the same as the tsp unit in the desired amount, but the two units are related as they both measure volume. The unit mL can easily be converted to tsp using the equivalent measurement 5 mL = 1 tsp. Therefore, the dosage strength is set up with the mL unit in the numerator and the equivalent measurement 1 tsp = 5 mL is added to the equation as a conversion factor.

Now apply the final steps: cancel the units and solve for *x*.

	Ordered Amount	×	Dosage Strength	×	Conversion Factor	=	Desired Amount	
Setup:	$\dfrac{125\ mg}{1}$	×	$\dfrac{5\ mL}{250\ mg}$	×	$\dfrac{1\ tsp}{5\ mL}$	=	x tsp	Set up the equation. Determine the setup of the conversion factors.
Solve:	$\dfrac{125\ \cancel{mg}}{1}$	×	$\dfrac{5\ \cancel{mL}}{250\ \cancel{mg}}$	×	$\dfrac{1\ tsp}{5\ \cancel{mL}}$	=	x tsp	Cancel the units of measurement. Check the remaining units.

$$\frac{125 \times 5 \times 1}{1 \times 250 \times 5} = x\ tsp$$

$$\frac{625}{1250} = 0.5\ tsp$$

Solve for x.

WORKING WITH MULTIPLE CONVERSION FACTORS

In some calculations, the nurse will need to convert multiple units of measurement to solve the problem. When multiple conversions are required, conversion factors can be set up one at a time until all the unnecessary units cancel. The first conversion factor is the dosage strength. The order of the other conversion factors does not matter.

Example 1:

The physician orders Vibramycin syrup 0.125 g PO twice daily for a patient who is going home from the hospital. The pharmacy sends the following bottle of Vibramycin. How many teaspoons will the nurse instruct the patient to take? (See Fig. 7-6.)

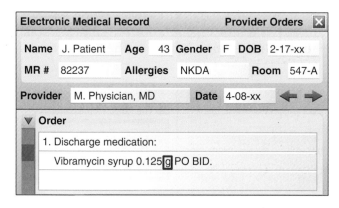

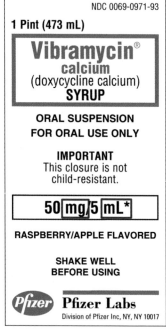

Figure 7-6. Physician's order for Vibramycin syrup.

To solve this problem, begin by applying the first three steps:

- **First,** write in the ordered amount.
- **Second,** write in the desired amount.
- **Third,** set up the dosage strength as the first conversion factor.

The metric units are not the same (g and mg), and the mL and tsp units are not the same. In addition to the dosage strength, two additional conversion factors are needed. The metric equivalent measurement of 1,000 mg = 1 g and the household equivalent 1 tsp = 5 mL are used.

Now apply the final steps: cancel the units and solve for *x*.

| $\dfrac{\text{Ordered}}{\text{Amount}}$ | $\times$ | $\dfrac{\text{Dosage}}{\text{Strength}}$ | $\times$ | $\dfrac{\text{Conversion}}{\text{Factor}}$ | $\times$ | $\dfrac{\text{Conversion}}{\text{Factor}}$ | $=$ | $\dfrac{\text{Desired}}{\text{Amount}}$ |

Setup: $\dfrac{0.125\ \text{g}}{1} \times \dfrac{5\ \text{mL}}{50\ \text{mg}} \times \dfrac{1000\ \text{mg}}{1\ \text{g}} \times \dfrac{1\ \text{tsp}}{5\ \text{mL}} = x\ \text{tsp}$ → Set up the equation. Determine the setup of the conversion factors.

Solve: $\dfrac{0.125\ \cancel{g}}{1} \times \dfrac{5\ \cancel{mL}}{50\ \cancel{mg}} \times \dfrac{1000\ \cancel{mg}}{1\ \cancel{g}} \times \dfrac{1\ \text{tsp}}{5\ \cancel{mL}} = x\ \text{tsp}$ → Cancel the units of measurement. Check the remaining units.

$$\dfrac{0.125 \times 5 \times 1000 \times 1}{1 \times 50 \times 1 \times 5} = x\ \text{tsp}$$

$$\dfrac{625}{250} = 2.5\ \text{tsp}$$

Solve for **x.**

Example 2:

The physician orders Vibramycin oral suspension 0.075 g PO twice daily. The pharmacy sends the following bottle of Vibramycin oral suspension and a measuring spoon that measures in teaspoons and tablespoons. How many Tbs will the nurse instruct the patient to take per dose? (See Fig. 7-7.)

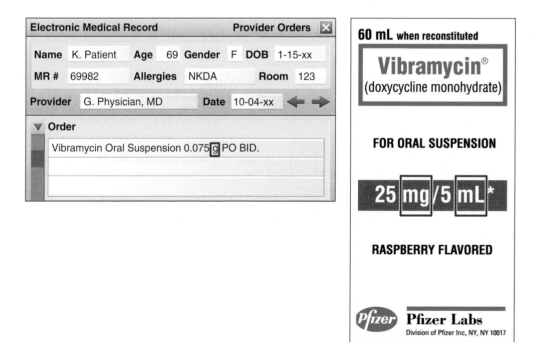

Figure 7-7. Physician's order for Vibramycin oral suspension.

To solve this problem, begin by applying the first three steps:

■ **First,** write in the ordered amount.
■ **Second,** write in the desired amount.
■ **Third,** set up the dosage strength as the first conversion factor.

$$\frac{\text{Ordered}}{\text{Amount}} \times \frac{\text{Dosage}}{\text{Strength}} = \frac{\text{Desired}}{\text{Amount}}$$

$$\frac{0.075 \boxed{g}}{1} \times \frac{5 \boxed{mL}}{25 \boxed{mg}} = x \boxed{Tbs}$$

In this problem, there are multiple units of measurement that need to be converted. The metric units are not the same (g and mg), and the mL and Tbs units are not the same. In addition to the dosage strength, three additional conversion factors are needed. Once the conversion factors are in the setup, the final steps can be applied: cancel the units and solve for x.

$$\frac{\text{Ordered}}{\text{Amount}} \times \frac{\text{Dosage}}{\text{Strength}} \times \frac{\text{Conversion}}{\text{Factor}} \times \frac{\text{Conversion}}{\text{Factor}} \times \frac{\text{Conversion}}{\text{Factor}} = \frac{\text{Desired}}{\text{Amount}}$$

Setup: $\dfrac{0.075\,g}{1} \times \dfrac{5\,mL}{25\,mg} \times \dfrac{1000\,mg}{1\,g} \times \dfrac{1\,tsp}{5\,mL} \times \dfrac{1\,Tbs}{3\,tsp} = x\ Tbs$ — Set up the equation. Determine the setup of the conversion factors.

Solve: $\dfrac{0.075\,\cancel{g}}{1} \times \dfrac{5\,\cancel{mL}}{25\,\cancel{mg}} \times \dfrac{1000\,\cancel{mg}}{1\,\cancel{g}} \times \dfrac{1\,\cancel{tsp}}{5\,\cancel{mL}} \times \dfrac{1\,Tbs}{3\,\cancel{tsp}} = x\ Tbs$ — Cancel the units of measurement. Check the remaining units.

$$\frac{0.075 \times 5 \times 1000 \times 1 \times 1}{1 \times 25 \times 1 \times 5 \times 3} = x\ Tbs$$

$$\frac{375}{375} = 1\ Tbs$$

Solve for **x.**

Working With Conversions for Other Clinical Calculations

In addition to drug dosage calculations, dimensional analysis can be used to solve a variety of other clinical calculations. These types of problems usually include:

■ the conversion of units within the household system such as teaspoon to tablespoon and tablespoon to ounce
■ the conversion of household to metric equivalent measurements such as pound to kilogram, mL to ounce, and inch to centimeter

In these types of problems, there is no dosage strength from a drug label to use as a conversion factor. Instead, the household and metric equivalencies are used as conversion factors in the setup.

CONVERSIONS WITHIN THE HOUSEHOLD SYSTEM FOR OTHER CLINICAL CALCULATIONS

If a unit of measurement from the household system needs to be converted to another household unit, a conversion table is used to identify the equivalent measurements.

Example 1:

The patient measures $1\frac{1}{2}$ tsp of medication in an oral dosing spoon. How many Tbs of medication has the patient measured?

This example requires a conversion between two household units, tsp and Tbs. The equivalent measurement of 3 tsp = 1 Tbs is used as the conversion factor in the setup.

$$\frac{\text{Ordered}}{\text{Amount}} \times \frac{\text{Conversion}}{\text{Factor}} = \frac{\text{Desired}}{\text{Amount}}$$

Setup: $\dfrac{1.5 \text{ tsp}}{1} \times \dfrac{1 \text{ Tbs}}{3 \text{ tsp}} = x \text{ Tbs}$ — Set up the equation. Determine the setup of the conversion factors.

Solve: $\dfrac{1.5 \,\cancel{\text{tsp}}}{1} \times \dfrac{1 \text{ Tbs}}{3 \,\cancel{\text{tsp}}} = x \text{ Tbs}$ — Cancel the units of measurement. Check the remaining units.

$\dfrac{1.5 \times 1}{1 \times 3} = x \text{ Tbs}$

$\dfrac{1.5}{3} = 0.5 \text{ Tbs}$ — Solve for x.

Example 2:

A patient takes 6 tablespoons of nutritional supplement. How many oz does the patient receive?

This example requires a conversion between two household units, Tbs and oz. The equivalent measurement of 2 Tbs = 1 oz is used as the conversion factor in the setup.

$$\frac{\text{Ordered}}{\text{Amount}} \times \frac{\text{Conversion}}{\text{Factor}} = \frac{\text{Desired}}{\text{Amount}}$$

Setup: $\dfrac{6 \text{ Tbs}}{1} \times \dfrac{1 \text{ oz}}{2 \text{ Tbs}} = x \text{ oz}$ — Set up the equation. Determine the setup of the conversion factor.

Solve: $\dfrac{6 \,\cancel{\text{Tbs}}}{1} \times \dfrac{1 \text{ oz}}{2 \,\cancel{\text{Tbs}}} = x \text{ oz}$ — Cancel the units of measurement. Check the remaining units.

$\dfrac{6 \times 1}{1 \times 2} = x \text{ oz}$

$\dfrac{6}{2} = 3 \text{ oz}$ — Solve for x.

CONVERSIONS BETWEEN THE HOUSEHOLD AND METRIC SYSTEMS FOR OTHER CLINICAL CALCULATIONS

The next example involves a conversion between a household and a metric unit of measurement for a clinical application other than a dosage calculation.

Example 1:

A patient weighs 143 lb. How many kg does the patient weigh?

This example requires a conversion between the household unit of measurement (lb) and the metric unit of measurement (kg). To convert from lb to kg, the equivalent measurement 1 kg = 2.2 lb is used as the conversion factor in the setup.

$$\frac{\text{Ordered}}{\text{Amount}} \times \frac{\text{Conversion}}{\text{Factor}} = \frac{\text{Desired}}{\text{Amount}}$$

Setup: $\dfrac{143\ \text{lb}}{1} \times \dfrac{1\ \text{kg}}{2.2\ \text{lb}} = x\ \text{kg}$ ⟶ Set up the equation. Determine the setup of the conversion factor.

Solve: $\dfrac{143\ \cancel{\text{lb}}}{1} \times \dfrac{1\ \text{kg}}{2.2\ \cancel{\text{lb}}} = x\ \text{kg}$ ⟶ Cancel the units of measurement. Check the remaining units.

$\dfrac{143 \times 1}{1 \times 2.2} = x\ \text{kg}$

$\dfrac{143}{2.2} = 65\ \text{kg}$

⟶ Solve for **x**.

APPLY LEARNED KNOWLEDGE 7-3

Add conversion factor(s) to the setup of the following problems. Solve for x.

1. The patient is to receive 500 mcg of a medication subcut now. The pharmacy sends a dose of the medication labeled 2.5 mg in 1 mL. How many mL should the nurse administer?

Setup: $\dfrac{500\ \text{mcg}}{1} \times \dfrac{1\ \text{mL}}{2.5\ \text{mg}} \times \boxed{} = x\ \text{mL}$

Conversion factor: _____

Administer: _____

2. The order is for 1 g of a medication PO BID. The pharmacy sends the medication labeled 200 mg in 5 mL. How many mL should the nurse administer?

Setup: $\dfrac{1\ \text{g}}{1} \times \boxed{} \times \boxed{} = x\ \text{mL}$

Dosage Strength: _____

Conversion factor: _____

Administer: _____

Continued

APPLY LEARNED KNOWLEDGE 7-3—cont'd

3. The patient is to receive 750 mg of a drug PO daily. The drug bottle is labeled 0.5 g in 5 mL. How many Tbs will the patient receive?

Setup: $\dfrac{750 \text{ mg}}{1} \times \dfrac{5 \text{ mL}}{0.5 \text{ g}} \times \boxed{} \times \boxed{} = \boldsymbol{x}$ Tbs

Conversion factor: _____

Conversion factor: _____

Administer: _____

4. The physician orders 75 mcg of a drug IM daily. The drug is available in a vial labeled 0.5 mg in 5 mL. How many mL will the patient receive?

Setup: $\dfrac{75 \text{ mcg}}{1} \times \boxed{} \times \boxed{} = \boldsymbol{x}$ mL

Dosage Strength: _____

Conversion factor: _____

Administer: _____

5. The patient is to receive 80 mg of a drug PO daily. The drug is labeled 0.4 g in 1 oz. How many mL will the patient receive?

Setup: $\dfrac{80 \text{ mg}}{1} \times \dfrac{1 \text{ oz}}{0.4 \text{ g}} \times \boxed{} \times \boxed{} = \boldsymbol{x}$ mL

Conversion factor: _____

Conversion factor: _____

Administer: _____

CLINICAL REASONING 7-1
The patient tells the home care nurse that he is taking 1 Tbs of Griseofulvin Oral Suspension every morning. Is the patient taking the correct amount of medication? Provide a rationale for your answer.

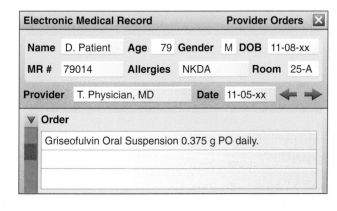

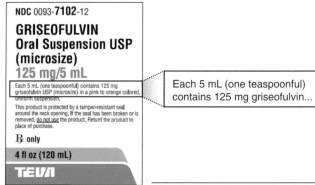

Each 5 mL (one teaspoonful) contains 125 mg griseofulvin...

In summary, the nurse can use dimensional analysis to solve all math problems encountered in the clinical area. The dosage strength of the medication is set up as a conversion factor, and additional conversion factors from a conversion table can be used as needed. The same steps are used in solving all dimensional analysis problems: write in the ordered amount and the desired amount, and set up conversion factors so that the unnecessary units of measurement cancel.

Developing Competency

Write the dosage strength of each medication as a conversion factor.

1.

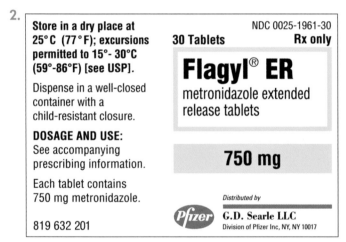

_____

2.

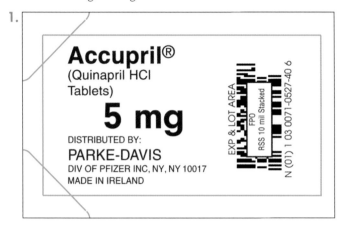

_____

3.

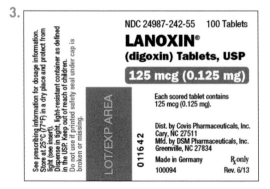

_____

Review the information and determine whether the nurse has set up the problem correctly.

4. A drug is labeled 0.1 mg per 10 mL. The doctor has ordered 0.25 mg of the drug. How many mL shall the nurse give to the patient? The nurse sets up the problem to calculate the dose:

$$\frac{0.25 \text{ mg}}{1} \times \frac{10 \text{ mL}}{0.1 \text{ mg}} = x \text{ mL} \quad \underline{\hspace{2cm}}$$

5. A medication has 350 grams in each tablet. The doctor has ordered 700 grams PO daily. How many tablets will the patient receive daily? The nurse sets up the problem to calculate the dose:

$$\frac{700\ g}{1} \times \frac{350\ g}{1\ tablet} = x\ tablet \qquad \underline{\hspace{2cm}}$$

Set up a dimensional analysis equation and solve each problem.

6. The label on the medication container states 0.25 g tablets. The patient is to receive 0.125 g each morning. How many tablets will the patient receive? _____

_____

7. The patient is to receive 8.75 mg of a medication. The pharmacy sends the medication to the nurse in a container labeled 2.5 mg/mL. How many mL will the patient receive? _____

_____

8. The medication is available in 0.05 mg scored pills. The order is for 0.125 mg. How many pills will the patient receive? _____

_____

Review the information and answer each question.

9. The patient tells the nurse that he takes 12 mL of Ceftin four times daily. How many mg does the patient receive per dose?

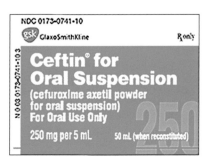

10. The pharmacy sends the nurse the following bottle of PrednisoLONE Oral Solution. The order is to administer 0.03g PO daily. How many tsp will the patient receive?

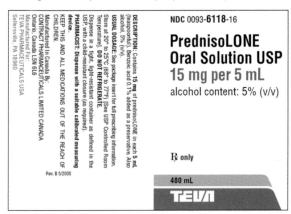

11. The patient is to receive 6 mg of IV morphine q.4h as needed for severe pain. How many mL will the nurse give per dose?

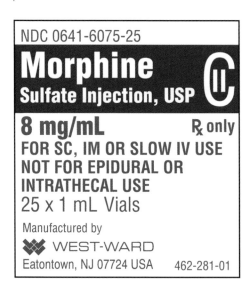

12. The doctor orders granisetron 450 mcg IV 30 minutes prior to chemotherapy. The nurse has the following vials of granisetron. How many mL will the nurse give to the patient?

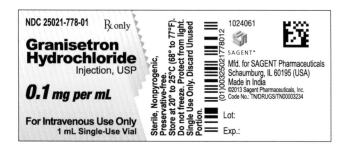

13. The patient is to receive 350 mg of a medication. The medication is labeled 250 mg in 15 mL. How many ounces will the nurse administer?   _____

14. The physician's order is for 0.01 g PO each morning. How many tablets will the nurse instruct the patient to take?

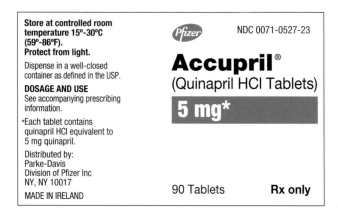

15. The patient is to drink 2,000 mL of water daily. Bottled water is available in 400 mL size. How many bottles will the patient need to drink daily?   _____

16. The pharmacy sends the nurse the following medication. How many capsules will the nurse give to the patient if the physician's order is for calcitriol 1.5 mcg p.o. daily?

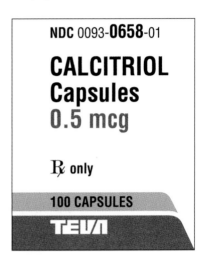

NDC 0093-**0658**-01

CALCITRIOL
Capsules
0.5 mcg

℞ only

100 CAPSULES

TEVA

_____

17. The nurse is to give 6.25 mg of carvedilol PO twice a day. How many tablets of carvedilol will the patient receive each day?

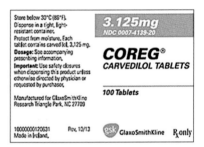

Store below 30°C (86°F).
Dispense in a tight, light-
resistant container.
Protect from moisture. Each
tablet contains carvedilol, 3.125 mg.
Dosage: See accompanying
prescribing information.
Important: Use safety closures
when dispensing this product unless
otherwise directed by physician or
requested by purchaser.

Manufactured for GlaxoSmithKline
Research Triangle Park, NC 27709

10000000120631   Rev. 10/13
Made in Ireland.

3.125mg
NDC 0007-4139-20

COREG®
CARVEDILOL TABLETS

100 Tablets

gsk GlaxoSmithKline   ℞ only

_____

18. The nurse practitioner orders 60 mg of Fluoxetine oral suspension PO daily for the patient. The pharmacy sends the following bottle of Fluoxetine. How many tsp will the patient receive?

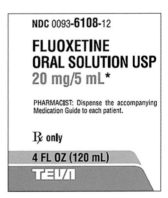

NDC 0093-**6108**-12

FLUOXETINE
ORAL SOLUTION USP
20 mg/5 mL*

PHARMACIST: Dispense the accompanying
Medication Guide to each patient.

℞ only

4 FL OZ (120 mL)

TEVA

_____

19. The order is for METHYLPREDnisolone Acetate 30 mg IM now. The pharmacy sends the following vial of METHYLPREDnisolone Acetate. How many mL will the nurse administer?

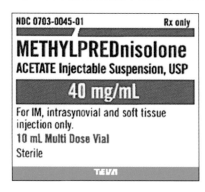

NDC 0703-0045-01   Rx only

METHYLPREDnisolone
ACETATE Injectable Suspension, USP

40 mg/mL

For IM, intrasynovial and soft tissue
injection only.
10 mL Multi Dose Vial
Sterile

TEVA

---

20. The following is the medication order: Give 0.75 g of Cephalexin oral suspension PO q12h. The following bottle of Cephalexin is available. How many oz will the nurse administer to the patient with each dose?

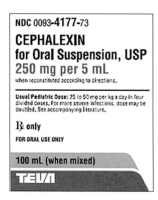

NDC 0093-4177-73

CEPHALEXIN
for Oral Suspension, USP
250 mg per 5 mL
when reconstituted according to directions.

Usual Pediatric Dose: 25 to 50 mg per kg a day in four
divided doses. For more severe infections, dose may be
doubled. See accompanying literature.

℞ only

FOR ORAL USE ONLY

100 mL (when mixed)

TEVA

Formula Method

Define the key components of the formula D, H, and Q.

Correctly place the D, H, and Q to set up the formula.

Discuss dosage strength and how it is used to set up a dosage calculation formula.

Solve drug dosage calculation problems using the formula method.

The medication administration process involves many members of the healthcare team: the physician prescribes the medication, the pharmacist dispenses the medication, and the nurse gives the medication to the patient. As the healthcare professional who administers the medication, the nurse has the responsibility to verify the ordered dose.

Safe medication administration requires that before giving any medication, the nurse must validate the **dosage.** Sometimes a calculation is required to determine how much of the medication to give. One method of solving a dosage calculation is to use a formula. The formula method can be used to solve some drug dosage calculations, but it cannot be used to solve complex calculations that required multiple steps.

The Formula

Here is the dosage calculation **formula:**

$$\frac{\textbf{Desired dose}}{\textbf{dose on Hand}} \times \textbf{Quantity} = \textbf{\textit{x}} \text{ (amount to give)} \qquad \text{or} \qquad \frac{D}{H} \times Q = \textbf{\textit{x}}$$

This formula must be memorized, and the nurse must know what each letter of the formula represents.

D = Desired: ordered dose of medication

H = Have: dose on hand; dose available from the pharmacy that is written on drug label

Q = Quantity: dosage form of the drug (tablet, capsule, amount of liquid) and the quantity of the dosage form

x = Unknown: the answer to the problem; the amount of medication to administer

Information Needed to Set Up the Formula

To calculate a drug dosage using the formula method, the nurse uses two sources of information:

- the ordered dose of medication from the physician's order
- the dosage strength from the drug label

THE ORDERED DOSE [(D)]

The physician who prescribes the medication specifies the drug name, dose, route, and frequency or time of administration. The ordered **dose** contains the **strength** of the medication (a number) with a **unit of measurement.** Here is an example of a physician's order for a medication on the electronic medical record:

The ordered dose is the D in the formula, which is placed in the numerator of the fraction: $\dfrac{D}{H} \times Q = \textbf{\textit{x}}$

Electronic Medical Record		Provider Orders ☒
Name L. Patient	**Age** 59 **Gender** F **DOB** 11-10-xx	
MR # 12345	**Allergies** NKDA	**Room** 317-B
Provider M. Physician, MD	**Date** 4-08-xx ⬅ ➡	

▽ **Order**

Flagyl 500 mg PO q.6h for 7 days.

D
Ordered Dose:
Strength of the medication
(number with unit of measurement)

THE DOSAGE STRENGTH FROM THE DRUG LABEL [(H) AND (Q)]

The pharmacy supplies the medication and the nurse identifies specific information from the drug label needed to set up the dosage calculation. In reviewing the drug label, the nurse will identify the following:

- the strength of the medication (a number with the unit of measurement)
- the **dosage form** in which the medication is available (the number of capsules, tablets, etc., the solid oral dosage form) or the specific volume of liquid (oral or parenteral liquid dosage form) that contains the strength of the medication).

The strength of the medication and the dosage form are called the **dosage strength** of the medication. Look at each part of the medication label in Figure 8-1.

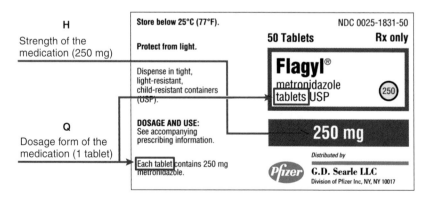

Figure 8-1. Information on the drug label: the dosage strength.

■ **Third,** write in the Q (quantity and dosage form of the medication). The fraction in the formula is multiplied by the Q to solve for the unknown (x).

$$\frac{500 \text{ mg (D)}}{250 \text{ mg (H)}} \times 1 \text{ tablet (Q)} = x$$

■ **Forth,** write in the unknown (x) with the correct unit of measurement. The unit of measurement of the unknown answers the question in the problem, in this case, "How many tablets will the nurse administer to the patient?"

$$\frac{500 \text{ mg}}{250 \text{ mg}} \times 1 \text{ tablet} = x \text{ tablet (x)}$$

■ **Fifth,** check the units of measurement and cancel the like units. The units in the fractional part of the formula must be the same so that they will cancel each other. If the units are not the same, a conversion must be done. Conversions are discussed at the end of this chapter.

$$\frac{500 \,\cancel{\text{mg}}}{250 \,\cancel{\text{mg}}} \times 1 \text{ tablet} = x \text{ tablet}$$

> In multiplication of fractions, if the unit of measurement in a numerator is the same as the unit of measurement in a denominator, the units cancel each other.

■ **Sixth,** solve for x.
- Divide the numerator (D) by the denominator (H), and multiply by Q.
- The answer has the same unit of measurement as the x in the original equation.
- Think critically: Does the answer make sense?

$\frac{D}{H}$	$\times$	Q	=	x	
Setup: $\frac{500 \text{ mg}}{250 \text{ mg}}$	$\times$	1 tablet	=	*x* tablet ⟶	Check the setup of the D, H, and Q (units match).
Solve: $\frac{500 \,\cancel{\text{mg}}}{250 \,\cancel{\text{mg}}}$	$\times$	1 tablet	=	*x* tablet ⟶	Cancel the units of measurement.
$\frac{500}{250}$	$\times$	1 tablet	=	*x* tablet	Solve for **x**. Check that the unit of measurement in the answer is the same as that in the **x**.
2	$\times$	1	=	2 tablets	

Here is another example of how to set up and solve a dosage calculation using the formula method. Notice how the six steps are used to solve the problem in this example:

The order is to give Vibramycin oral suspension 80 mg PO twice daily. How many mL of Vibramycin will the nurse administer in each dose?

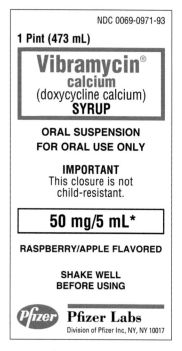

Steps to set up and solve the drug dosage problem:

■ **First,** write in the D (ordered dose).
  • The D is placed in the numerator of the fraction.
■ **Second,** write in the H (dose on hand).
  • The H is part of the dosage strength of the medication. It is placed in the denominator of the fraction.
■ **Third,** write in the Q (quantity and form of the medication).
  • The Q is the amount and dosage form of the medication (part of the dosage strength).
■ **Fourth,** write in the unknown (*x*).
  • The unknown, *x*, has the unit of measurement that is asked for in the problem (e.g., "How many mL?").
■ **Fifth,** check the units and cancel the like units.
  • If the units of measurement in the numerator and denominator of the fraction are the same, no conversion is needed.
■ **Sixth,** solve for *x*.

$$\frac{D}{H} \times Q = x$$

Setup: $\frac{80 \text{ mg}}{50 \text{ mg}} \times 5 \text{ mL} = x \text{ mL}$ ⟶ Check the setup of the D, H, and Q (units match).

Solve: $\frac{80 \cancel{\text{ mg}}}{50 \cancel{\text{ mg}}} \times 5 \text{ mL} = x \text{ mL}$ ⟶ Cancel the units of measurement.

$\frac{80}{50} \times 5 \text{ mL} = x \text{ mL}$

$1.6 \times 5 = 8 \text{ mL}$

Solve for **x**. Check that the unit of measurement in the answer is the same as that in the **x**.

APPLY LEARNED KNOWLEDGE 8-2

Write the formula to set up the problems below, then solve each problem.

1. The MD orders 50 mg of Aldactone PO daily. How many tablets will the nurse administer?

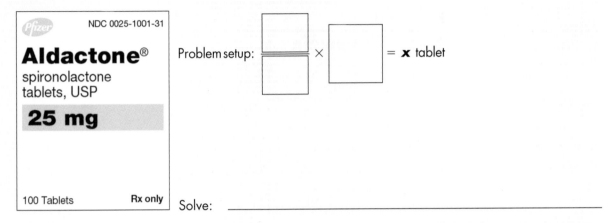

Problem setup: ⬚/⬚ × ⬚ = **x** tablet

Solve: _____

2. The order is for 750 mg of Cefdinir oral suspension PO q. AM. How many mL will the nurse administer?

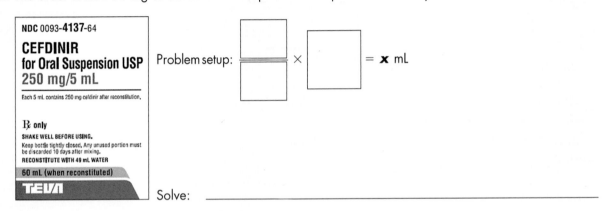

Problem setup: ⬚/⬚ × ⬚ = **x** mL

Solve: _____

3. The patient is to receive 25 mg Catopril PO q.12h. How many tablets will the nurse instruct the patient to take with each dose?

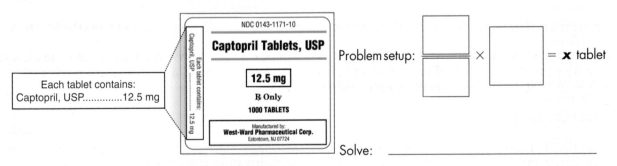

Problem setup: ⬚/⬚ × ⬚ = **x** tablet

Solve: _____

APPLY LEARNED KNOWLEDGE 8-2—cont'd

4. The order is for Bumetanide 0.6 mg IV now. How many mL will the nurse administer?

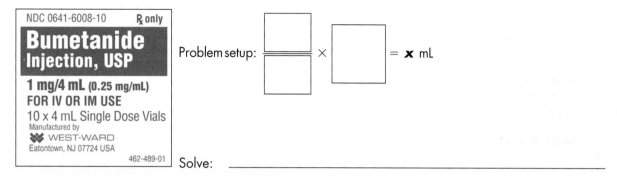

Problem setup: ☐/☐ × ☐ = **x** mL

Solve: _____

5. The MD orders Vibramycin oral suspension 200 mg PO daily. How many mL will the nurse administer?

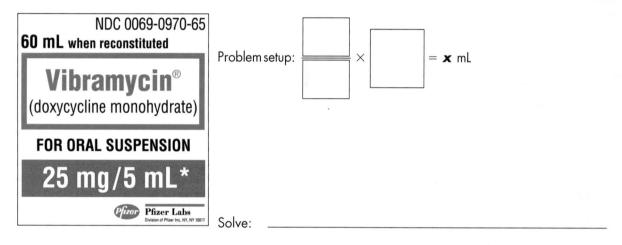

Problem setup: ☐/☐ × ☐ = **x** mL

Solve: _____

Setting Up the Formula When the Units of Measurement Are Not the Same

In the examples presented, the units of measurement in the fraction $\dfrac{D}{H}$ have been the same. But in many dosage calculations, the medication order is in one unit of measurement, and the pharmacy provides the drug with a different unit of measurement. To solve a dosage calculation when there are different units of measurement, a **conversion** is needed.

Working With Conversions Within the Metric System

If a unit of measurement from the metric system needs to be converted to another unit of measurement within the metric system, the metric line is used to **convert** to the equivalent unit of measurement. To promote safety in medication administration, it is recommended that the units of measurement be converted toward the unit on the drug label (the H). That way, the answer has the same unit of measurement as the drug that the nurse has available from the pharmacy.

Example 1:

The physician orders Enalaprilat 625 mcg IV stat. The nurse has the following vial of Enalaprilat (Fig. 8-3). How many mL will the nurse administer to the patient?

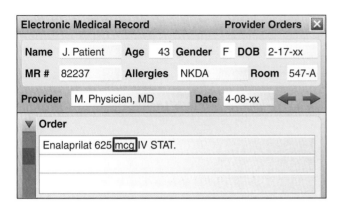 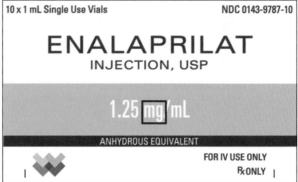

Figure 8-3. Physician's order for Enalaprilat Injection.

To solve this problem, begin by applying the first five steps:

- **First,** write in the D.
- **Second,** write in the H.
- **Third,** write in the Q.
- **Fourth,** write in the unknown (*x*) with the correct unit of measurement.
- **Fifth,** check the units of measurement and cancel the like units.

$$\frac{625 \; \boxed{mcg}}{1.25 \; \boxed{mg}} \times 1 \; mL = \textbf{\textit{x}} \; mL$$

The units of measurement in the fraction are not the same. A conversion is required so that the units in the fraction cancel.

In this example, mcg is the unit of measurement from the physician's order (D) and mg is the unit of measurement from the drug label (H). To convert from mcg (the starting place) to mg (the desired place), move the decimal point three places to the left.

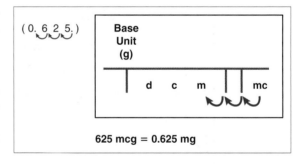

Once the conversion is complete and the units in the fraction are the same, the like units can cancel.

$$\frac{0.625 \; \boxed{mg}}{1.25 \; \boxed{mg}} \times 1 \; mL = \textbf{\textit{x}} \; mL$$

$$\frac{0.625 \; \cancel{mg}}{1.25 \; \cancel{mg}} \times 1 \; mL = \textbf{\textit{x}} \; mL$$

Now apply the final step: solve for *x*.

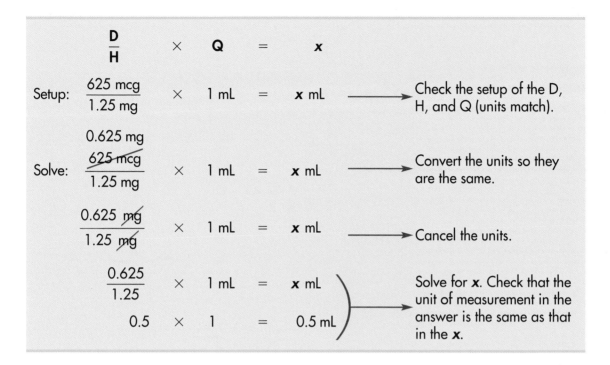

Example 2:

The physician orders Cleocin 0.375 g IM q.12h. The nurse has the following vial of Cleocin. How many mL will the nurse administer to the patient? (Fig. 8-4.)

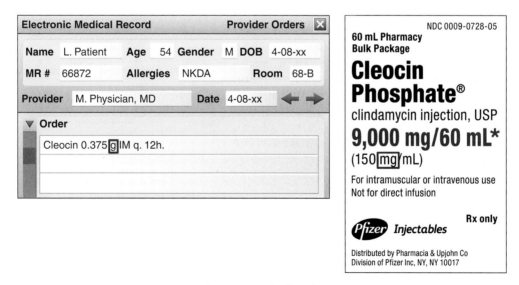

Figure 8-4. Physician's order for Cleocin Injection.

To solve this problem, begin by applying the first five steps. There are two equivalent dosage strengths listed on the drug label. For simplicity, use the smaller numbers.

- ■ **First,** write in the D.
- ■ **Second,** write in the H.
- ■ **Third,** write in the Q.
- ■ **Fourth,** write in the unknown (*x*) with the correct unit of measurement.
- ■ **Fifth,** check the units of measurement and cancel the like units.

$$\frac{0.375 \boxed{g}}{150 \boxed{mg}} \times 1 \text{ mL} = \boldsymbol{x} \text{ mL}$$

The units of measurement in the fraction are not the same. A conversion is required so that the units in the fraction can cancel.

In this example, g is the unit of measurement from the physician's order (D) and mg is the unit of measurement from the drug label (H). To convert from g (the starting place) to mg (the desired place), move the decimal point three places to the right.

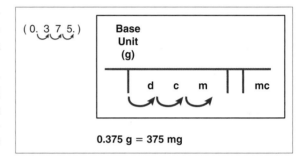

0.375 g = 375 mg

$$\frac{\overset{375 \boxed{mg}}{\cancel{0.375\, g}}}{150 \boxed{mg}} \times 1 \text{ mL} = \boldsymbol{x} \text{ mL}$$

Once the conversion is complete and the units in the fraction are the same, the like units can cancel.

$$\frac{375 \cancel{mg}}{150 \cancel{mg}} \times 1 \text{ mL} = \boldsymbol{x} \text{ mL}$$

Now apply the final step: solve for *x*.

$\dfrac{\mathbf{D}}{\mathbf{H}}$	×	**Q**	=	**x**	
Setup: $\dfrac{0.375 \text{ g}}{150 \text{ mg}}$	×	1 mL	=	**x** mL	→ Check the setup of the D, H, and Q (units match).
Solve: $\dfrac{\overset{375 \text{ mg}}{\cancel{0.375\, g}}}{150 \text{ mg}}$	×	1 mL	=	**x** mL	→ Convert the units so they are the same.
$\dfrac{375 \cancel{mg}}{150 \cancel{mg}}$	×	1 mL	=	**x** mL	→ Cancel the units.
$\dfrac{375}{150}$	×	1 mL	=	**x** mL	Solve for **x**. Check that the unit of measurement in the answer is the same as that in the **x**.
2.5	×	1	=	2.5 mL	

APPLY LEARNED KNOWLEDGE 8-3

Convert the units of measurement in the problems and solve for **x***.*

1. $\dfrac{0.25 \text{ g}}{500 \text{ mg}} \times 1 \text{ pill} = \textbf{x} \text{ pill}$

_____
_____
_____
_____

2. $\dfrac{0.625 \text{ g}}{25 \text{ mg}} \times 1 \text{ mL} = \textbf{x} \text{ mL}$

_____
_____
_____
_____

3. $\dfrac{0.096 \text{ mg}}{32 \text{ mcg}} \times 1 \text{ capsule} = \textbf{x} \text{ capsule}$

_____
_____
_____

4. $\dfrac{500 \text{ mg}}{0.2 \text{ g}} \times 1 \text{ tsp} = \textbf{x} \text{ tsp}$

_____
_____
_____
_____

5. $\dfrac{4000 \text{ mg}}{2.5 \text{ g}} \times 1 \text{ oz} = \textbf{x} \text{ oz}$

_____
_____
_____
_____

Working With Conversions Between the Metric and the Household Systems

Sometimes the nurse needs to convert between metric and household units of measurement. In this case, the metric and household equivalent measurements are used. See Table 8-1.

Table 8-1. Conversion Tables of Commonly Used Metric and Household Equivalents

METRIC EQUIVALENT MEASUREMENTS
1 g = 1,000 mg
1 mg = 1,000 mcg
1 mcg = 0.001 mg
1 kg = 1000 g
1 L = 1,000 mL
1 mm = 0.001 m

HOUSEHOLD UNIT OF MEASUREMENT	HOUSEHOLD EQUIVALENT	METRIC EQUIVALENT
1 tablespoon	3 tsp	15 mL
1 teaspoon	—	5 mL
1 ounce	6 tsp, 2 Tbs	30 mL
1 glass	6 oz	180 mL
	8 oz	240 mL
1 cup	6 oz	180 mL
	8 oz	240 mL
—	2.2 lb	1 kg
—	1 in	2.54 cm

The following is an example of a problem requiring a metric-to-household conversion. The physician orders 125 mg of Cefdinir oral suspension PO two times a day for the patient who is to be discharged home (Fig. 8-5). The pharmacy dispenses the medication with a dosing spoon that measures in tsp. How many tsp should the nurse instruct the patient to take with each dose?

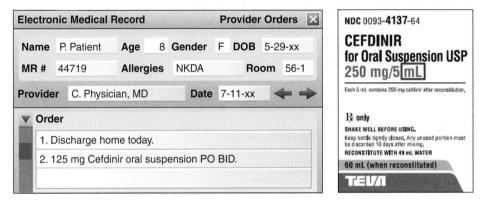

Figure 8-5. Physician's order for Cefdinir oral suspension.

To solve this problem, begin by applying the first five steps:

- **First,** write in the D.
- **Second,** write in the H.
- **Third,** write in the Q.
- **Fourth,** write in the unknown (*x*) with the correct unit of measurement.
- **Fifth,** check the units of measurement and cancel the like units.

$$\frac{125\ \cancel{mg}}{250\ \cancel{mg}} \times 5\ \boxed{mL} = \textbf{\textit{x}}\ \boxed{tsp}$$

The units of measurement in the fraction cancel as they are the same (mg). However, the mL unit in Q is not the same as the tsp unit in the unknown. A conversion needs to be done before the problem can be solved. The unit mL can easily be converted to tsp using the equivalent measurement 5 mL = 1 tsp.

$$\frac{125\ mg}{250\ mg} \times \frac{1\ tsp}{\cancel{5\ mL}} = \textbf{\textit{x}}\ tsp$$

Now apply the final step: solve for *x*.

	$\dfrac{D}{H}$	×	Q	=	x	
Setup:	$\dfrac{125\ mg}{250\ mg}$	×	5 mL	=	**x** tsp	Check the setup of the D, H, and Q (units match).
Solve:	$\dfrac{125\ mg}{250\ mg}$	×	$\dfrac{1\ tsp}{\cancel{5\ mL}}$	=	**x** tsp	Convert the units so they are the same.
	$\dfrac{125\ \cancel{mg}}{250\ \cancel{mg}}$	×	1 tsp	=	**x** tsp	Cancel the units.
	0.5	×	1 tsp	=	0.5 tsp	Solve for **x**. Check that the unit of measurement in the answer is the same as that in the **x**.

Working With Multiple Conversion Factors

In some calculations, the nurse will need to convert multiple units of measurement before solving the problem. See the example in Figure 8-6. The physician orders Vibramycin oral suspension 0.075 g PO twice daily. The pharmacy sends the following bottle of Vibramycin oral suspension and a measuring spoon that measures in teaspoons.

How many tsp will the nurse instruct the patient to take per dose?

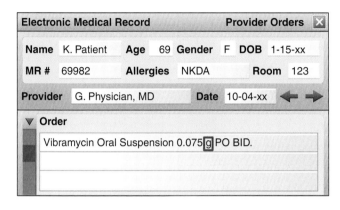
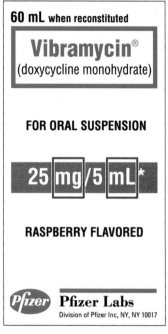

Figure 8-6. Physician's order for Vibramycin oral suspension.

To solve this problem, begin by applying the first five steps:

- **First,** write in the D.
- **Second,** write in the H.
- **Third,** write in the Q.
- **Fourth,** write in the unknown (*x*) with the correct unit of measurement.
- **Fifth,** check the units of measurement and cancel the like units.

$$\frac{0.075 \boxed{g}}{25 \boxed{mg}} \times 5 \boxed{mL} = \boxed{x} \boxed{tsp}$$

The metric units in the fraction are not the same (g and mg), and the mL and tsp units are not the same. Two conversions are needed.

First, convert the metric units. In this example, g is the unit of measurement from the physician's order (D), and mg is the unit of measurement from the drug label (H). To convert from g (the starting place) to mg (the desired place), move the decimal point three places to the right.

(0. 0 7 5.)

Base Unit (g)				
	d	c	m		mc

0.075 g = 75 mg

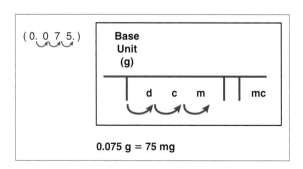

$$\frac{\cancel{0.075\ g}\ \ 75\boxed{mg}}{25\boxed{mg}} \times 5\ mL = \boldsymbol{x}\ tsp$$

Next, convert the metric unit mL to the household unit tsp. The equivalent measurement 1 tsp = 5 mL is used.

$$\frac{75\ \boxed{mg}}{25\ \boxed{mg}} \times 1\ \boxed{tsp} \times \cancel{5\ mL} = x\ \boxed{tsp}$$

Cancel the units of measurement in the fraction.

$$\frac{75\ \cancel{mg}}{25\ \cancel{mg}} \times 1\ tsp = x\ tsp$$

Now apply the final step: solve for *x*.

$$\frac{D}{H} \times Q = x$$

Setup: $\dfrac{0.075\ g}{25\ mg} \times 5\ mL = x\ tsp$ ⟶   Check the setup of the D, H, and Q (units match).

Solve: $\dfrac{\overset{75\ mg}{\cancel{0.075\ g}}}{25\ mg} \times \dfrac{1\ tsp}{\cancel{5\ mL}} = x\ tsp$ ⟶   Convert the units so they are the same.

$\dfrac{75\ \cancel{mg}}{25\ \cancel{mg}} \times 1\ tsp = x\ tsp$ ⟶   Cancel the units.

$3 \times 1\ tsp = 3\ tsp$ ⟶   Solve for *x*. Check that the unit of measurement in the answer is the same as that in the *x*.

APPLY LEARNED KNOWLEDGE 8-4

1. The patient is to receive 500 mcg of a medication subcut now. The pharmacy sends a dose of the medication labeled 2.5 mg in 1 mL. How many mL should the nurse administer?

Setup: _____

Administer: _____

2. The order is for 1 g of a medication PO bid. The pharmacy sends the medication labeled 200 mg in 5 mL. How many mL should the nurse administer?

Setup: _____

Administer: _____

APPLY LEARNED KNOWLEDGE 8-4—cont'd

3. The patient is to receive 750 mg of a drug PO daily. The drug bottle is labeled 0.5 g in 15 mL. How many Tbs will the patient receive?

Setup: _____

Administer: _____

4. The physician orders 75 mcg of a drug IM daily. The drug is available in a vial labeled 0.5 mg in 5 mL. How many mL will the patient receive?

Setup: _____

Administer: _____

5. The patient is to receive 80 mg of a drug PO daily. The drug is labeled 0.4 g in 1 oz. How many mL will the patient receive?

Setup: _____

Administer: _____

CLINICAL REASONING 8-1
The patient tells the home care nurse that he is taking 1 Tbs of Griseofulvin Oral Suspension every morning. Is the patient taking the correct amount of medication? Provide a rationale for your answer.

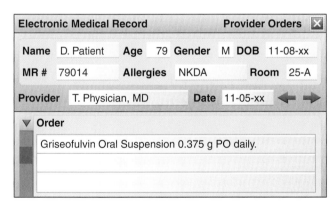

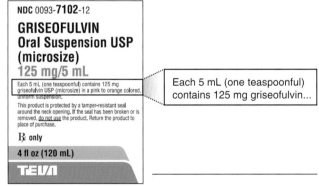

Electronic Medical Record	Provider Orders ☒
Name D. Patient **Age** 79 **Gender** M **DOB** 11-08-xx	
MR # 79014 **Allergies** NKDA **Room** 25-A	
Provider T. Physician, MD **Date** 11-05-xx ⬅ ➡	
▼ **Order**	
Griseofulvin Oral Suspension 0.375 g PO daily.	

NDC 0093-7102-12
GRISEOFULVIN
Oral Suspension USP
(microsize)
125 mg/5 mL
Each 5 mL (one teaspoonful) contains 125 mg griseofulvin USP (microsize) in a pink to orange colored, uniform suspension.
This product is protected by a tamper-resistant seal around the neck opening. If the seal has been broken or is removed, do not use the product. Return the product to place of purchase.
℞ only
4 fl oz (120 mL)
TEVA

Each 5 mL (one teaspoonful) contains 125 mg griseofulvin...

In summary, the nurse can use the formula $\dfrac{D}{H} \times Q = x$ to solve many dosage calculation problems encountered in the clinical area. The information on the drug label (the dosage strength) and the ordered medication are used to set up the formula for a dosage calculation. The same steps are used to solve the formula: check the units of measurement, convert if necessary so that the units in the fraction are the same and the units in the Q and the unknown are the same, cancel the units, and solve for the x (the unknown).

Developing Competency

Write the dosage strength of each medication. Fill in the formula.

1.

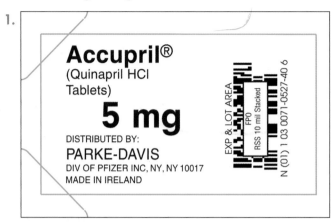

ordered
amount ☐ × ☐ = **x** tablet

_____

2.

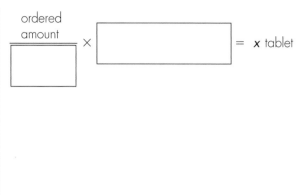

ordered
amount ☐ × ☐ = **x** tablet

_____

3.

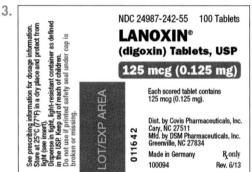

ordered
amount ☐ × ☐ = **x** tablet

_____

Review the information and determine whether the nurse has set up each problem correctly.

4. A drug is labeled 0.1 mg per 10 mL. The doctor has ordered 0.25 mg of the drug. How many mL should

the nurse give to the patient? The nurse sets up the problem to calculate the dose: $\dfrac{0.25 \text{ mg}}{0.1 \text{ mg}} \times 10 \text{ mL} = x \text{ mL}$

_____

5. A medication has 350 grams in each tablet. The doctor has ordered 700 grams PO daily. How many tablets

will the patient receive daily? The nurse sets up the problem to calculate the dose: $\dfrac{350 \text{ mg}}{700 \text{ g}} \times 1 \text{ tablet} = x \text{ tablet}$

_____

Set up a formula and solve each problem.

6. The label on the medication container states 0.25 g tablets. The patient is to receive 0.125 g each morning. How many tablets will the patient receive?   _____

7. The patient is to receive 8.75 mg of a medication. The pharmacy sends the medication to the nurse in a container labeled 2.5 mg/mL. How many mL will the patient receive?   _____

8. The medication is available in 0.05 mg scored pills. The order is for 0.125 mg. How many pills will the patient receive?   _____

9. The patient tells the nurse that he takes 12 mL of Ceftin four times daily. How many mg does the patient receive per dose?

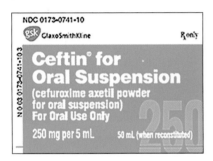

10. The pharmacy sends the nurse the following bottle of PrednisoLONE Oral Solution. The order is to administer 0.03g PO daily. How many tsp will the patient receive?

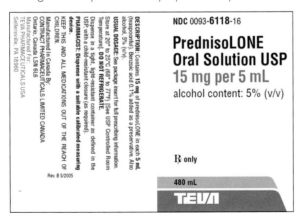

11. The patient is to receive 6 mg of IV morphine q.4h as needed for severe pain. How many mL will the nurse give per dose?

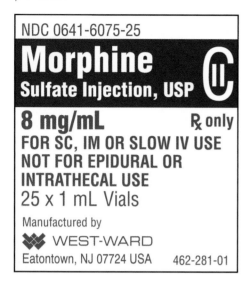

12. The doctor orders granisetron 450 mcg IV 30 minutes prior to chemotherapy. The nurse has the following vials of granisetron. How many mL will the nurse give to the patient?

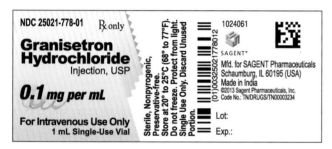

13. The patient is to receive 350 mg of a medication. The medication is labeled 250 mg in 15 mL. How many ounces will the nurse administer? _____

14. The physician's order is for 0.01 g PO each morning. How many tablets will the nurse instruct the patient to take?

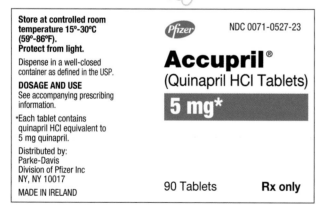

15. The patient is to drink 2,000 mL of water daily. Bottled water is available in 400 mL size. How many bottles will the patient need to drink daily? _____

16. The pharmacy sends the nurse the following medication. How many capsules will the nurse give to the patient if the physician's order is for calcitriol 1.5 mcg PO daily?

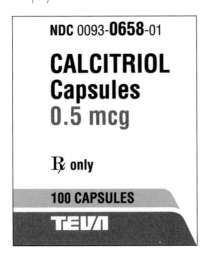

NDC 0093-**0658**-01

CALCITRIOL
Capsules
0.5 mcg

℞ only

100 CAPSULES

TEVA

_____

17. The nurse is to give 6.25 mg of carvedilol PO twice a day. How many tablets of carvedilol will the patient receive each day?

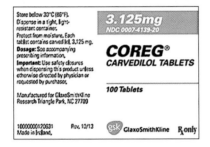

Store below 30°C (86°F).
Dispense in a tight, light-
resistant container.
Protect from moisture. Each
tablet contains carvedilol, 3.125 mg.
Dosage: See accompanying
prescribing information.
Important: Use safety closures
when dispensing this product unless
otherwise directed by physician or
requested by purchaser.

Manufactured for GlaxoSmithKline
Research Triangle Park, NC 27709

10000000120631   Rev. 10/13
Made in Ireland.

3.125mg
NDC 0007-4139-20

COREG®
CARVEDILOL TABLETS

100 Tablets

gsk GlaxoSmithKline   ℞ only

_____

18. The nurse practitioner orders 60 mg of fluoxetine oral suspension PO daily for the patient. The pharmacy sends the following bottle of fluoxetine. How many tsp will the patient receive?

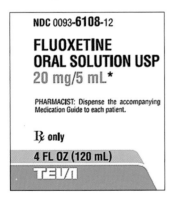

NDC 0093-**6108**-12

FLUOXETINE
ORAL SOLUTION USP
20 mg/5 mL*

PHARMACIST: Dispense the accompanying
Medication Guide to each patient.

℞ only

4 FL OZ (120 mL)

TEVA

_____

19. The order is for METHYLPREDnisolone Acetate 30 mg IM now. The pharmacy sends the following vial of METHYLPREDnisolone. How many mL will the nurse administer?

NDC 0703-0045-01   Rx only

METHYLPREDnisolone
ACETATE Injectable Suspension, USP

40 mg/mL

For IM, intrasynovial and soft tissue injection only.
10 mL Multi Dose Vial
Sterile

TEVA

_____

20. The following is the medication order: Give 0.75 g of cephalexin oral suspension PO q.12h. The following bottle of cephalexin is available. How many oz will the nurse administer to the patient?

NDC 0093-**4177**-73

CEPHALEXIN
for Oral Suspension, USP
250 mg per 5 mL
when reconstituted according to directions.

Usual Pediatric Dose: 25 to 50 mg per kg a day in four divided doses. For more severe infections, dose may be doubled. See accompanying literature.

℞ only
FOR ORAL USE ONLY

100 mL (when mixed)
TEVA

_____

Methods of Calculation

Unit Review—Evaluate for Clinical Decision Making

*For each question, use your clinical judgment to determine whether the nurse's decision is **Correct** or **Incorrect**. For incorrect problems, write the correct answer.*

Nurse's Action

Nurse's Decision

1. The medication order is to give Digoxin 0.25 mg PO daily. The nurse gives two of the following tablets to the patient.

Correct	Incorrect	Answer: _____
✓	✗	

NDC 0143-1240-01

Digoxin Tablets, USP

125 mcg (0.125 mg)

℞ Only
6505-00-449-0321
100 TABLETS

Manufactured by:
West-Ward Pharmaceutical Corp.
Eatontown, NJ 07724

2. The doctor's order is for 0.3 g of Amoxicillin PO q.8h. The nurse plans to administer 6 mL of the drug per dose from the following bottle.

Correct	Incorrect	Answer: _____

NDC 0143-9889-15

**AMOXICILLIN
POWDER FOR ORAL
SUSPENSION, USP**

250 mg / 5 mL

Rx Only
150 mL (when reconstituted)
Dye free

Distributed by
West-ward Pharmaceutical Corp.
Eatontown, NJ 07724

 pg 536

Nurse's Action

3. The doctor orders 2.5 mg of Clemastine fumarate syrup twice daily. The nurse calculates the dose and gives the patient 2.5 mL of the drug. *incd*

```
NDC 0093-0309-12

CLEMASTINE
FUMARATE Syrup
0.5 mg/5 mL*

Each 5 mL (teaspoonful) contains:
Clemastine                    0.5 mg*
Alcohol                       5.5%
*(present as clemastine fumarate 0.67 mg)

℞ only

120 mL

TEVA
```

4. The following is the medication order: Give 80 mg of Vibramycin PO daily. The nurse administers 15 mL of the drug. *incd*

```
NDC 0069-0970-65

60 mL when reconstituted

Vibramycin®
(doxycycline monohydrate)

FOR ORAL SUSPENSION

25 mg/5 mL*

RASPBERRY FLAVORED

Pfizer  Pfizer Labs
Division of Pfizer Inc, NY, NY 10017
```

5. The nurse is to administer Ceftin oral suspension 75 mg PO twice daily. The nurse gives the patient 3 mL of Ceftin per dose.

```
NDC 0173-0740-00

gsk GlaxoSmithKline          ℞ only

Ceftin® for
Oral Suspension
(cefuroxime axetil powder
for oral suspension)
For Oral Use Only

125 mg per 5 mL    100 mL (when reconstituted)
```

Nurse's Decision

3.

Correct	Incorrect	Answer: _____
	✓	

4.

Correct	Incorrect	Answer: _____
	✓	

5.

Correct	Incorrect	Answer: _____
✓		

Nurse's Action

Nurse's Decision

6. The patient tells the nurse that she takes two tablets of Lanoxin daily. The order is for Lanoxin 0.125 mg daily. The nurse advises the patient to continue with the same dose of Lanoxin.

Correct	Incorrect	Answer: _____
✓		

```
NDC 24987-240-55    100 Tablets
LANOXIN®
(digoxin) Tablets, USP
62.5 mcg (0.0625 mg)

Each tablet contains
62.5 mcg (0.0625 mg).

Dist. by Covis Pharmaceuticals, Inc.
Cary, NC 27511
Mfd. by DSM Pharmaceuticals, Inc.
Greenville, NC 27834
Made in Germany        R only
100089                 Rev. 3/13
011629
```

7. The ordered dose of Granisetron HCl is 650 mcg IV now. The nurse gives 0.65 mL of Granisetron to the patient.

Correct	Incorrect	Answer: _____
	✗	

```
NDC 25021-778-01
Granisetron
Hydrochloride
Injection, USP
0.1 mg per mL*
SAGENT
Discover Injectables Excellence™
```

8. The doctor orders Mesna 250 mg IV at the start of chemotherapy. The nurse calculates the dosage and draws up 2.5 mL of Mesna in the syringe.

Correct	Incorrect	Answer: _____
✗		

```
NDC 25021-201-10        R only
MESNA
INJECTION
1 g per 10 mL
(100 mg per mL)
SAGENT™        For IV Use
               10 mL Multi-Dose Vial
LATEX-FREE
Sterile, Nonpyrogenic.
Each mL contains: 100 mg of mesna,
0.25 mg of edetate disodium, sodium
hydroxide to adjust the pH to (6.5 to
7.4) and q.s. with Water for Injection.
10.4 mg of benzyl alcohol added
as a preservative.
Usual Dosage: See insert for dosing
information.
Store at 20° to 25°C (68° to 77°F).
[See USP Controlled
Room Temperature].
```

9. MD order: 3 mg of drug X daily
Dosage strength: 1.5 mg/5 mL
The patient takes 2 teaspoons of drug X every morning. The nurse advises the patient to continue with the same dose of drug X.

Correct	Incorrect	Answer: _____
✗		

Nurse's Action

10. MD order:

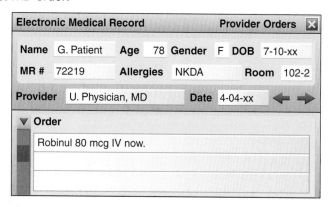

Pharmacy sends:

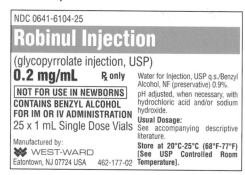

The nurse calculates the dosage and draws up 4 mL of Robinul in the syringe.

Nurse's Decision

Correct	Incorrect	Answer: _____
	X	

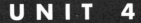

UNIT 4

Administration of Medications

Safe medication administration requires the nurse to apply the Six Rights of Medication Administration, including validation of the right drug and route, accurate calculation of the dosage, and selection of the most appropriate calibrated measuring device. This unit provides you with the clinical reasoning skills essential to the calculation of oral and parenteral medications dosages.

 APPLICATION TO NURSING PRACTICE

The nurse uses the patient's electronic medication administration record and the drug label to calculate the dosage.

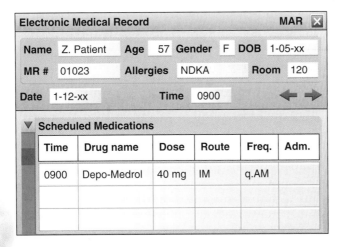

Electronic Medical Record				MAR ⊠
Name Z. Patient **Age** 57 **Gender** F **DOB** 1-05-xx				
MR # 01023 **Allergies** NDKA **Room** 120				
Date 1-12-xx **Time** 0900 ← →				

▼ Scheduled Medications

Time	Drug name	Dose	Route	Freq.	Adm.
0900	Depo-Medrol	40 mg	IM	q.AM	

For IM, intrasynovial and soft tissue injection only. NOT for IV use.
DOSAGE AND USE: See accompanying prescribing information. Shake well immediately before using.
Distributed by
Pharmacia & Upjohn Co
Division of Pfizer Inc
New York, NY 10017

NDC 0009-3475-01
1 mL Single-Dose Vial
Depo-Medrol®
(methylprednisolone acetate injectable suspension, USP)
80 mg/mL
Rx only

To safely administer the medication, the nurse uses clinical reasoning to answer questions such as:

- *Is the dosage I am about to administer correct?*
- *Which syringe accurately measures the ordered dose?*
- *Which needle length and gauge are most appropriate for the ordered route?*

149

CHAPTER 9

Calculating Oral Medication Doses

LEARNING OUTCOMES

Describe the enteral routes of medication administration.

Identify equipment used in the administration of oral medications.

Calculate drug dosage problems for oral administration.

The administration of medications is a part of the clinical responsibilities of the practicing nurse. Safe medication administration includes practices that minimize medication errors, such as the preparation of medications in a distraction-free environment, and allowing sufficient time to carry out the Six Rights of Medication Administration.

In the preparation of medications, the nurse begins by applying the first three rights of medication administration: the right drug, the right dose, and the right route. Once the nurse has determined the right dose of medication, the nurse then selects the most appropriate equipment that will safely and accurately administer the medication.

Routes of Medication Administration

Medications are introduced into the body through nonparenteral and parenteral routes. Medications introduced into the body by mouth (oral route), applied directly to the surfaces of the body such as the skin or mucous membrane (topical route), or inhaled (respiratory) are examples of **nonparenteral** routes. **Parenteral** administration of a medication indicates that the medication is delivered into the body by injection. Medications given intramuscularly (into a muscle) or intravenously (into a vein) are two examples of the administration of medications via the parenteral route.

The oral route is part of the gastrointestinal tract. Beginning with the mouth, the gastrointestinal tract includes the stomach, the intestines, and the rectum. The oral route allows for medications to be swallowed or to be placed under the tongue (sublingual) or between the gum and the inner lining of the cheek (buccal) to dissolve. Medications may be also administered into the gastrointestinal tract through feeding tubes. Feeding tubes such as the nasogastric tube, gastrostomy tube, and jejunostomy tube are placed directly into the gastrointestinal tract and provide a means for giving nutrition and medications. The administration of nutrition or medications into the gastrointestinal tract is referred to as **enteral** nutrition or enteral medication administration. "Enteral" indicates that the medication or nutrition will pass through the digestive process of the gastrointestinal tract (Table 9-1).

Table 9-1. Enteral Routes of Medication Administration

ENTERAL ROUTES	ADMINISTRATION INTO GASTROINTESTINAL TRACT
• Oral (PO)	• By mouth/orally
• Buccal (buc)	• Between the gums and inner lining of the cheek
• Sublingual (SL)	• Under the tongue
• Common feeding tubes	
• Nasogastric tube	• Tube that is introduced from the nose into the stomach
• Gastrostomy tube	• Tube directly into the stomach for feeding
• Jejunostomy tube	• Tube directly into the jejunum for feeding
• Rectal (PR)	• Into the rectum

Solid Oral Medications

Oral medications come in various solid forms. The most common forms include tablets and capsules. **Tablets** contain the drug's active ingredient in a compressed form and come in a variety of shapes and sizes. A variation of the tablet is the caplet. The **caplet** is small and has a smooth covering that makes it easier to swallow. Tablets may be scored or have an enteric coating.

■ **Scored tablets** have indented lines. A scored tablet may be broken along the indented line. Each part of the tablet will contain an equal amount of the active ingredient of the drug.

■ **Enteric coating (EC)** is a special covering on the tablet that allows the tablet to be dissolved and absorbed in a particular place in the gastrointestinal tract. Tablets with enteric coating should not be crushed or broken (see Fig. 9-1).

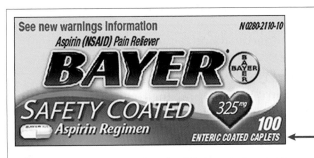

Figure 9-1. Enteric-coated caplet. (Used under license from Bayer.)

Capsules have a gelatin-like covering that holds the powdered form of the drug. Softgel capsules are a variation of the capsule used specifically for liquid or oil-based drug ingredients.

Some capsules contain tiny beads or pellets that are dissolved and released over time, allowing the drug's active ingredient to enter into the bloodstream at a slower and steadier rate. Drug labels identify time-released medications in various formats. Table 9-2 lists examples of words and abbreviations on drug labels associated with time-released medications. Both capsules and tablets with time-released ingredients should be administered whole and should not be crushed or chewed (see Fig. 9-2).

Table 9-2. Words and Abbreviations Associated With Time-Released Medications

WORD	ABBREVIATION(S)
Controlled-release	CR
Continuous-release	Contin
Extended-release	ER, XR, or XL
Sustained-action	SA
Sustained-release	SR
Time-release	TR

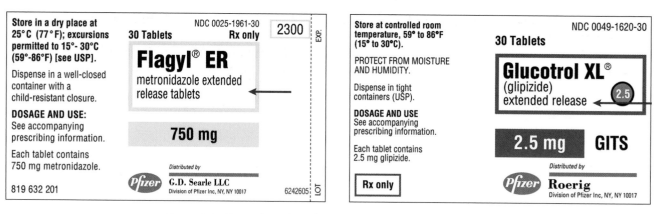

Figure 9-2. Time-released medications identified on the drug label.

Liquid Oral Medications

Liquid medications are supplied in a variety of mixtures that combine the drug in a liquid. The most common type of mixtures consists of elixirs, syrups, and suspensions. An **elixir** is a mixture of the drug mixed with water, alcohol, and flavored subtances, whereas a **syrup** contains the drug in a viscous liquid preparation consisting largely of purified water and sucrose or a sugar substitute for a more pleasant taste. A **suspension** is a liquid that contains small particles of the drug that cannot be dissolved. The particles from the suspension will settle to the bottom if left standing for a period of time, so suspensions need to be shaken well before administering a dose.

Powdered Medication for Oral Administration

Powdered medications require special preparation prior to administering the ordered dose to the patient. In the preparation and administration of powdered medications, the nurse needs to consider these three key points:

■ the instructions for mixing the powdered medication and the dosage strength
■ proper storage of the reconstituted medication
■ labeling the oral medication bottle after reconstitution

PREPARATION OF THE POWDERED MEDICATION AND THE DOSAGE STRENGTH

Powdered oral medications must be mixed just before administration. This process, called **reconstitution,** involves mixing the powder with a liquid so that the powdered medication can be administered. Powdered medications for oral administration are mostly reconstituted with tap or distilled water. To correctly obtain the dosage strength of the drug, the nurse needs to follow the reconstitution directions as listed on the drug label because reconstitution directions will vary for each powdered medication. For example in Figure 9-3,

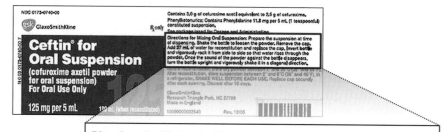

Directions for Mixing Oral Suspension: Prepare the suspension at time of dispensing. Shake the bottle to loosen the powder. Remove the cap. Add **37 mL** of water for reconstitution and replace the cap. Invert the bottle and vigorously rock it from side to side so that water rises through the powder. Once the sound of the powder against the bottle disappears, turn the bottle upright and vigorously shake it in a diagonal direction.

Figure 9-3. Directions for mixing of Ceftin for Oral Suspension 125 mg/5 mL.

notice that the dosage strength of 125 mg/5 mL is obtained after mixing Ceftin for oral suspension with 37 mL of water.

In the Ceftin for Oral Suspension 250 mg per 5 mL (Fig. 9-4), the nurse adds 19 mL of water to arrive at the dosage strength. In the Cephalexin for Oral Suspension (Fig. 9-5), the nurse adds 71 mL of water to arrive at the dosage strength of 250 mg/5 mL.

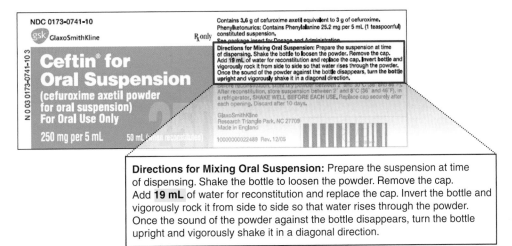

Directions for Mixing Oral Suspension: Prepare the suspension at time of dispensing. Shake the bottle to loosen the powder. Remove the cap. Add **19 mL** of water for reconstitution and replace the cap. Invert the bottle and vigorously rock it from side to side so that water rises through the powder. Once the sound of the powder against the bottle disappears, turn the bottle upright and vigorously shake it in a diagonal direction.

Figure 9-4. Directions for mixing of Ceftin for Oral Suspension 250 mg/5 mL.

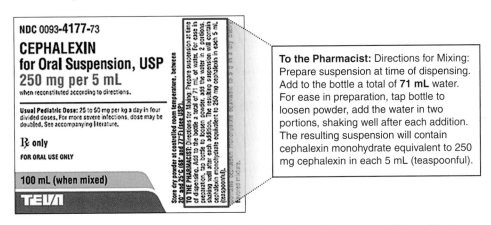

To the Pharmacist: Directions for Mixing: Prepare suspension at time of dispensing. Add to the bottle a total of **71 mL** water. For ease in preparation, tap bottle to loosen powder, add the water in two portions, shaking well after each addition. The resulting suspension will contain cephalexin monohydrate equivalent to 250 mg cephalexin in each 5 mL (teaspoonful).

Figure 9-5. Directions for mixing of Cephalexin for Oral Suspension 250 mg/5 mL.

Adding more or less water affects the amount of the drug's active ingredient in each dose. Therefore, the nurse must be aware that obtaining the dosage strength, as indicated on the drug label of the powdered medication, is completely dependent on following the directions for reconstitution as listed on the label.

PROPER STORAGE OF THE RECONSTITUTED MEDICATION

After reconstitution, the nurse needs to identify the storage information specific for the reconstituted drug and not the storage information for the powdered drug. For example, in Figure 9-4, the storage information listed on the Ceftin for Oral Suspension indicates, "Store constituted suspension in refrigerator." For Vibramycin 25 mg/mL (Fig. 9-6), the storage information includes, "This prescription, when in suspension, will maintain its potency for two weeks when kept at room temperature." Proper storage of the reconstituted drug will help to ensure that the physical, chemical, and therapeutic properties of the drug are maintained.

LABELING THE ORAL MEDICATION BOTTLE AFTER RECONSTITUTION

Because reconstituted oral medications contain several doses, the nurse who initially mixes the medication will write the following information on the bottle:

04/21/xx
1200
VN. RN

▪ the date the medication was reconstituted

▪ the time the medication was reconstituted

▪ the initials of the nurse.

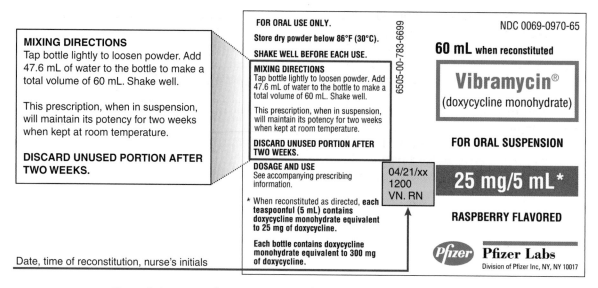

MIXING DIRECTIONS
Tap bottle lightly to loosen powder. Add 47.6 mL of water to the bottle to make a total volume of 60 mL. Shake well.

This prescription, when in suspension, will maintain its potency for two weeks when kept at room temperature.

DISCARD UNUSED PORTION AFTER TWO WEEKS.

FOR ORAL USE ONLY.
Store dry powder below 86°F (30°C).
SHAKE WELL BEFORE EACH USE.

MIXING DIRECTIONS
Tap bottle lightly to loosen powder. Add 47.6 mL of water to the bottle to make a total volume of 60 mL. Shake well.

This prescription, when in suspension, will maintain its potency for two weeks when kept at room temperature.

DISCARD UNUSED PORTION AFTER TWO WEEKS.

DOSAGE AND USE
See accompanying prescribing information.

* When reconstituted as directed, **each teaspoonful (5 mL) contains** doxycycline monohydrate equivalent to 25 mg of doxycycline.

Each bottle contains doxycycline monohydrate equivalent to 300 mg of doxycycline.

6505-00-783-6699

NDC 0069-0970-65

60 mL when reconstituted

Vibramycin®
(doxycycline monohydrate)

FOR ORAL SUSPENSION

25 mg/5 mL*

RASPBERRY FLAVORED

Pfizer **Pfizer Labs**
Division of Pfizer Inc, NY, NY 10017

04/21/xx
1200
VN. RN

Date, time of reconstitution, nurse's initials

Figure 9-6. Mixing directions, storage information, and labeling information.

This communication provides a standard format to assist in the administration of subsequent doses. It is the responsibility of every nurse who administers a subsequent dose to verify the expiration date of the reconstituted drug. This can be determined by identifying the time period when the reconstituted drug will need to be discarded, such as "Discard unused portion after 2 weeks." This indicates that all subsequent doses must be administered within the 2-week time period. The Vibramycin label (see Fig. 9-6) highlights the mixing directions, storage information, and the labeling information.

Some healthcare facilities require the nurse to write the date when the medication will expire after it has been reconstituted instead of the date of reconstitution. The nurse must be aware of the specific policies and procedures of the facility to ensure compliance, proper documentation, and appropriate written communication.

 It is important to inform patients and family that a reconstituted drug maintains its therapeutic effectiveness when stored according to the manufacturer's recommendations and used within the recommended time period.

Interpreting Oral Liquid Medication Orders

Liquid medications can be ordered by a specific dose or by the amount to be administered (Fig. 9-7). When the amount of a medication is ordered, the nurse will simply measure the ordered amount in the appropriate measuring device.

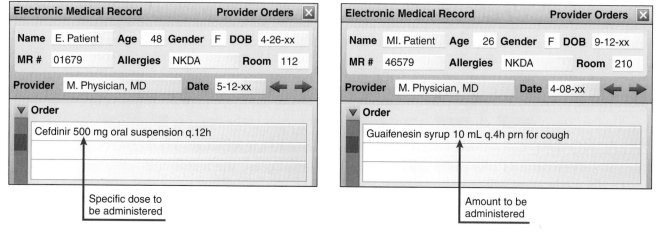

Electronic Medical Record		Provider Orders ✕
Name E. Patient	**Age** 48 **Gender** F	**DOB** 4-26-xx
MR # 01679	**Allergies** NKDA	**Room** 112
Provider M. Physician, MD		**Date** 5-12-xx ⬅ ➡

▼ **Order**

Cefdinir 500 mg oral suspension q.12h

Specific dose to be administered

Electronic Medical Record		Provider Orders ✕
Name MI. Patient	**Age** 26 **Gender** F	**DOB** 9-12-xx
MR # 46579	**Allergies** NKDA	**Room** 210
Provider M. Physician, MD		**Date** 4-08-xx ⬅ ➡

▼ **Order**

Guaifenesin syrup 10 mL q.4h prn for cough

Amount to be administered

Figure 9-7. Medications ordered by specific dose or by amount to be administered.

When a specific dose is ordered, the nurse uses the dosage strength listed on the drug label to determine the amount of medication to give. For example, in the cefdinir 500 mg oral suspension q.12h order, the nurse receives the following drug from the pharmacy (Fig. 9-8). After reconstitution, the nurse can solve for the dose using any of the methods of calculation.

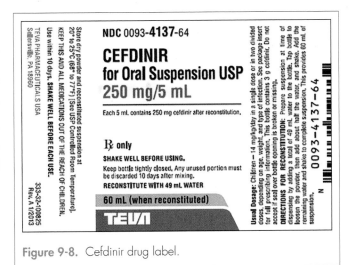

Figure 9-8. Cefdinir drug label.

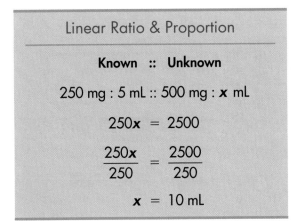

Linear Ratio & Proportion

Known :: Unknown

$$250 \text{ mg} : 5 \text{ mL} :: 500 \text{ mg} : x \text{ mL}$$

$$250x = 2500$$

$$\frac{250x}{250} = \frac{2500}{250}$$

$$x = 10 \text{ mL}$$

Fractional Ratio & Proportion

Known = Unknown

$$\frac{250 \text{ mg}}{5 \text{ mL}} \diagdown\!\!\!\!\diagup \frac{500 \text{ mg}}{x \text{ mL}}$$

$$250x = 2500$$

$$\frac{250x}{250} = \frac{2500}{250}$$

$$x = 10 \text{ mL}$$

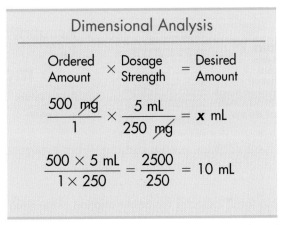

Dimensional Analysis

$$\frac{\text{Ordered}}{\text{Amount}} \times \frac{\text{Dosage}}{\text{Strength}} = \frac{\text{Desired}}{\text{Amount}}$$

$$\frac{500 \text{ mg}}{1} \times \frac{5 \text{ mL}}{250 \text{ mg}} = x \text{ mL}$$

$$\frac{500 \times 5 \text{ mL}}{1 \times 250} = \frac{2500}{250} = 10 \text{ mL}$$

Formula Method

$$\frac{D}{H} \times Q = x$$

$$\frac{500 \text{ mg}}{250 \text{ mg}} \times 5 \text{ mL} = x \text{ mL}$$

$$\frac{500}{250} \times 5 \text{ mL} = x \text{ mL}$$

$$2 \times 5 \text{ mL} = 10 \text{ mL}$$

The nurse administers 10 mL to the patient.

APPLY LEARNED KNOWLEDGE 9-1

Use the drug labels (a–f) to answer the following questions.

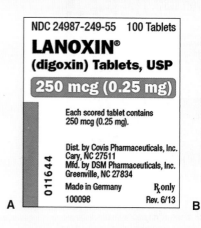

NDC 24987-249-55　100 Tablets

LANOXIN®
(digoxin) Tablets, USP

250 mcg (0.25 mg)

Each scored tablet contains
250 mcg (0.25 mg).

Dist. by Covis Pharmaceuticals, Inc.
Cary, NC 27511
Mfd. by DSM Pharmaceuticals, Inc.
Greenville, NC 27834

011644

Made in Germany　R only
100098　Rev. 6/13

A

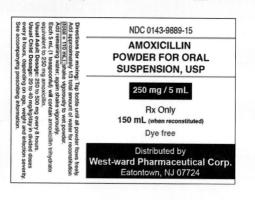

NDC 0143-9889-15

AMOXICILLIN
POWDER FOR ORAL
SUSPENSION, USP

250 mg / 5 mL

Rx Only
150 mL (when reconstituted)
Dye free

Distributed by
West-ward Pharmaceutical Corp.
Eatontown, NJ 07724

B

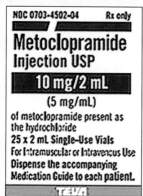

NDC 0703-4502-04　Rx only

Metoclopramide
Injection USP

10 mg/2 mL

(5 mg/mL)

of metoclopramide present as
the hydrochloride
25 x 2 mL Single-Use Vials
For Intramuscular or Intravenous Use
Dispense the accompanying
Medication Guide to each patient.

TEVA

C

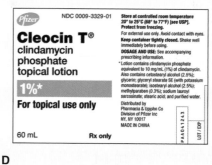

Pfizer　NDC 0009-3329-01

Cleocin T®
clindamycin
phosphate
topical lotion

1%*

For topical use only

60 mL　Rx only

D

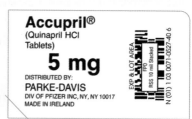

Accupril®
(Quinapril HCl
Tablets)

5 mg

DISTRIBUTED BY:
PARKE-DAVIS
DIV OF PFIZER INC, NY, NY 10017
MADE IN IRELAND

E

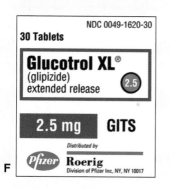

NDC 0049-1620-30

30 Tablets

Glucotrol XL®
(glipizide)
extended release　**2.5**

2.5 mg　**GITS**

Distributed by
Pfizer　**Roerig**
Division of Pfizer Inc, NY, NY 10017

F

1. Which drug label indicates the administration of the drug through the enteral route?

   a a,b,ef

2. Which drug label indicates a time-released drug?　*F*

3. Which drug label indicates that the drug may be safely broken in half?

   A

4. Which drug label will need to have the nurse's initials, date, and time written on the drug label?

   b (b/c Black Box Warning)

5. Which drug label(s) are not administered via the enteral route?

   C D

Measuring Devices Used to Administer Oral Medications

The equipment used for the administration of medications includes calibrated devices and household measuring devices (see Table 9-3).

Table 9-3. Measuring Devices for Administration of Oral Medications

MEASURING DEVICE	USES
Medicine Cup (Highlighting the most commonly used metric and household units for measuring volume.) 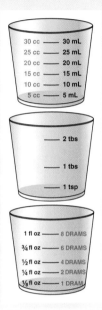	• Container to hold solid oral medications such as tablets, capsules, etc. • Measuring device calibrated in various measuring units. Most commonly used units to measure volume include: milliliter (mL) teaspoon, tablespoon (tsp, Tbs) fluid ounce (fl oz) **Note:** The measuring units found on the medicine cup that are no longer used in clinical practice include: cubic centimeter (cc) dram (dr)
Oral Syringe 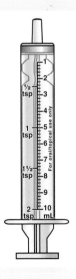	• Measuring device, available in various sizes, ranging from 3 mL to 10 mL capacity. Tip of syringe designed for ease in the administration of oral medications. An oral syringe is needleless.

Continued

Table 9-3. Measuring Devices for Administration of Oral Medications—*cont'd*

MEASURING DEVICE	USES
Cylindrical Dosing Spoon 2 10 tsp mL 1½ 7½ tsp mL 1 5 tsp mL ¾ ½ 2½ tsp mL ¼	• Measuring device, calibration lines measure from 1 mL to 10 mL of medication. Also includes the equivalent household measurement for teaspoon (tsp). Designed with a spoon end shape for ease in the administration of oral medications.
Calibrated Dropper 5 mL 4 mL 3 mL 2 mL 1 mL	• Size of calibrated dropper varies. May measure from 1 mL to 5 mL of medication. Designed to facilitate the administration of oral medications, especially useful for children.

In deciding which measuring device to use, the nurse considers the total amount of liquid medication that needs to be administered and then selects the measuring device that most accurately measures the liquid amount. The most frequently used measuring device in clinical practice is the medicine cup. Because liquids tend to curve at the edges of certain containers, it is important to read the liquid measurement at the **meniscus** level or at the horizontal center of the liquid and not from the outer edges of the cup (see Fig. 9-9).

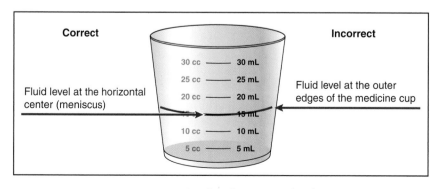

Figure 9-9. Reading the meniscus level.

The following five examples show how measuring devices are selected.

1. The nurse has an order to administer 20 mL of cough syrup. The medicine cup can measure 20 mL accurately.

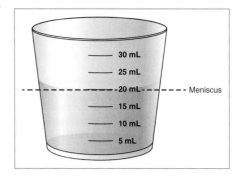

2. The nurse has an order to administer 2 Tbs of an antacid. The medicine cup can measure 2 Tbs accurately.

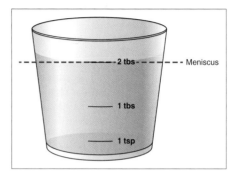

3. The nurse has an order to administer 1.5 tsp of an antibiotic. The cylindrical dosing spoon or an oral syringe can measure 1.5 tsp accurately.

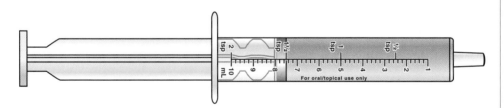

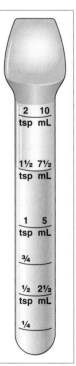

4. The nurse has an order to administer 1 mL of an antibiotic for a 4-year-old child. The calibrated medicine dropper can measure 1 mL accurately.

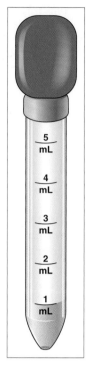

5. The nurse measures 0.5 oz of juice. The medicine cup can measure 0.5 oz accurately.

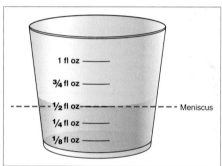

Working With Drug Dosage Calculations With the Same Unit of Measurement

In the calculations of drug dosages, the nurse will identify the unit of measurement from the

■ MD order (medication order)

■ medication sent by pharmacy.

If the units of measurement are the same in the MD order and on the medication label, the nurse sets up the problem and solves for the amount to give to the patient.

For example:

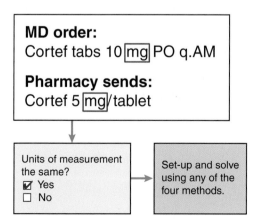

Linear Ratio & Proportion

Known :: Unknown

5 mg : 1 tablet :: 10 mg : **x** tablet

$$5x = 10$$

$$\frac{5x}{5} = \frac{10}{5}$$

$$x = 2 \text{ tablets}$$

Dimensional Analysis

$$\underset{\text{Amount}}{\text{Ordered}} \times \underset{\text{Strength}}{\text{Dosage}} = \underset{\text{Amount}}{\text{Desired}}$$

$$\frac{10 \text{ mg}}{1} \times \frac{1 \text{ tablet}}{5 \text{ mg}} = x \text{ tablets}$$

$$\frac{10 \times 1 \text{ tablet}}{1 \times 5} = \frac{10}{5} = 2 \text{ tablets}$$

Fractional Ratio & Proportion

Known = Unknown

$$\frac{5 \text{ mg}}{1 \text{ tablet}} \quad \frac{10 \text{ mg}}{x \text{ tablet}}$$

$$5x = 10$$

$$\frac{5x}{5} = \frac{10}{5}$$

$$x = 2 \text{ tablets}$$

Formula Method

$$\frac{D}{H} \times Q = x$$

$$\frac{10 \text{ mg}}{5 \text{ mg}} \times 1 \text{ tablet} = x \text{ tablets}$$

$$\frac{10}{5} \times 1 = x \text{ tablets}$$

$$2 \times 1 = 2 \text{ tablets}$$

The nurse will administer 2 tablets.

APPLY LEARNED KNOWLEDGE 9-2

Calculate the amount to give to the patient using the method of your choice for the following problems.

1. **MD orders:** Lasix 40 mg tab PO q.AM
   Pharmacy sends: Lasix 10 mg/tablet

   How many tablet(s) will the nurse give? _____

   _____

   _____

2. **MD orders:** Dilantin 250 mg oral suspension bid.
   Pharmacy sends: Dilantin oral suspension 125 mg/5 mL

   How many mL will the nurse give? _____

   Fill in the amount to administer in the medicine cup.

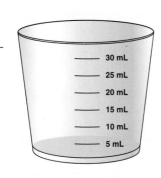

Continued

APPLY LEARNED KNOWLEDGE 9-2—cont'd

3. **MD orders:** Paxil HCl 15 mg PO bid.
   Pharmacy sends: Paxil 10 mg scored tablets

   How many tablet(s) will the nurse give? _____

   _____

   _____

4. **MD orders:** Glyburide 7.5 mg PO q.AM and q.PM
   Pharmacy sends: Glyburide 5 mg scored tablets

   How many tablet(s) will the nurse give? _____

   _____

   _____

5. **MD orders:** Naprosyn SR 500 mg tablets PO q.12h prn migraine headache
   Pharmacy sends: Naprosyn SR 250 tablets

   How many tablet(s) will the nurse give? _____

Working With Drug Dosage Calculations Requiring Conversion Within the Metric System

If the metric units of measurement in the medication order and in the drug label are different, the nurse needs to convert the metric units so that they are the same. In ratio and proportion and formula methods, the metric line may used to convert the metric units. In the dimensional analysis method, a conversion factor is used.

USING THE METRIC LINE TO CONVERT THE METRIC UNITS

Calculations requiring conversion within the metric system can be solved by working with the metric line to convert from one unit of measurement to another. When using the metric line, recall the following steps:

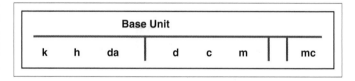

Step 1: Identify the starting place on the metric line (unit of measurement from the MD order).

Step 2: Identify the desired place on the metric line (unit of measurement from drug label).

Step 3: Convert to the desired place on the metric line by moving decimal point.

The steps can be applied using the following two examples.

Example 1:

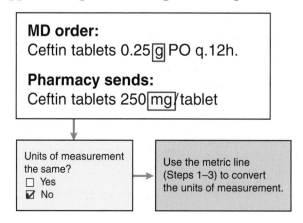

In Example #1, gram (g) is the unit of measurement from the MD order and milligram (mg) is the unit of measurement from the drug label. To convert from the base unit place (the starting place) to the milli place (the desired place), move the decimal point from left to right three places: 0.25 g (0. 2 5 0) equals 250 mg. Now the problem can be solved.

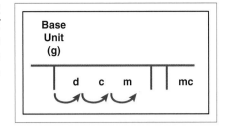

USING A CONVERSION FACTOR IN DIMENSIONAL ANALYSIS

To set up the problem in Example #1 using dimensional analysis, the nurse recalls the conversion factor of 1,000 mg = 1 g. Now the problem can be solved.

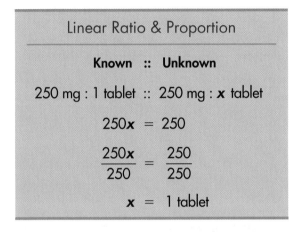

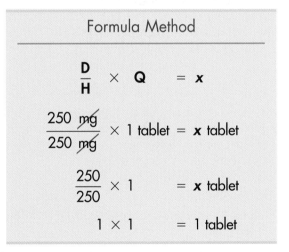

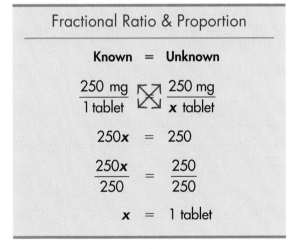

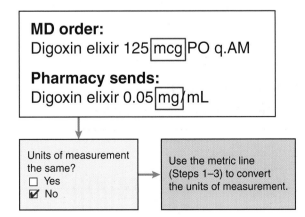

The nurse will administer 1 tablet.

Example 2:

MD order:
Digoxin elixir 125 mcg PO q.AM

Pharmacy sends:
Digoxin elixir 0.05 mg/mL

Units of measurement the same?
☐ Yes
☑ No

Use the metric line (Steps 1–3) to convert the units of measurement.

In Example 2, if using the metric line to convert, microgram (mcg) is the unit of measurement from the drug order and milligram (mg) is the unit of measurement from the drug label. Because the amount, 125, is a whole number, add a decimal point after the whole number. To convert from "mcg" (the starting place) to the "mg" (the desired place), move the decimal point from right to left three places, so that 125 mcg (0 . 1 2 5.) equals 0.125 mg. Now the problem can be solved.

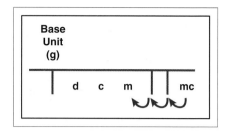

To set up the problem in Example #2 using dimensional analysis, the nurse recalls the conversion factor of 1,000 mcg = 1 mg. Now the problem can be solved.

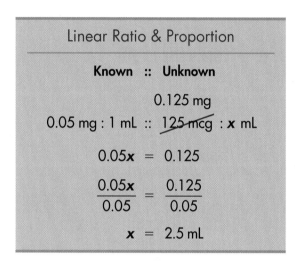

Linear Ratio & Proportion

Known :: Unknown

$$0.125 \text{ mg}$$
$$0.05 \text{ mg} : 1 \text{ mL} :: 125 \text{ mcg} : x \text{ mL}$$

$$0.05x = 0.125$$

$$\frac{0.05x}{0.05} = \frac{0.125}{0.05}$$

$$x = 2.5 \text{ mL}$$

Dimensional Analysis

$$\frac{\text{Ordered}}{\text{Amount}} \times \frac{\text{Dosage}}{\text{Strength}} \times \frac{\text{Conversion}}{\text{Factor}} = \frac{\text{Desired}}{\text{Amount}}$$

$$\frac{125 \text{ mcg}}{1} \times \frac{1 \text{ mL}}{0.05 \text{ mg}} \times \frac{1 \text{ mg}}{1000 \text{ mcg}} = x \text{ mL}$$

$$\frac{125 \times 1 \text{ mL} \times 1}{1 \times 0.05 \times 1000} = \frac{125}{50} = 2.5 \text{ mL}$$

Fractional Ratio & Proportion

Known = Unknown

$$\frac{0.05 \text{ mg}}{1 \text{ mL}} \underset{\nwarrow \searrow}{\overset{\nearrow \swarrow}{\times}} \frac{\overset{0.125 \text{ mg}}{125 \text{ mcg}}}{x \text{ mL}}$$

$$0.05x = 0.125$$

$$\frac{0.05x}{0.05} = \frac{0.125}{0.125}$$

$$x = 2.5 \text{ mL}$$

Formula Method

$$\frac{D}{H} \times Q = x$$

$$\frac{\overset{0.125 \text{ mg}}{125 \text{ mcg}}}{0.05 \text{ mg}} \times 1 \text{ mL} = x \text{ mL}$$

$$\frac{0.125}{0.05} \times 1 = x \text{ mL}$$

$$2.5 \times 1 = 2.5 \text{ mL}$$

 Because the nurse will administer the ordered dose from the drug sent by the pharmacy, it is safer to convert unlike units of measurement to the unit of measurement listed on the drug label. The "g" from the MD order is converted to "mg" so that the nurse works with the unit of measurement found on the drug label.

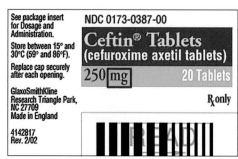

MD order:
Ceftin 0.5 g
tabs PO now

See package insert for Dosage and Administration.
Store between 15° and 30°C (59° and 86°F).
Replace cap securely after each opening.

GlaxoSmithKline
Research Triangle Park, NC 27709
Made in England

4142817
Rev. 2/02

NDC 0173-0387-00
Ceftin® Tablets
(cefuroxime axetil tablets)
250 mg   20 Tablets

R̠ only

Use the metric line to convert 0.5 g to 500 mg.

The nurse can now calculate the number of tablets to administer to the patient.

APPLY LEARNED KNOWLEDGE 9-3

Use the physician's orders and the medication sent by pharmacy to answer the following questions.

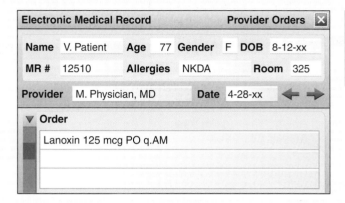

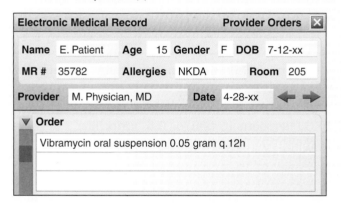

Pharmacy sends:
Lanoxin 0.25 mg
scored tablets.

1. Do the units of measurement need to be converted?   ☐ Yes   ☐ No

2. How many tablet(s) of Lanoxin will the nurse administer? _____

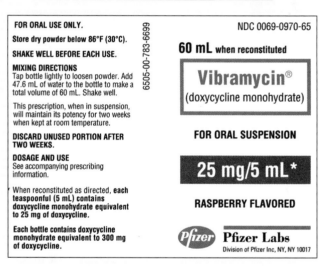

FOR ORAL USE ONLY.

Store dry powder below 86°F (30°C).

SHAKE WELL BEFORE EACH USE.

MIXING DIRECTIONS
Tap bottle lightly to loosen powder. Add 47.6 mL of water to the bottle to make a total volume of 60 mL. Shake well.

This prescription, when in suspension, will maintain its potency for two weeks when kept at room temperature.

DISCARD UNUSED PORTION AFTER TWO WEEKS.

DOSAGE AND USE
See accompanying prescribing information.

When reconstituted as directed, **each teaspoonful (5 mL) contains doxycycline monohydrate equivalent to 25 mg of doxycycline.**

Each bottle contains doxycycline monohydrate equivalent to 300 mg of doxycycline.

6505-00-783-6699

NDC 0069-0970-65

60 mL when reconstituted

Vibramycin®
(doxycycline monohydrate)

FOR ORAL SUSPENSION

25 mg/5 mL*

RASPBERRY FLAVORED

Pfizer **Pfizer Labs**
Division of Pfizer Inc, NY, NY 10017

3. Calculate the amount of Vibramycin oral suspension to be administered per dose to the patient.

_____

4. Fill in the medicine cup with the ordered amount of Vibramycin.

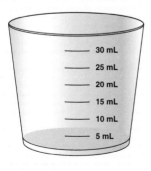

_____ 30 mL
_____ 25 mL
_____ 20 mL
_____ 15 mL
_____ 10 mL
_____ 5 mL

Continued

APPLY LEARNED KNOWLEDGE 9-3 — cont'd

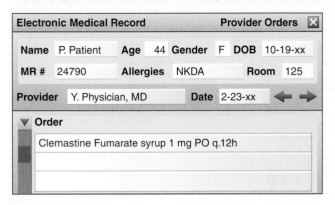

Electronic Medical Record   **Provider Orders** ☒

Name	P. Patient	**Age**	44	**Gender**	F	**DOB** 10-19-xx

MR # 24790   **Allergies** NKDA   **Room** 125

Provider Y. Physician, MD   **Date** 2-23-xx ⬅ ➡

▼ **Order**

Clemastine Fumarate syrup 1 mg PO q.12h

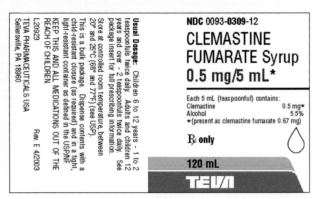

Usual Dosage: Children 6 to 12 years - 1 to 2 teaspoonfuls twice daily. Adults and children 12 years and over - 2 teaspoonfuls twice daily. See package insert for full prescribing information.

Store at controlled room temperature, between 20° and 25°C (68° and 77°F) (see USP).

This is a bulk package. Dispense contents with a child-resistant closure (as required) and in a tight, light-resistant container as defined in the USP/NF.

KEEP THIS AND ALL MEDICATIONS OUT OF THE REACH OF CHILDREN.

TEVA PHARMACEUTICALS USA
Sellersville, PA 18960

L20923

Rev. E 4/2003

NDC 0093-0309-12

CLEMASTINE FUMARATE Syrup 0.5 mg/5 mL*

Each 5 mL (teaspoonful) contains:
Clemastine   0.5 mg*
Alcohol   5.5%
*(present as clemastine fumarate 0.67 mg)

℞ only

120 mL

TEVA

5. How many mL of Clemastine Fumarate syrup will the nurse administer? _____

Calculations Requiring Conversion Within the Household System

Sometimes the nurse needs to convert the household units of measurement to equivalent household measurements. To work with the household system, the nurse recalls the household units and the standard equivalent household measurements:

■ 1 tablespoon (T, tbs) **is equivalent to** 3 teaspoons (t, tsp), or 0.5 ounce (oz)

■ 2 tablespoons (T, tbs), 6 teaspoons (t, tsp), **is equivalent to** 1 ounce (oz)

In the following two examples, the standard equivalent household measurements are used to solve the problem.

Example 1:

The physician orders 1 ounce of aluminum hydroxide.

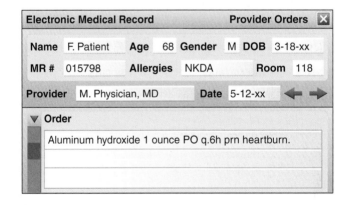

Electronic Medical Record   **Provider Orders** ☒

Name	F. Patient	**Age**	68	**Gender**	M	**DOB** 3-18-xx

MR # 015798   **Allergies** NKDA   **Room** 118

Provider M. Physician, MD   **Date** 5-12-xx ⬅ ➡

▼ **Order**

Aluminum hydroxide 1 ounce PO q.6h prn heartburn.

How many tablespoons will the nurse give?

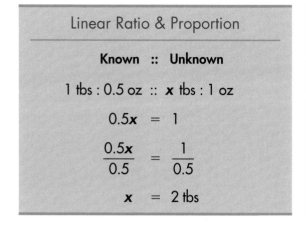

Linear Ratio & Proportion

Known :: Unknown

1 tbs : 0.5 oz :: **x** tbs : 1 oz

0.5**x** = 1

$\dfrac{0.5x}{0.5} = \dfrac{1}{0.5}$

x = 2 tbs

Dimensional Analysis

$\dfrac{\text{Ordered}}{\text{Amount}} \times \dfrac{\text{Conversion}}{\text{Factor}} = \dfrac{\text{Desired}}{\text{Amount}}$

$\dfrac{1\ \cancel{oz}}{1} \times \dfrac{1\ \text{tbs}}{0.5\ \cancel{oz}} = x\ \text{tbs}$

$\dfrac{1 \times 1\ \text{tbs}}{1 \times 0.5} = \dfrac{1}{0.5} = 2\ \text{tbs}$

Fractional Ratio & Proportion

Known = Unknown

$\dfrac{1\ \text{tbs}}{0.5\ \text{oz}} \diagdown\!\!\!\diagup \dfrac{x\ \text{tbs}}{1\ \text{oz}}$

0.5**x** = 1

$\dfrac{0.5x}{0.5} = \dfrac{1}{0.5}$

x = 2 tbs

Formula Method

$\dfrac{D}{H} \times Q = x$

$\dfrac{1\ \cancel{oz}}{0.5\ \cancel{oz}} \times 1\ \text{tbs} = x\ \text{tbs}$

$\dfrac{1}{0.5} \times 1 = x\ \text{tbs}$

$2 \times 1 = 2\ \text{tbs}$

Example 2:

The physician orders 2 T (tablespoon) of guaifenesin syrup.

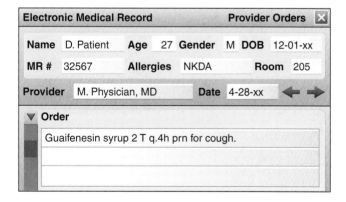

Electronic Medical Record	Provider Orders ✕

Name D. Patient   **Age** 27 **Gender** M **DOB** 12-01-xx

MR # 32567   **Allergies** NKDA   **Room** 205

Provider M. Physician, MD   **Date** 4-28-xx ← →

▼ **Order**

Guaifenesin syrup 2 T q.4h prn for cough.

What is the equivalent measurement in teaspoons?

Linear Ratio & Proportion

Known :: Unknown

3 tsp : 1 T :: **x** tsp : 2 T

$1x = 6$

$$\frac{1x}{1} = \frac{6}{1}$$

$x = 6$ tsp

Dimensional Analysis

$$\frac{\text{Ordered}}{\text{Amount}} \times \frac{\text{Conversion}}{\text{Factor}} = \frac{\text{Desired}}{\text{Amount}}$$

$$\frac{2\,\cancel{T}}{1} \times \frac{3\text{ tsp}}{1\,\cancel{T}} = x\text{ tsp}$$

$$\frac{2 \times 3\text{ tsp}}{1 \times 1} = \frac{6}{1} = 6\text{ tsp}$$

Fractional Ratio & Proportion

Known = Unknown

$$\frac{3\text{ tsp}}{1\text{ T}} \bowtie \frac{x\text{ tsp}}{2\text{ T}}$$

$1x = 6$

$$\frac{1x}{1} = \frac{6}{1}$$

$x = 6$ tsp

Formula Method

$$\frac{D}{H} \times Q = x$$

$$\frac{2\,\cancel{T}}{1\,\cancel{T}} \times 3\text{ tsp} = x\text{ tsp}$$

$$\frac{2}{1} \times 3 = x\text{ tsp}$$

$$2 \times 3 = 6\text{ tsp}$$

Two tablespoons is equivalent to six teaspoons.

Knowing the standard equivalent household measurements helps the nurse to inform patients and families how to safely administer ordered doses using equivalent household measurements.

 When converting within the household system, a mathematical calculation is not absolutely necessary. The problem can be solved by recalling the equivalent measurement such as 2 Tbs equals 1 oz. However, a mathematical calculation provides a good method for double-checking the calculations.

APPLY LEARNED KNOWLEDGE 9-4

Use the physician's orders and the MAR to answer the following questions.

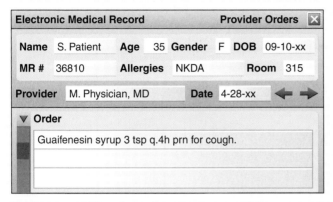

Electronic Medical Record — **Provider Orders** ☒

Name S. Patient   **Age** 35 **Gender** F **DOB** 09-10-xx

MR # 36810   **Allergies** NKDA   **Room** 315

Provider M. Physician, MD   **Date** 4-28-xx ← →

▼ **Order**

Guaifenesin syrup 3 tsp q.4h prn for cough.

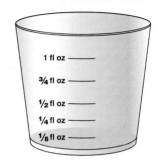

1 fl oz ——
¾ fl oz ——
½ fl oz ——
¼ fl oz ——
⅛ fl oz ——

1. How many Tbs of guaifenesin syrup will the nurse give? _____

2. How many oz of guaifenesin syrup will the nurse give? _____

3. Fill in the medicine cup with the ordered amount of guaifenesin syrup.

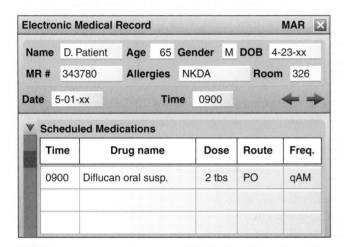

Electronic Medical Record — **MAR** ☒

Name D. Patient   **Age** 65 **Gender** M **DOB** 4-23-xx

MR # 343780   **Allergies** NKDA   **Room** 326

Date 5-01-xx   **Time** 0900   ← →

▼ **Scheduled Medications**

Time	Drug name	Dose	Route	Freq.
0900	Diflucan oral susp.	2 tbs	PO	qAM

4. How many teaspoons of Diflucan susp will the nurse give? _____

5. How many ounces are equivalent to 2 Tbs of Diflucan susp? _____

Calculations Requiring Conversion Between the Household System and the Metric System

Liquid medications may be measured using the household measurements or the equivalent metric measurements. To convert between the household measurements and the equivalent metric measurements, the nurse simply recalls the metric equivalents for common household measurements:

HOUSEHOLD UNIT OF MEASUREMENT USED IN CLINICAL PRACTICE	METRIC EQUIVALENTS
Tablespoon	15 mL
Teaspoon	5 mL
Ounce	30 mL
Glass (6 oz)	180 mL
(8 oz)	240 mL
Cup (6 oz)	180 mL
(8 oz)	240 mL

The following two examples show how the household measurements are used with the metric equivalents.

Example 1:

The physician orders 0.5 ounce of aluminum magnesium.

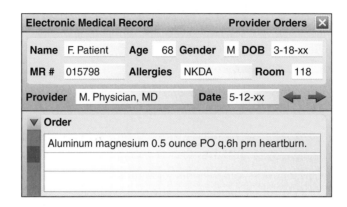

How many mL will the nurse administer to the patient?

Linear Ratio & Proportion

Known :: Unknown

1 oz : 30 mL :: 0.5 oz : **x** mL

$$1x = 15$$

$$\frac{1x}{1} = \frac{15}{1}$$

$$x = 15 \text{ mL}$$

Dimensional Analysis

$$\frac{\text{Ordered}}{\text{Amount}} \times \frac{\text{Conversion}}{\text{Factor}} = \frac{\text{Desired}}{\text{Amount}}$$

$$\frac{0.5 \text{ oz}}{1} \times \frac{30 \text{ mL}}{1 \text{ oz}} = x \text{ mL}$$

$$\frac{0.5 \times 30 \text{ mL}}{1 \times 1} = \frac{15}{1} = 15 \text{ mL}$$

Fractional Ratio & Proportion

Known = Unknown

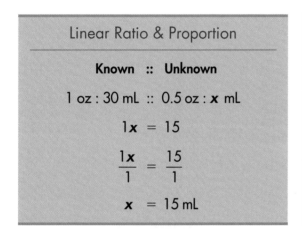

$$\frac{30 \text{ mL}}{1 \text{ oz}} \qquad \frac{x \text{ mL}}{0.5 \text{ oz}}$$

$$1x = 15$$

$$\frac{1x}{1} = \frac{15}{1}$$

$$x = 15 \text{ mL}$$

Formula Method

$$\frac{D}{H} \times Q = x$$

$$\frac{0.5 \text{ oz}}{1 \text{ oz}} \times 30 \text{ mL} = x \text{ mL}$$

$$\frac{0.5}{1} \times 30 = x \text{ mL}$$

$$0.5 \times 30 = 15 \text{ mL}$$

The nurse will administer 15 mL.

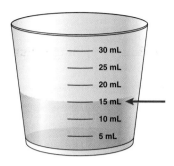

Example 2:

The patient drinks two 8-ounce glasses of water. How many mL did the patient drink? This problem can be set up as follows:

Linear Ratio & Proportion
Known :: Unknown
8 oz : 240 mL :: 16 oz : **x** mL
$8x = 3840$
$\dfrac{8x}{8} = \dfrac{3840}{8}$
$x = 480$ mL

Dimensional Analysis
$\dfrac{\text{Ordered}}{\text{Amount}} \times \dfrac{\text{Conversion}}{\text{Factor}} = \dfrac{\text{Desired}}{\text{Amount}}$
$\dfrac{16\ \cancel{oz}}{1} \times \dfrac{240\ \text{mL}}{8\ \cancel{oz}} = x\ \text{mL}$
$\dfrac{16 \times 240\ \text{mL}}{1 \times 8} = \dfrac{3840}{8} = 480\ \text{mL}$

Fractional Ratio & Proportion
Known = Unknown
$\dfrac{240\ \text{mL}}{8\ \text{oz}} \bowtie \dfrac{x\ \text{mL}}{16\ \text{oz}}$
$8x = 3840$
$\dfrac{8x}{8} = \dfrac{3840}{8}$
$x = 480$ mL

Formula Method
$\dfrac{\textbf{D}}{\textbf{H}} \times \textbf{Q} = \textbf{x}$
$\dfrac{16\ \cancel{oz}}{8\ \cancel{oz}} \times 240\ \text{mL} = x\ \text{mL}$
$\dfrac{16}{8} \times 240 = x\ \text{mL}$
$2 \times 240 = 480\ \text{mL}$

The nurse calculated that the patient drank 480 mL.

Calculations Requiring Multiple Conversions

Liquid medication orders may require conversions of units within the metric system and use of metric and household equivalent measurements before the problem can be solved. The metric line and household equivalent measurements, or conversion factors are used to convert the units so that they are the same.

Example:

Conversion of metric units and use of metric and household equivalents to arrive at the answer.

> **MD orders:**
>
> Amoxicillin oral suspension 0.5 g q.AM
>
> **Pharmacy sends:**
>
> Amoxicillin oral suspension 250 mg/5 mL

How many teaspoons will the nurse instruct the patient to take?

To solve, the nurse needs to

- convert the metric units of measurement or use a conversion factor.
- use the household equivalent measurement 5 mL = 1 tsp to answer the question, "How many teaspoons will the nurse instruct the patient to take?"

Linear Ratio & Proportion

Known :: Unknown

$$1 \text{ tsp} \quad 500 \text{ mg}$$

$$250 \text{ mg} : 5 \text{ mL} :: 0.5 \text{ g} : x \text{ tsp}$$

$$250x = 500$$

$$\frac{250x}{250} = \frac{500}{250}$$

$$x = 2 \text{ tsp}$$

Dimensional Analysis

$$\frac{\text{Ordered}}{\text{Amount}} \times \frac{\text{Dosage}}{\text{Strength}} \times \frac{\text{Conversion}}{\text{Factor}} \times \frac{\text{Conversion}}{\text{Factor}} = \frac{\text{Desired}}{\text{Amount}}$$

$$\frac{0.5 \text{ g}}{1} \times \frac{5 \text{ mL}}{250 \text{ mg}} \times \frac{1000 \text{ mg}}{1 \text{ g}} \times \frac{1 \text{ tsp}}{5 \text{ mL}} = x \text{ tsp}$$

$$\frac{0.5 \times 5 \times 1000 \times 1 \text{ tsp}}{1 \times 250 \times 1 \times 5} = \frac{2500}{1250} = 2 \text{ tsp}$$

Fractional Ratio & Proportion

Known = Unknown

$$\frac{250 \text{ mg}}{5 \text{ mL}} \quad \underset{1 \text{ tsp}}{\nearrow\kern-1.2em\diagdown} \quad \frac{\overset{500 \text{ mg}}{0.5 \text{ g}}}{x \text{ tsp}}$$

$$250x = 500$$

$$\frac{250x}{250} = \frac{500}{250}$$

$$x = 2 \text{ tsp}$$

Formula Method

$$\frac{D}{H} \times Q = x$$

$$\frac{\overset{500 \text{ mg}}{0.5 \text{ g}}}{250 \text{ mg}} \times 5 \text{ mL} = x \text{ mL}$$

$$\frac{500}{250} \times 5 \text{ mL} = x \text{ mL}$$

$$2 \times 5 \text{ mL} = 10 \text{ mL}$$

[To convert mL to tsp, the nurse recalls the equivalent measurement, 5 mL = 1 tsp. Therefore, 10 mL = 2 tsp.]

The nurse calculated 2 tsp as the final answer for this problem.

CLINICAL REASONING 9-1

The nurse is assigned to an adult patient who routinely takes a daily dose of levothyroxine 0.075 mg PO. Before administering the drug, the nurse uses a drug reference book and reads the following drug information:

> ***PO (Adults):*** *Hypothyroidism—50 mcg as a single dose initially; may be ↑ q.2–3 wk; usual maintenance dose is 75 to 125 mcg/day.*

The nurse decides to hold the medication and question the ordered dose. Is the nurse's decision correct?

In summary, the administration of oral medications includes understanding the enteral routes, reading medication labels, following the instructions for the reconstitution of liquid medications, and using the household and metric units of measurement in the conversion of units. Using appropriate calibrated devices for the administration of oral liquid medications helps to provide the patient with the correct dose. The nurse must always promote safety in the preparation and administration of medications. This includes proper labeling of liquid medications used for multiple doses to ensure appropriate written communication and avoid administration of expired medications.

Developing Competency

Use the information provided to answer questions 1 through 5.

1. How many mL of erythromycin ethylsuccinate will the nurse administer? _____

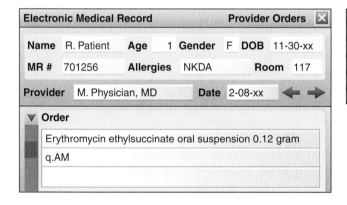

2. The nurse receives a bottle of Amoxicillin and Clavulanate Potassium for Oral Suspension from the pharmacy. What is the total amount of water the nurse will add to reconstitute the Amoxicillin and Clavulanate Potassium for Oral Suspension? _____

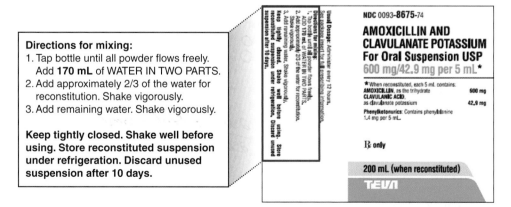

3. What is the total amount (mL) of Amoxicillin and Clavulanate Potassium for Oral Suspension in the bottle after reconstitution? _____

4. The reconstituted medication must be shaken each time before the administration of a dose. ❑ Yes ❑ No

5. **MD orders:** Amoxicillin and Clavulanate Potassium for Oral Suspension 600 mg/42.9 mg 2 tsp PO bid.

To administer the medication, the nurse needs to clarify the dosage strength. ❑ Yes ❑ No

In the following questions, calculate the ordered dose using the method of your choice.

6. MD orders: Ceftin Oral Suspension 375 mg PO bid.

Pharmacy sends: Ceftin Oral Suspension 125 mg/5 mL

How many tsp will the nurse give? **3 5mL = 1 TSP**

The most appropriate measuring device to administer this dose is the:

a. medicine cup.
b. 5 mL oral syringe.
c. 10 mL oral syringe.

$$= \frac{375}{125} \times 5mL$$

$$= \frac{75}{25} \times 1 = 15mL$$

$$=$$

7. MD orders: Nitrostat 0.6 mg SL now.

Pharmacy sends: Nitrostat 0.3 mg tablets

How many tablet(s) will the nurse give? **two**

To properly administered the ordered dose, the nurse will:

a. give the tablet(s) orally with water.
b. place the tablet(s) between the gum and the cheek.
c. place the tablet(s) under the tongue.

8. MD orders: Naprosyn SR 500 mg PO q.12h prn migraine headache.

Pharmacy sends: Naprosyn SR 250 tablets

How many tablet(s) will the nurse give? **2**

Which of the following best describes the appropriate administration of this drug? The tablet:

a. may be chewed.
b. active ingredient is released slowly.
c. is placed under the tongue.

9. After reconstituting the fluconazole oral suspension, the nurse will include which of the following on the drug label? (Select all that apply.)

a. Total amount of reconstituted drug
b. Dosage strength of the drug
c. Time of reconstitution
d. Nurse's initials
e. Date of reconstitution

10. Cefdinir for Oral Suspension 250 mg is ordered. Pharmacy sends the following drug. Which of the following applies to the administration of this ordered dose? (Select all that apply.)

a. One tsp will be administered.
b. The bottle needs to be shaken well.
c. 2.5 mL will be administered.
d. 2 mL will be administered.
e. It is for enteral use only.

$$\frac{250}{250} \times 5mL = 5mL$$

11. Albuterol sulfate syrup 1 mg is ordered. Pharmacy sends the following drug with a dropper calibrated at the 0.5 mL and 1 mL markings. Which of the following apply to the administration of this ordered dose? (Select all that apply.)

a. 1 mL will be administered.
b. The medicine cup can also be used to measure this dose.
c. The drug needs to be reconstituted.
d. A conversion is not necessary.
e. It is for enteral use only.

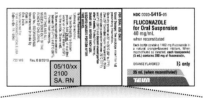

NDC 0093-0661-16

ALBUTEROL SULFATE Syrup

2 mg/5 mL

℞ only

Each 5 mL (1 teaspoonful) contains albuterol sulfate 2.4 mg, equivalent to 2 mg albuterol.

Usual Dosage: See package insert for full prescribing information.

Store at 20° to 25°C (68° to 77°F) [See USP Controlled Room Temperature].

This is a bulk package. Dispense in a tight, light-resistant container as defined in the USP, with a child-resistant closure (as required).

KEEP THIS AND ALL MEDICATIONS OUT OF THE REACH OF CHILDREN.

Manufactured in Canada By:
CONTRACT PHARMACEUTICALS LIMITED CANADA
Ontario, Canada L5N 6L6
Manufactured For:
TEVA PHARMACEUTICALS USA
Sellersville, PA 18960

473 mL

TEVA

12. Use the PrednisoLONE Oral Solution drug label to answer the following questions.

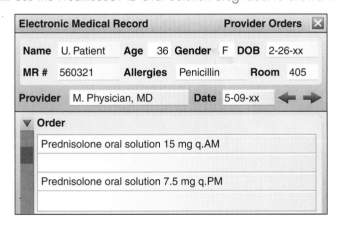

Electronic Medical Record   **Provider Orders** ☒

Name U. Patient   Age 36 Gender F DOB 2-26-xx

MR # 560321   Allergies Penicillin   Room 405

Provider M. Physician, MD   Date 5-09-xx ← →

▼ Order

Prednisolone oral solution 15 mg q.AM

Prednisolone oral solution 7.5 mg q.PM

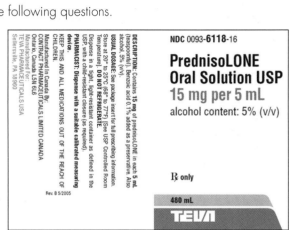

NDC 0093-6118-16

PrednisoLONE Oral Solution USP

15 mg per 5 mL

alcohol content: 5% (v/v)

DESCRIPTION: Contains **15 mg** of prednisoLONE in each 5 mL (teaspoonful). Benzoic acid 0.1% added as a preservative. Also alcohol, 5% (v/v).

USUAL DOSAGE: See package insert for full prescribing information. Store at 20° to 25°C (68° to 77°F) [See USP Controlled Room Temperature]. **DO NOT REFRIGERATE.**

Dispense in a tight, light-resistant container as defined in the USP, with a child-resistant closure (as required).

PHARMACIST: Dispense with a suitable calibrated measuring device.

KEEP THIS AND ALL MEDICATIONS OUT OF THE REACH OF CHILDREN.

Manufactured in Canada By:
CONTRACT PHARMACEUTICALS LIMITED CANADA
Ontario, Canada L5N 6L6
Manufactured For:
TEVA PHARMACEUTICALS USA
Sellersville, PA 18960

Rev. 8 5/2005

℞ only

480 mL

TEVA

How many mL of PrednisoLONE Oral Solution will the nurse administer to the patient q.AM? ___5 mL___

How many mL of PrednisoLONE Oral Solution will the nurse administer to the patient q.PM? ___2.5 mL___

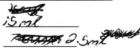

13. Use the Fluconazole for Oral Suspension drug label to determine the amount of water the nurse will add for reconstitution of the drug. _____

NDC 0093-5415-05

FLUCONAZOLE for Oral Suspension

40 mg/mL

when reconstituted

Each bottle contains 1400 mg fluconazole in a natural orange-flavored mixture. When reconstituted as directed, each teaspoonful (5 mL) contains 200 mg of fluconazole.

ORANGE FLAVORED   ℞ only

35 mL (when reconstituted)

TEVA

05/10/xx
2100
SA. RN

FOR ORAL USE ONLY

Usual Dosage: See package insert for full prescribing information. Store dry powder at 20° to 25°C (68° to 77°F) [See USP Controlled Room Temperature]. Store reconstituted suspension between 25°C (77°F) and 2°C (36°F) and **discard unused portion after 2 weeks.** Protect from freezing.

SHAKE WELL BEFORE EACH USE.

DISCARD UNUSED PORTION AFTER TWO WEEKS.

Which of the following best describes the action of the nurse who is preparing to administer the 0900 dose of Fluconazole for Oral Suspension on 5/23/xx? (Select all that apply.)

a. The nurse may store the drug in the refrigerator.
b. The nurse may use this reconstituted drug.
c. The nurse needs to reconstitute a new bottle of fluconazole.

14. Use the Lanoxin drug label to calculate the ordered dose: Lanoxin tablet 0.125 mg PO qAM. How many tablet(s) will the nurse administer?

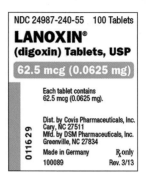

NDC 24987-240-55   100 Tablets

LANOXIN®
(digoxin) Tablets, USP

62.5 mcg (0.0625 mg)

Each tablet contains
62.5 mcg (0.0625 mg).

Dist. by Covis Pharmaceuticals, Inc.
Cary, NC 27511
Mfd. by DSM Pharmaceuticals, Inc.
Greenville, NC 27834
Made in Germany   R only
100089   Rev. 3/13

011629

15. Use the provider's orders and Calcitriol label to determine the ordered dose. How many Calcitriol capsule(s) will the nurse administer to the patient? _____

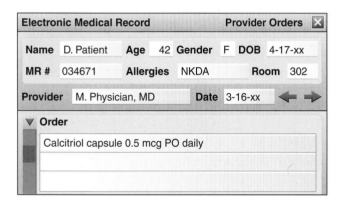

Electronic Medical Record		Provider Orders ✕
Name D. Patient	**Age** 42 **Gender** F **DOB** 4-17-xx	
MR # 034671	**Allergies** NKDA	**Room** 302
Provider M. Physician, MD	**Date** 3-16-xx	← →

▼ **Order**

Calcitriol capsule 0.5 mcg PO daily

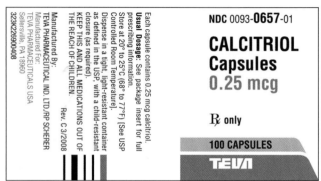

Manufactured By:
TEVA PHARMACEUTICAL IND. LTD./RP SCHERER
Manufactured For:
TEVA PHARMACEUTICALS USA
Sellersville, PA 18960
323K22690Q408

Each capsule contains 0.25 mcg calcitriol.
Usual Dosage: See package insert for full
prescribing information.
Store at 20° to 25°C (68° to 77°F) [See USP
Controlled Room Temperature].
Dispense in a tight, light-resistant container
as defined in the USP, with a child-resistant
closure (as required).
KEEP THIS AND ALL MEDICATIONS OUT OF
THE REACH OF CHILDREN.   Rev. C 3/2008

NDC 0093-**0657**-01

CALCITRIOL
Capsules
0.25 mcg

R only

100 CAPSULES

TEVA

16. The medication order is for Coreg 6.25 mg PO q.12h. The nurse finds the following drugs in the patient's medication drawer.

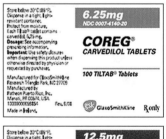

Store below 30°C (86°F).
Dispense in a tight, light-
resistant container.
Protect from moisture.
Each Tiltab® tablet contains
carvedilol, 6.25 mg.
Dosage: See accompanying
prescribing information.
Important: Use safety closures
when dispensing this product unless
otherwise directed by physician or
requested by purchaser.

6.25mg
NDC 0007-4140-20

COREG®
CARVEDILOL TABLETS

100 TILTAB® Tablets

Manufactured for GlaxoSmithKline
Research Triangle Park, NC 27709
Manufactured by
Patheon Puerto Rico, Inc.
Manati, PR 00674, USA
100000000058854   Rev. 8/08
Made in Ireland.   gsk GlaxoSmithKline   R only

For the morning dose, the nurse is correct in:
a. administering one tablet of the 6.25 mg dose.
b. administering one-half tablet of the 12.5 mg dose.

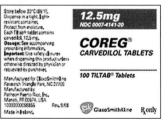

Store below 30°C (86°F).
Dispense in a tight, light-
resistant container.
Protect from moisture.
Each Tiltab® tablet contains
carvedilol, 12.5 mg.
Dosage: See accompanying
prescribing information.
Important: Use safety closures
when dispensing this product unless
otherwise directed by physician or
requested by purchaser.

12.5mg
NDC 0007-4141-20

COREG®
CARVEDILOL TABLETS

100 TILTAB® Tablets

Manufactured for GlaxoSmithKline
Research Triangle Park, NC 27709
Manufactured by
Patheon Puerto Rico, Inc.
Manati, PR 00674, USA
100000000058855   Rev. 8/08
Made in Ireland.   gsk GlaxoSmithKline   R only

17. The medication order is for metformin 0.5 g PO q.AM. The nurse finds the following drugs in the patient's medication drawer.

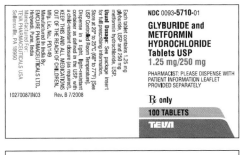

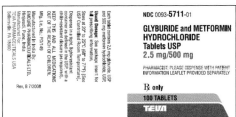

The nurse is most correct in:
a. administering two tablets of the 1.25 mg/250 mg dose.
b. administering one tablet of the 2.5 mg/500 mg dose.
c. calling the pharmacist.

18. Penicillin V Potassium oral solution 100 mg PO q.6h is ordered. How many mL will the nurse administer to the patient?

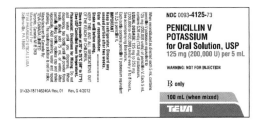

_____

19. Ceftin oral suspension 250 mg is ordered q.8h. On May 16, the nurse is preparing to give the 5:00 p.m. dose and finds the patient's medication in the refrigerator.

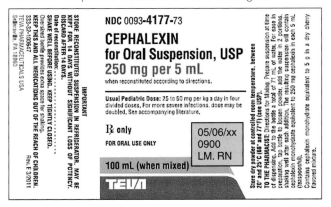

Which action by the nurse is most appropriate?
a. Administer 5 mL.
b. Discard expired bottle.
c. Clarifying the drug with the pharmacist.

20. Vibramycin syrup 150 mg PO is ordered. How many tsp will the nurse instruct the patient to take?

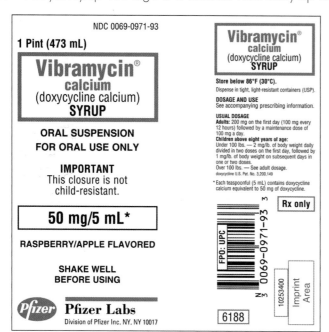

CHAPTER 10

Syringes and Needles

LEARNING OUTCOMES

Describe the parts of a syringe and a needle.

Identify the zero line and the calibration lines on syringes commonly used in clinical practice.

Choose the correct syringe and fill line for a variety of drug doses.

Choose the appropriate syringe to administer parenteral medications.

Many medications are administered by a route other than the oral route. The term **parenteral** is used to indicate routes other than the oral or gastrointestinal route. Common parenteral routes include the **intradermal** route (**ID**—under the skin or dermis), the **subcutaneous** route (**subcut**—into the subcutaneous tissue), the **intramuscular** route (**IM**—into the muscle), and the **intravenous** route (**IV**—directly into the vein).

Parenteral medications are administered using a syringe, a device used to inject medications into a body tissue or into a vein. The choice of syringe and needle size is determined by the nurse and is based on the properties of the medication and the route of administration. Nurses must choose the appropriate syringe and needle, accurately read the calibration lines on the syringe, and draw up the correct amount of medication into the syringe.

The Parts of a Syringe

To work with syringes, the nurse must know the parts of a syringe (Fig. 10-1).

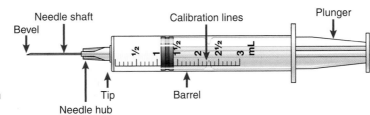

Figure 10-1. The main parts of a syringe.

Syringes have three main parts: the needle, the barrel of the syringe, and the plunger.

● The shaft of the needle has a sharp slanted end (called a **bevel**) that enables it to easily penetrate the skin and body tissues. The hub of the needle attaches to the tip of the syringe.

● The body of the syringe that holds the medication is called the **barrel.** The barrel of the syringe is marked with **calibration lines** that measure medication doses in mL. Depending on the size of the syringe, each calibration line measures from 0.01 to 1 mL of medication.

● The rubber-tipped cylinder called the **plunger** fills and empties the syringe.

Using the Plunger to Measure the Amount of Medication in a Syringe

The amount of medication in the syringe is measured by looking at the proximal end of the plunger, which is the end closest to the tip of the syringe. The rubber section on the proximal end has two rings. Measurement of medication is made at the first ring (the one closest to the tip of the syringe), as shown in Figure 10-2. The first ring of the plunger must cover the desired calibration line for accurate measurement (Fig. 10-3).

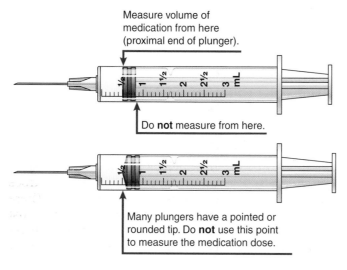

Figure 10-2. Measuring medication volume by looking at the proximal end of the plunger.

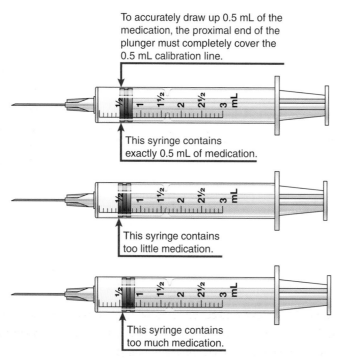

Figure 10-3. Measuring medication doses accurately.

The Calibration Lines on a Syringe

To accurately measure medication in a syringe, the nurse reads the calibration lines on the barrel of the syringe. Calibration lines vary according to the size of the syringe. For example, the calibration lines on the 1 mL syringe measure hundredths of a milliliter (0.01 mL), whereas the calibration lines on the 3 mL syringe measure tenths of milliliter (0.1 mL). Regardless of the size of the syringe or the value of the calibration lines, the first line on all syringes is the zero line.

THE ZERO LINE

The **zero line,** the first line on the barrel of the syringe, represents the starting point when there is no medication in the syringe. The zero line takes into account that a small volume of medication is contained in the needle, hub, and tip of the syringe (called **dead space**). It is important for the nurse to differentiate between the zero line and the first calibration line on the syringe (Fig. 10-4).

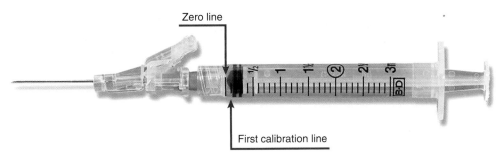

Figure 10-4. Zero line on a syringe.

READING CALIBRATION LINES ON A SYRINGE

Syringes measure very small amounts of liquid medication, such as tenths or hundredths of a milliliter. Accuracy in measurement is essential when working with syringes. Nurses do not measure between calibration lines or estimate when measuring medications. There is no need to memorize what the calibration lines measure on each type of syringe. Most nurses can carefully examine the calibration lines on a syringe and determine the measurements visually. Table 10-1 provides a clinical application to show the importance of calibration lines.

Table 10-1. The Importance of Calibration Lines on a Syringe

CLINICAL SITUATION	SYRINGE	CLINICAL DECISION-MAKING
After calculating a drug dosage, Nurse A prepares 0.4 mL of medication in the syringe. Nurse A shows the syringe to Nurse B to verify the dose. Nurse B validates that the syringe contains 0.4 mL of medication.	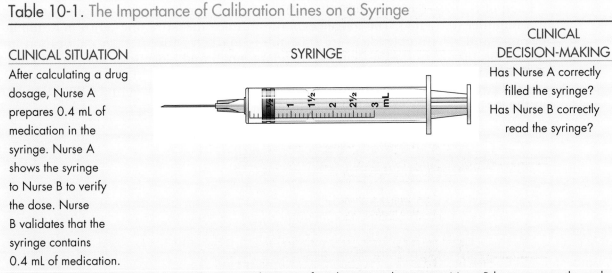	Has Nurse A correctly filled the syringe? Has Nurse B correctly read the syringe?

Discussion: Nurse A has not correctly measured 0.4 mL of medication in the syringe. Nurse B has not correctly read the calibration lines on the filled syringe. The zero line must be read as "0," and not as the 0.1 syringe calibration line. Nurse B should tell Nurse A that there is not enough medication in the syringe.

Choosing the Correct Syringe

There are many different types and sizes of syringes for the nurse to select. The nurse makes the choice of a syringe by the volume of medication to be given. The syringes most frequently used in clinical practice include the 3 mL syringe, the 1 mL or tuberculin syringe, and the insulin syringes. Other available syringes include the 5, 6, 10, 12, 20, 30, 50, and 60 mL syringes.

THE 3 ML SYRINGE

The 3 mL syringe is the most commonly used syringe in clinical practice because it can measure most parenteral medication doses that are ordered. The 3 mL syringe is used for medications administered by all of the parenteral routes (Fig. 10-5).

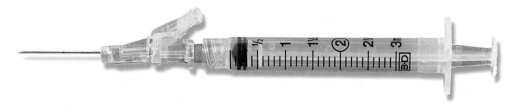

Figure 10-5. 3 mL Safety Glide syringe from Becton Dickinson.

Look at the calibration lines on the 3 mL syringe. In the 3 mL syringe, each shorter calibration line measures one-tenth of a milliliter (0.1 mL). Every ¹/₂ mL is marked with a longer calibration line and is numbered from ¹/₂ mL to 3 mL.

THE 1 ML OR TUBERCULIN SYRINGE

A tuberculin or TB syringe gets its name from its original use: administration of tuberculin skin tests. This is a small-volume syringe that measures hundredths of a milliliter (0.01 mL). The nurse may choose a 1 mL syringe if the measurement of very small doses of medication is required or if a medication dose is contained in hundredths of a milliliter. Look at the calibration lines on the 1 mL syringe in Figure 10-6.

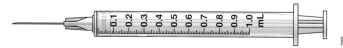

Figure 10-6. The 1 mL or tuberculin syringe.

Each of the shorter calibration lines on the 1 mL syringe represent one-hundredth of a milliliter (0.01 mL). The longer calibration lines measure one-tenth of a milliliter (0.1 mL) and are numbered. Every 0.05 mL is marked with a longer calibration line. The calibration lines on the 1 mL syringe are small and close together. Great care is needed in reading the calibration lines on this syringe. Figure 10-7 shows an enlargement of part of the 1 mL syringe barrel. In the enlargement, the actual calibration lines on the syringe appear in black numbers.

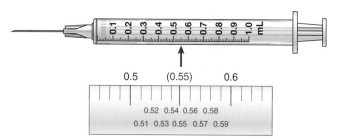

Figure 10-7. Close-up of the calibration lines on a 1 mL syringe.

The calibration lines on the 1 mL syringe have a number for every tenth of a milliliter. On some 1 mL syringes, **leading zeros** are not included and the 1 mL calibration line has a **trailing zero** (Fig. 10-8). It is important that the nurse recognize the numbers on a 1 mL syringe as decimal fractions and not whole numbers.

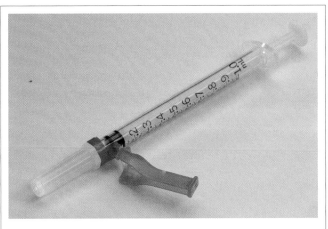

Figure 10-8. Smith Medical 1 mL syringe with no preceding zeros.

 Some TB syringes have two sets of calibration lines: one measuring mL, and one measuring minims, a unit of measurement from the apothecary system. The Institute for Safe Medication Practices (ISMP) has included the minim on the **List of Error-Prone Abbreviations, Symbols, and Dose Designations.** ISMP and other organizations recommend that the apothecary system no longer be used for prescribing drugs. If the nurse finds a syringe with both minim and mL calibration lines, it is essential to double-check that the correct calibration lines are used to measure the dose.

Many syringe manufacturers now put only the mL calibration lines on the syringe.

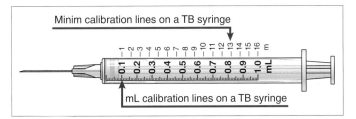

APPLY LEARNED KNOWLEDGE 10-1

Choose the correct syringe for the medication dose ordered. Shade in the syringe with the correct dose.

1. The nurse is to administer 1.2 mL of medication.

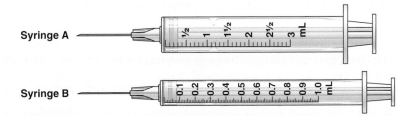

2. The nurse is to administer 0.4 mL of medication.

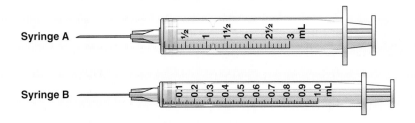

Continued

APPLY LEARNED KNOWLEDGE 10-1 — cont'd

3. The order is for 15 mg, which is contained in 0.15 mL.

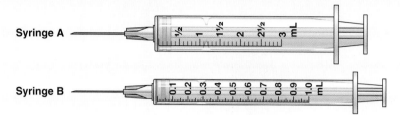

4. The nurse is to administer 1 mL of medication.

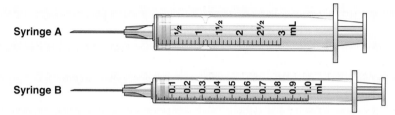

5. The nurse is to administer 0.25 mL of medication.

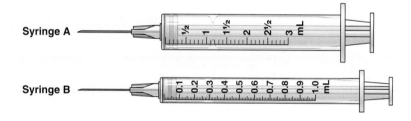

THE 5 AND 10 ML SYRINGES

The 5 mL and 10 mL syringes can be used to measure doses of medication larger than 3 mL and are most often used to prepare and administer IV medications (Fig. 10-9).

With these syringes, each small calibration line measures 0.2 mL. Every whole mL is marked by a longer calibration line and is numbered. Other syringe sizes available include the 6 mL and the 12 mL syringe. Although not as frequently used in clinical practice, these syringes have the same calibration line measurements as the 5 mL and 10 mL syringe.

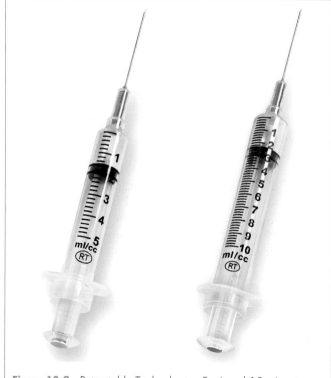

Figure 10-9. Retractable Technologies 5 mL and 10 mL syringes.

Some syringes in clinical practice still use cubic centimeters (cc) as the calibration measurement. Some have "cc/mL" written on the syringe. Milliliters (mL) and cubic centimeters (cc) are equivalent measurements. But because the term "cc" can be mistaken for "U" (units) in medication orders and documentation, national safety guidelines now recommend the use of the term "mL" in the patient care setting.

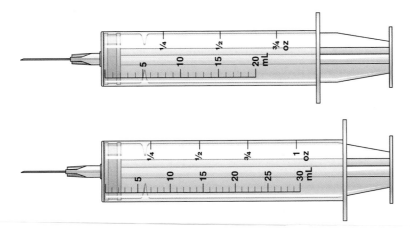

Figure 10-10. The 20 mL and 30 mL syringes.

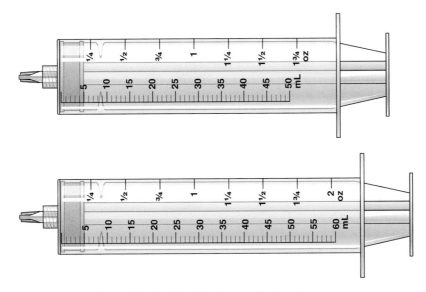

Figure 10-11. The 50 mL and 60 mL syringes.

THE 20, 30, 50, AND 60 ML SYRINGES

The 20, 30, 50, and 60 mL syringes can be used for administration of large volumes of IV medication and for other clinical uses. These syringes have two sets of calibration lines: mL and ounce. On the mL side, each small calibration line measures 1 mL, and every fifth mL has a longer calibration line and is numbered. The calibration lines on the other side of the syringe barrel measure ounces (Figs. 10-10 and 10-11).

APPLY LEARNED KNOWLEDGE 10-2

Determine whethr the statement is True or False. If the statement is false, write a rationale explaining the reason.

1. The only difference between a 1 mL and a 3 mL syringe is the difference in volume.　　T　　F

_____

2. A TB syringe can measure the following volume of medication: 0.38 mL.　　T　　F

_____

3. A 3 mL syringe can measure the following volume of medication: 2.4 mL.　　T　　F

_____

4. A 1 mL syringe will measure a small amount of medication with greater accuracy
than will a 3 mL syringe.　　T　　F

_____

5. A 5 mL syringe can measure ounces.　　T　　F

_____

INSULIN SYRINGES

One additional type of syringe, the insulin syringe, is only used to administer the drug insulin. The insulin syringe measures units of insulin, not mL, and it cannot be used for any other medications. See Figure 10-12. The administration of insulin and insulin syringes are covered in Chapter 13, Administration of Insulin.

PREFILLED SYRINGES OR CARTRIDGES

Drug manufacturers supply certain drugs in prefilled syringes or syringe cartridges. A **prefilled syringe** has a needle and plunger (Figs. 10-13). A **syringe cartridge** needs a special holder (usually with a plunger) to administer the medication (Figs. 10-14).

The prefilled syringe or syringe cartridge may be completely filled with medication, or it may have empty space to allow for adding a second medication to the syringe. Like all syringes, calibration lines enable the measurement of the ordered dose.

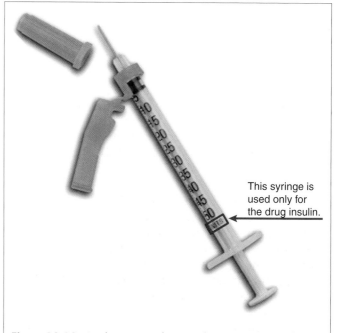

This syringe is used only for the drug insulin.

Figure 10-12. Insulin syringe showing the measurement of units, not mL.

When using a prefilled syringe or cartridge, the nurse must calculate the ordered dose prior to the administration of the medication. The prefilled syringe contains a certain volume of medication. The nurse may administer the exact amount in the prefilled syringe. Or, if the ordered dose is contained in a smaller volume of medication, the nurse may need to discard some of the medication. The exact dose must be in the syringe prior to administration of the medication.

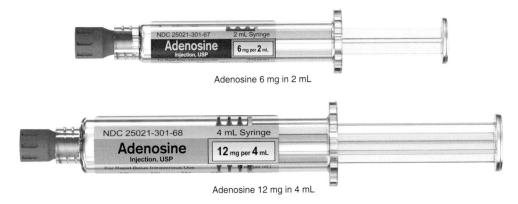

Adenosine 6 mg in 2 mL

Adenosine 12 mg in 4 mL

Figure 10-13. Prefilled syringes.

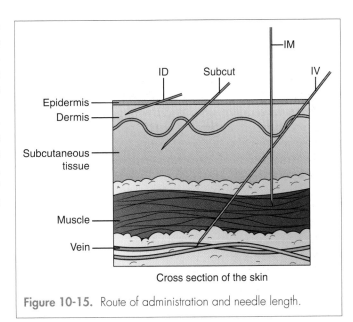

Prefilled cartridge

Cartridge holder

Figure 10-14. Prefilled syringe cartridge and holder.

Numbering System for Needles

Parenteral medications are injected into a variety of body tissues. The nurse must decide what needle size is most appropriate to administer the medication to the patient. Every needle has two measurement numbers: the first number refers to the length of the needle and the second number refers to the **gauge** of the needle.

NEEDLE LENGTH

Needles vary in length so that the injected medication can reach the desired tissue. The route of administration, injection site, and the size of the patient determine the length of needle. For example, the more superficial that the injection is, the shorter the needle used. An injection deep into the muscle requires a longer needle. Large patients may need a longer needle to deliver the medication to the desired tissue (Fig. 10-15).

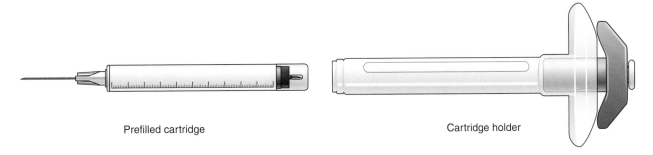

Cross section of the skin

Figure 10-15. Route of administration and needle length.

The length of a needle is measured in inches. Standard needles come in a variety of lengths, from 5/16 inch to 2 inches (Fig. 10-16).

NEEDLE GAUGE

Needle gauge is a measurement of the diameter of a needle and is described by a number followed by a "G" (gauge). Standard gauge numbers range from 16G (a very large needle gauge) to 31G (a very small needle gauge). See Figure 10-17.

The determination of needle gauge requires the nurse to consider the viscosity of the medication, the ease of withdrawing and administering the medication, and recommended needle gauges for various injection sites and routes. Taking these factors into consideration, the nurse also considers the smallest needle gauge for the comfort of the patient.

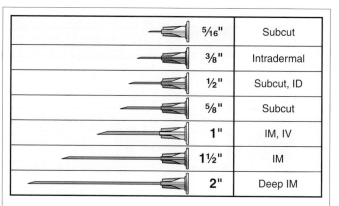

	5/16"	Subcut
	3/8"	Intradermal
	1/2"	Subcut, ID
	5/8"	Subcut
	1"	IM, IV
	1½"	IM
	2"	Deep IM

Figure 10-16. Standard needle lengths.

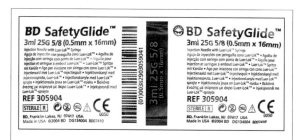

Needle Gauge	Cross Section of Needle Diameter	Uses
31G, 30G, 29G, 28G, 27G, 26G	°	Common needle gauges used for subcutaneous and intradermal injections
25G	○	Standard needle gauge for most subcutaneous injections
23G, 22G, 21G	○	Standard needle gauge for most IM injections
19G, 18G	○	Can be used for IV medication preparation

Figure 10-17. Standard needle gauges.

Syringes and Needles Commonly Used in Clinical Practice

Syringe manufacturers package syringes and needles together so that commonly used syringe and needle combinations are readily available (Figs. 10-18, 10-19, and 10-20).

Prepackaged syringes and needles are a time-saving convenience for the nurse in the busy clinical setting. However, the nurse still needs to choose the most appropriate syringe and needle size for the individual patient and medication to be given. In some instances, the needle in a prepackaged syringe will need to be exchanged for a needle of a different size.

Figure 10-18. BD SafetyGlide syringe package: 3 mL 25G 5/8".

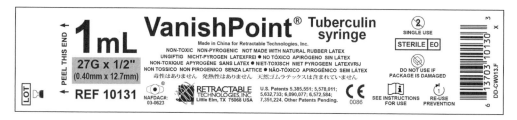

Figure 10-19. Retractable Technologies syringe package: 1 mL 27G ½".

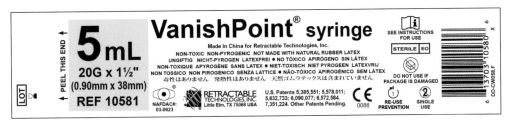

Figure 10-20. Retractable Technologies syringe package: 5 mL 20G 1½".

Color Coding on Syringes and Needles

Syringe manufacturers conform to standards from the International Organization for Standardization (ISO) and use standardized colors for needle hubs and syringe and needle packaging (ISO Standard 6009:1992). To ensure safe practice, the nurse should always double-check the syringe, the volume of medication, and the length and gauge of the needle.

APPLY LEARNED KNOWLEDGE 10-3

Choose the best syringe and needle to use in the situations below.

1. The nurse is to draw up a medication for subcutaneous injection. Which of the following is the most appropriate needle size for the nurse to choose?
   a. 27G 1"
   b. 25G 5/8"
   c. 22G 1½"
   d. 19G 1"

2. The nurse is to draw up 2.4 mL of medication for IM injection. The patient weighs 235 pounds. Which of the following is the best syringe and needle for the nurse to choose?
   a. 3 mL 27G ½"
   b. 3 mL 25G 5/8"
   c. 3 mL 23G 2"
   d. 3 mL 18G 1½"

3. The nurse in the allergy clinic prepares an intradermal injection. The dose is contained in 0.3 mL. Which syringe will the nurse choose?
   a. 3 mL 27G 1"
   b. 3 mL 25G 5/8"
   c. 1 mL 21G 1"
   d. 1 mL 26G ½"

4. The nurse draws up a viscous medication into a 3 mL syringe with an 18G 1" needle. The nurse changes the needle before giving the IM injection to the patient. Which of the following needles will the nurse choose for the IM injection?
   a. 27G 1"
   b. 25G 5/8"
   c. 22G 1½"
   d. 19G 1½"

5. The nurse is preparing 1 mL an intravenous medication for direct IV injection into the IV tubing. The medication is contained in a vial. The nurse is most correct to use which of the following to withdraw the medication?
   a. 1 mL 27G 3/8"
   b. 1 mL 25G 5/8"
   c. 3 mL 23G ½"
   d. 3 mL 19G 1"

CLINICAL REASONING 10-1

The nurse is visiting a patient who was discharged from the hospital yesterday. The patient's wife is to give her husband injections of 3,000 units of heparin subcut daily. The ordered dose is contained in 0.6 mL. During the visit, the nurse has the wife demonstrate drawing up heparin into the syringe. The wife shows the nurse the heparin medication and the following syringe:

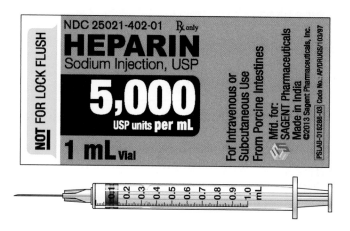

The nurse tells the wife that she needs to draw up more heparin into the syringe. Has the nurse evaluated the wife's return demonstration correctly? Provide a rationale for your answer.

In summary, the nurse considers the amount and route of medication ordered, the size of the patient, and the viscosity of the drug when making the choice of syringe and needle. The most important skill for the nurse to master is reading of the calibration lines on each syringe used.

Developing Competency

For questions 1 through 8, read the dose of medication measured in the syringes.

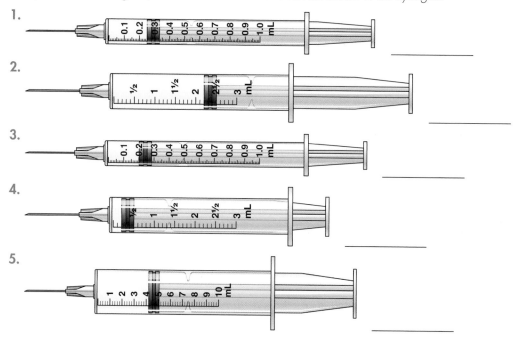

1.

2.

3.

4.

5.

6.

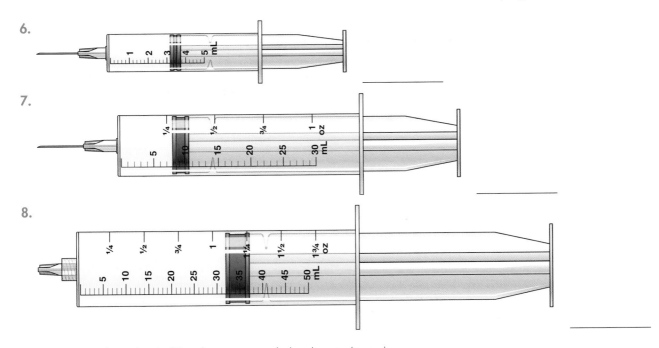

7.

8.

_____

For questions 9 through 16, fill in the syringe with the dose indicated.

9. 0.68 mL

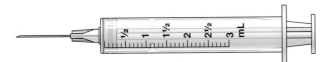

10. 0.5 mL

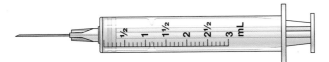

11. 1.8 mL

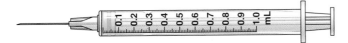

12. 2.2 mL

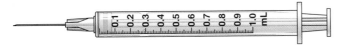

13. 0.33 mL

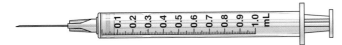

14. 3.2 mL

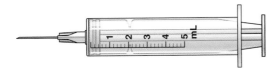

15. 18 mL

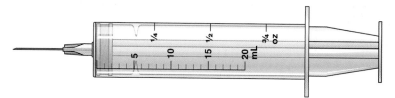

16. 6.8 mL

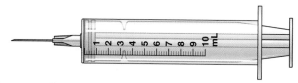

For questions 17 through 20, use the physician's order on the electronic medical record and the medication label to determine the amount to administer to the patient. Fill in the syringe with the correct amount.

17.

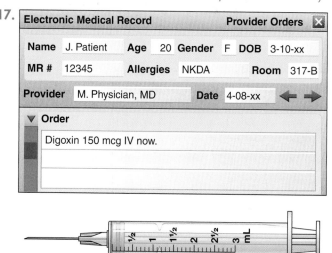

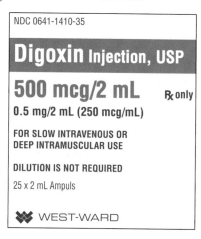

18.

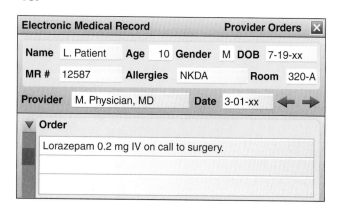

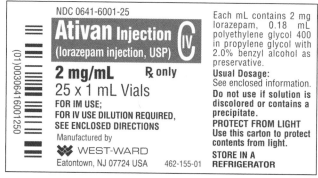

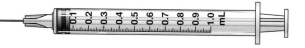

19.

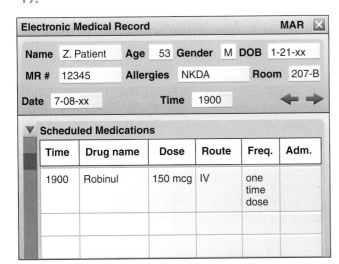

Time	Drug name	Dose	Route	Freq.	Adm.
1900	Robinul	150 mcg	IV	one time dose	

Electronic Medical Record — MAR

Name Z. Patient Age 53 Gender M DOB 1-21-xx
MR # 12345 Allergies NKDA Room 207-B
Date 7-08-xx Time 1900

▼ Scheduled Medications

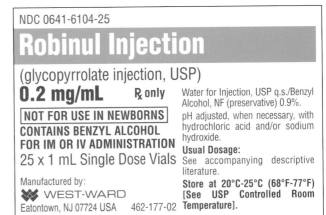

NDC 0641-6104-25

Robinul Injection

(glycopyrrolate injection, USP)

0.2 mg/mL ℞ only

NOT FOR USE IN NEWBORNS
CONTAINS BENZYL ALCOHOL
FOR IM OR IV ADMINISTRATION
25 x 1 mL Single Dose Vials

Water for Injection, USP q.s./Benzyl Alcohol, NF (preservative) 0.9%. pH adjusted, when necessary, with hydrochloric acid and/or sodium hydroxide.
Usual Dosage: See accompanying descriptive literature.
Store at 20°C-25°C (68°F-77°F) [See USP Controlled Room Temperature].

Manufactured by:
WEST-WARD
Eatontown, NJ 07724 USA 462-177-02

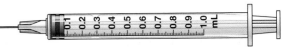

20.

Electronic Medical Record — Provider Orders

Name B. Patient Age 76 Gender M DOB 7-23-xx
MR # 12345 Allergies Sulfa Room 1330-A
Provider T. Physician, MD Date 1-10-xx

▼ Order

Enalaprilat 312.5 mcg IV q.6h.

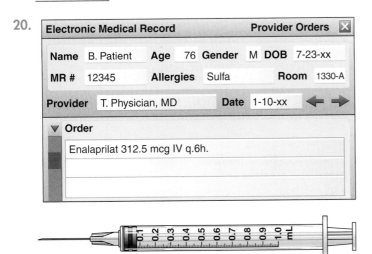

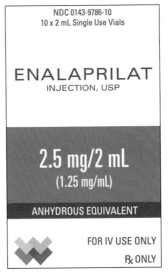

NDC 0143-9786-10
10 x 2 mL Single Use Vials

ENALAPRILAT

INJECTION, USP

2.5 mg/2 mL
(1.25 mg/mL)

ANHYDROUS EQUIVALENT

FOR IV USE ONLY
℞ ONLY

CHAPTER 11

Calculating Parenteral Medication Dosages

LEARNING OUTCOMES

Describe the parenteral routes of medication administration.

Solve parenteral medication dosage calculation problems.

Select the appropriate syringe and fill in the ordered amount.

The delivery of medications using routes other than the gastrointestinal tract is known as *parenteral* medication administration. In the clinical setting, use of the term "parenteral" generally refers to the administration of injectable medications. The most common parenteral routes used by the nurse for injections are the *subcutaneous (subcut),* the *intravenous (IV),* the *intramuscular (IM),* and the *intradermal (ID)* routes.

Topical and *inhalant* medications can also be considered parenteral, as these are given by routes other than the gastrointestinal tract (see Table 11-1). As usually no

Table 11-1. Common Parenteral Routes of Medication Administration

PARENTERAL MEDICATION ADMINISTRATION: COMMON INJECTABLE ROUTES	
• Subcutaneous (subcut)	Into the subcutaneous tissue; beneath the skin
• Intravenous (IV)	Within or into a vein
• Intramuscular (IM)	Within a muscle
• Intradermal (ID)	Within the dermis; under the skin
OTHER PARENTERAL MEDICATION ADMINISTRATION ROUTES	
• Intranasal	Within the nasal cavity
• Ophthalmic	On the tissue of the eye
• Intra-auricular (otic)	Into the ear
• Dermal	Applied on the skin or mucous membrane; local effect
• Transdermal	Applied to the skin surface; systemic effect
• Intravaginal	Into the vagina
• Inhalation	Inhaled through the mouth or nose into the respiratory tract for absorption

calculation is needed for administration of drugs by the topical or inhalation routes, the focus in this chapter is on calculating dosages for injectable parenteral medications.

The nurse's role in administering parenteral medications includes accurately interpreting the medication order, calculating the dosage, and drawing up the ordered amount using the appropriate syringe. These components of the Six Rights of Medication Administration form the basis for safe parenteral medication administration practice.

Types of Parenteral Drug Containers

Drug manufacturers package parenteral drugs for injection in prefilled syringes and cartridges, ampules, and vials (see Table 11-2). The prefilled syringe, prefilled cartridge, and ampule are for single doses of drugs. Drugs supplied in vials can be for single or multi-dose use.

Table 11-2. Parenteral Drug Containers

Prefilled syringe and prefilled cartridge	Prefilled syringes (with or without a needle) come from the manufacturer filled with medication, eliminating the need to draw up the medication into an empty syringe. Prefilled cartridges are similar, but need a special cartridge holder to administer the drug. Prefilled syringes and cartridges usually have 1 mL or 2 mL of space available so that another compatible drug can be added to the medication in the syringe. With a prefilled syringe or cartridge, the dose is calculated and any excess medication is discarded prior to administering the dose to the patient.	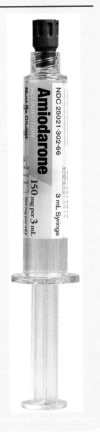

Continued

Table 11-2. Parenteral Drug Containers—cont'd

Ampule	An ampule is a glass container with a long narrow top that is snapped off to allow withdrawal of the medication. Ampules contain a single dose of medication. If the entire amount is not administered to the patient, the remaining drug must be discarded.	
Vial	A vial is a plastic or glass container that has a rubber stopper that is punctured for withdrawal of the medication. Drugs supplied in vials can be for single-dose use or multi-dose use. A multi-dose vial typically contains an antimicrobial preservative to help prevent the growth of bacteria.	

Parenteral Medication Orders and the Parenteral Medication Drug Label

Parenteral medications are ordered by the specific strength of medication to be administered, for example, the number of grams, milligrams, or micrograms (Fig. 11-1). The nurse uses the dosage strength listed on the drug label to calculate the number of mL of medication to give (Fig. 11-2).

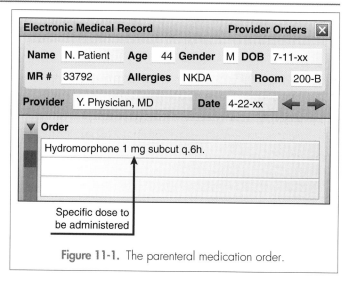

Figure 11-1. The parenteral medication order.

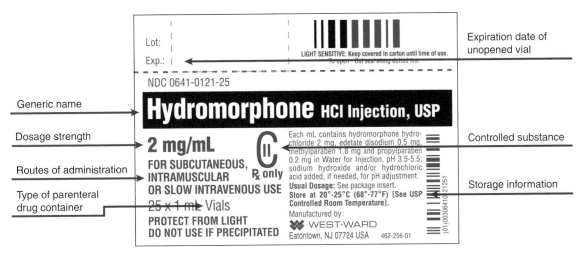

Figure 11-2. The parenteral drug label.

Drug Labels That List More Than One Dosage Strength

Some parenteral drug labels may list more than one dosage strength (Fig. 11-3). When more than one dosage strength is listed, the nurse can choose which dosage strength to use in the calculation.

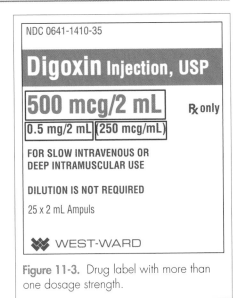

Figure 11-3. Drug label with more than one dosage strength.

The Expiration Date and the Beyond-Use Date of a Multi-Dose Vial

When using a multi-dose vial, the nurse needs to consider two dates: the expiration date of the drug and the beyond-use date.

■ The **expiration date** of the drug is determined by the manufacturer and is stamped on the drug package and/or drug label. This is the last day that an unopened vial can be used.

Once the vial cap is removed or the vial is punctured, the manufacturer's expiration date should be replaced with a new date, the beyond-use date.

■ The **beyond-use date,** the last date that an opened vial can be used, can be written on the drug label by the pharmacist or the nurse who opens the multi-dose vial. The Joint Commission, the organization that accredits hospitals and healthcare organizations, requires that multi-dose vials be discarded 28 days after first use unless the manufacturer specifies otherwise (shorter or longer). This date is based on research regarding the length of time that the sterility of the drug can be guaranteed.

 For many drugs, discarding the multi-dose vial when the beyond-use date has passed is not an issue as the drug is used up or the patient is discharged well before the 28-day limit. However, a few parenteral drugs that come in multi-dose vials, such as insulin, may remain on the clinical unit for use with multiple patients. With these multi-dose vials, the nurse needs to carefully check the beyond-use date. Many healthcare facilities have policies that state that if this date is not clearly written on the vial, the vial should be discarded. Also, if sterility is questioned or compromised then the multi-dose vial should be discarded regardless of the date.

Current Standards for Labeling the Multi-Dose Vial

The Joint Commission requires pharmacists in healthcare organizations to relabel multi-dose vials with a beyond-use date once the multi-dose vial is opened or punctured. To apply this requirement to nursing practice, it is recommended that the first time a multi-dose vial is used, the nurse should put the following information on the drug label: date and time the vial was opened, the initials of the nurse first using the vial, and the beyond-use or discard date of the vial (Fig. 11-4).

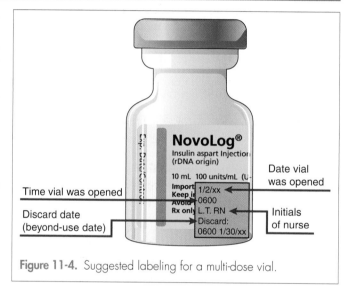

Figure 11-4. Suggested labeling for a multi-dose vial.

 Communicating and interpreting the beyond-use or discard date is a dual responsibility. The nurse who punctures the vial for the first time must write information that will enable the next nurse to evaluate whether the vial can be used for another dose. The nurse who next uses the vial must refer to the beyond-use or discard date before administering the dose.

 Some controversy exists around the issue of discarding multi-dose vials using the beyond-use date rather than the manufacturer's expiration date, as this may increase waste and the cost associated with it, and contribute to a drug shortage crisis. Research and surveys of healthcare providers are being conducted by organizations such as the Institute for Safe Medication Practices (ISMP) to determine best practices in this area. More nursing research needs to be done to standardize policies that will best promote patient safety with the use of multi-dose vials.

Choice of Syringe

If the parenteral medication is contained in an ampule or vial, the nurse must choose the syringe needed to administer the dose of medication. In deciding which syringe to use, the nurse considers the number of mL that need to be administered. Most parenteral medications for IM, subcut, and ID injection are manufactured so that the dose is contained in a volume less than 3 mL. Therefore, the most frequently used syringes are the 1 mL and 3 mL syringes. Doses of IV medications can be contained in volumes greater than 3 mL.

Considerations When Calculating and Rounding Parenteral Medication Dosages

Organizations concerned with patient safety, such as the ISMP and the Centers for Disease Control and Prevention (CDC), recommend that parenteral drugs be available in single-dose amounts. Drug manufacturers are now packaging many parenteral drugs so that the usual or recommended dose is contained in an ampule, vial, or prefilled syringe.

DOSAGE CALCULATIONS THAT COME OUT EVENLY

When a dosage calculation comes out evenly, for example, 0.25 mL or 1.5 mL, the nurse does not need to round the answer. The nurse should select the syringe that most accurately measures the calculated amount. For example, 0.25 mL can be measured in a 1 mL syringe, and 1.5 mL can be measured in a 3 mL syringe. This will ensure that the patient receives the most accurate dose of the medication.

DOSAGE CALCULATIONS THAT MUST BE ROUNDED

Sometimes parenteral dosage calculations result in an answer that does not come out evenly. Although the type of medication and clinical condition of the patient are always the nurse's priority, some general guidelines of rounding can be used when calculating parenteral medication dosages (Table 11-3).

Table 11-3. Suggested Rounding Guidelines for Parenteral Medication Dosages

CALCULATED DOSAGE AMOUNT	ROUNDING RULE	SYRINGE SELECTION
Less than 1 mL	Work the problem to the thousandth place (three places to the right of the decimal point) and round to the hundredths place.	Administer the dose in a 1 mL syringe.
	Example: The physician orders 30 mcg of medication. The medication has a dosage strength of 90 mcg/mL. The nurse solves the calculation to the thousandths place and arrives at an answer of 0.333 mL.	
	The nurse cannot measure 0.333 mL in a syringe. The answer to the calculation must be rounded so that it can be drawn up and administered. The nurse follows the rules of rounding and rounds the answer to the hundredths place: 0.33 mL. This amount can be drawn up and administered in a 1 mL syringe.	

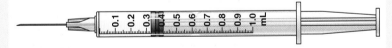

Greater than 1 mL	Work the problem to the hundredth place (two places to the right of the decimal point) and round to the tenths place.	Administer the dose in a 3 mL syringe.
	Example: The physician orders 500 mg of medication. The medication has a dosage strength of 300 mg/mL. The nurse solves the calculation to the hundredths place and arrives at an answer of 1.66 mL.	
	The nurse cannot measure 1.66 mL in a syringe. The answer to the calculation must be rounded so that it can be drawn up and administered. The nurse follows the rules of rounding and rounds the answer to the tenths place: 1.7 mL. This amount can be drawn up and administered in a 3 mL syringe.	

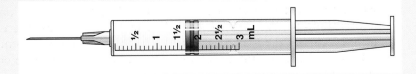

APPLY LEARNED KNOWLEDGE 11-1

Answer the following questions. Circle T if the statement is true. Circle F if the statement is false. Write a rationale for the correct answer.

1. The nurse calculates that the ordered dose of the drug is contained in 0.95 mL. The nurse is correct to round the answer to the calculation to 1 mL and administer the dose in a 3 mL syringe.

   T F _____

2. A prefilled syringe may have space to allow for the addition of another compatible parenteral medication.

   T F _____

3. The expiration date imprinted on the drug label is used by the nurse to determine whether a punctured multi-dose vial can be used to administer a dose of medication.

   T F _____

4. A single-dose vial can be used again provided that the second dose is administered to the same patient.

   T F _____

5. If the nurse found an opened multi-dose vial of medication that did not have any information written on the label, the nurse should label it with date, time, initials, and discard date after administering the dose to the patient.

   T F _____

Drug Dosage Calculations With the Same Unit of Measurement

In the calculation of drug dosages, the nurse identifies the unit of measurement from the

- ■ medication order.
- ■ drug label sent by the pharmacy.

If the medication order and the dosage strength from the drug label have the same unit of measurement, no conversion is needed and the problem can be set up and solved easily.

Example 1:

The order is for 0.625 mg of enalaprilat IV q.6h. The pharmacy sends the following vial of enalaprilat. How many mL will the nurse administer?

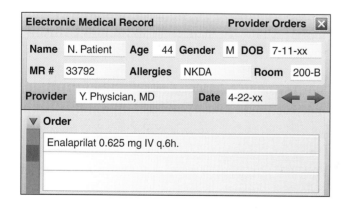

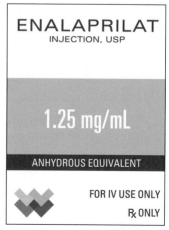

In this example:

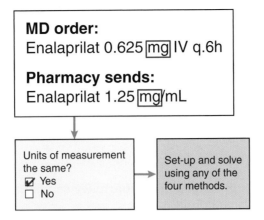

MD order:
Enalaprilat 0.625 mg IV q.6h

Pharmacy sends:
Enalaprilat 1.25 mg/mL

Units of measurement
the same?
☑ Yes
☐ No

Set-up and solve
using any of the
four methods.

Because the unit of measurement, mg, is the same in the medication order and on the enalaprilat drug label, no conversion is needed.

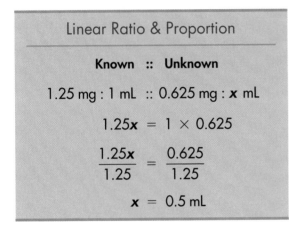

Linear Ratio & Proportion

Known :: Unknown

$$1.25 \text{ mg} : 1 \text{ mL} :: 0.625 \text{ mg} : x \text{ mL}$$

$$1.25x = 1 \times 0.625$$

$$\frac{1.25x}{1.25} = \frac{0.625}{1.25}$$

$$x = 0.5 \text{ mL}$$

Dimensional Analysis

$$\text{Ordered Amount} \times \text{Dosage Strength} = \text{Desired Amount}$$

$$\frac{0.625 \text{ mg}}{1} \times \frac{1 \text{ mL}}{1.25 \text{ mg}} = x \text{ mL}$$

$$\frac{0.625 \times 1 \text{ mL}}{1 \times 1.25} = \frac{0.625}{1.25} = 0.5 \text{ mL}$$

Fractional Ratio & Proportion

Known = Unknown

$$\frac{1.25 \text{ mg}}{1 \text{ mL}} = \frac{0.625 \text{ mg}}{x \text{ mL}}$$

$$1.25x = 1 \times 0.625$$

$$\frac{1.25x}{1.25} = \frac{0.625}{1.25}$$

$$x = 0.5 \text{ mL}$$

Formula Method

$$\frac{D}{H} \times Q = x$$

$$\frac{0.625 \text{ mg}}{1.25 \text{ mg}} \times 1 \text{ mL} = x \text{ mL}$$

$$\frac{0.625}{1.25} \times 1 \text{ mL} = x \text{ mL}$$

$$0.5 \times 1 \text{ mL} = 0.5 \text{ mL}$$

The nurse can choose either a 1 mL or a 3 mL syringe to administer 0.5 mL to the patient.

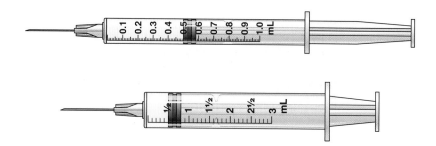

Example 2:

The MD orders Zantac 75 mg IV q.8h. The pharmacy sends the following vial of Zantac. How many mL will the nurse administer?

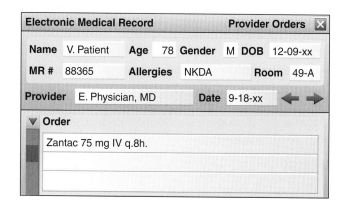

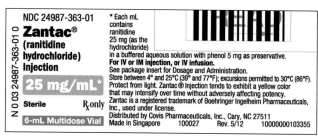

In this example:

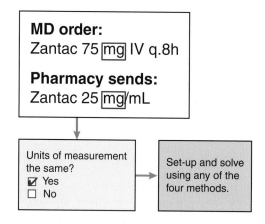

The unit of measurement in the medication order is mg. The dosage strength listed on the Zantac medication label is in mg. No conversion is needed.

Linear Ratio & Proportion

Known :: Unknown

$25 \text{ mg} : 1 \text{ mL} :: 75 \text{ mg} : x \text{ mL}$

$25x = 1 \times 75$

$$\frac{25x}{25} = \frac{75}{25}$$

$x = 3 \text{ mL}$

Dimensional Analysis

$$\underset{\text{Amount}}{\text{Ordered}} \times \underset{\text{Strength}}{\text{Dosage}} = \underset{\text{Amount}}{\text{Desired}}$$

$$\frac{75 \text{ mg}}{1} \times \frac{1 \text{ mL}}{25 \text{ mg}} = x \text{ mL}$$

$$\frac{75 \times 1 \text{ mL}}{1 \times 25} = \frac{75}{25} = 3 \text{ mL}$$

Fractional Ratio & Proportion

Known = Unknown

$$\frac{25 \text{ mg}}{1 \text{ mL}} \diagup\!\!\!\diagdown \frac{75 \text{ mg}}{x \text{ mL}}$$

$25x = 1 \times 75$

$$\frac{25x}{25} = \frac{75}{25}$$

$x = 3 \text{ mL}$

Formula Method

$$\frac{D}{H} \times Q = x$$

$$\frac{75 \text{ mg}}{25 \text{ mg}} \times 1 \text{ mL} = x \text{ mL}$$

$$\frac{75}{25} \times 1 \text{ mL} = x \text{ mL}$$

$$3 \times 1 \text{ mL} = 3 \text{ mL}$$

The nurse chooses a 3 mL syringe and administers 3 mL to the patient.

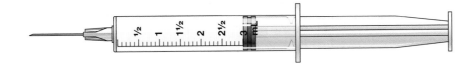

Calculating Parenteral Medication Dosages With Heparin

Some drugs are supplied in units of measurement that do not convert to any other unit of measurement. For example, the parenteral medication heparin is measured in "units." The "unit" measurement expresses the biological activity or potency of a drug and is the standard measurement for heparin. Heparin, an anticoagulant drug used to prevent blood clots, is a high alert medication with a great potential for patient harm (Fig. 11-5).

 Many healthcare organizations have standard safety protocols that nurses follow in relation to heparin administration, such as having another nurse independently double-check all heparin calculations and heparin doses prior to administration.

Heparin is commonly available in many concentrations, from 10 units/mL (used for flushing an IV line) to 40,000 units/mL (the higher concentrations are used in anticoagulant therapy). See Figure 11-6. The nurse must use great care in reading the label of any heparin medication to validate the concentration of heparin.

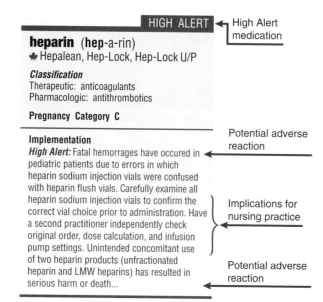

High Alert medication

Potential adverse reaction

Implications for nursing practice

Potential adverse reaction

Figure 11-5. Information about heparin from drug reference.

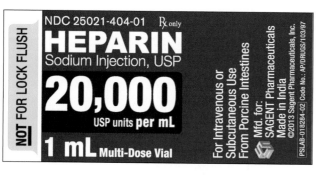

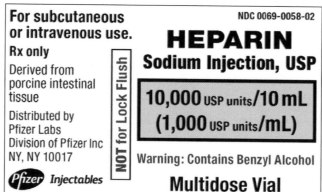

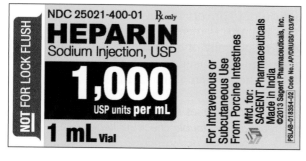

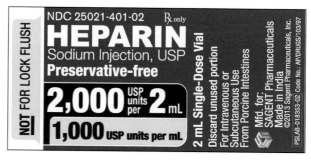

Figure 11-6. Variety of heparin concentrations.

When calculating dosages of heparin, the unit of measurement in the medication order and on the drug label will always match, and no conversion of units will be needed. See the following example.

Example:

The physician's order is for heparin sodium 4,000 units subcut daily. The pharmacy sends a vial of heparin sodium injection. How many mL will the nurse administer?

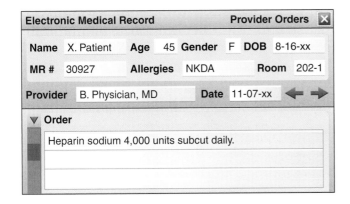
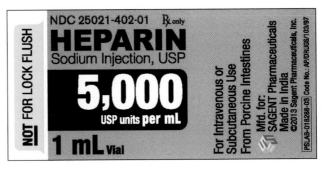

In this example:

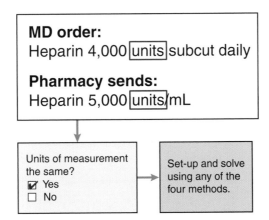

The units of measurement in the physician's order and the medication label are the same, so no conversion is needed.

Linear Ratio & Proportion

Known :: Unknown

5000 units : 1 mL :: 4000 units : x mL

$$5000x = 1 \times 4000$$

$$\frac{5000x}{5000} = \frac{4000}{5000}$$

$$x = 0.8 \text{ mL}$$

Dimensional Analysis

Ordered Amount	×	Dosage Strength	=	Desired Amount

$$\frac{4000 \text{ units}}{1} \times \frac{1 \text{ mL}}{5000 \text{ units}} = x \text{ mL}$$

$$\frac{4000 \times 1 \text{ mL}}{1 \times 5000} = \frac{4000}{5000} = 0.8 \text{ mL}$$

Fractional Ratio & Proportion

Known = Unknown

$$\frac{5000 \text{ units}}{1 \text{ mL}} \quad \frac{4000 \text{ units}}{x \text{ mL}}$$

$$5000x = 4000$$

$$\frac{5000x}{5000} = \frac{4000}{5000}$$

$$x = 0.8 \text{ mL}$$

Formula Method

$$\frac{D}{H} \times Q = x$$

$$\frac{4000 \text{ units}}{5000 \text{ units}} \times 1 \text{ mL} = x \text{ mL}$$

$$\frac{4000}{5000} \times 1 \text{ mL} = x \text{ mL}$$

$$0.8 \times 1 \text{ mL} = 0.8 \text{ mL}$$

The nurse chooses either a 1 mL or a 3 mL syringe and administers 0.8 mL to the patient.

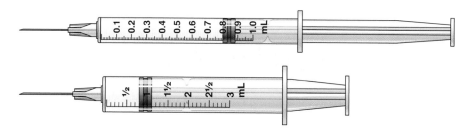

Differentiating Heparin From Other Anticoagulant Drugs

Other anticoagulant drugs (called low molecular weight heparins, or LMWHs) are used in clinical practice. These drugs are commonly ordered by their specific generic or trade name. One LMWH drug [dalteparin (Fragmin)] is ordered in IU (international units). Another LMWH drug [enoxaparin (Lovenox)] is ordered in mg. These types of anticoagulant drugs must not be confused with the drug heparin. The nurse must use great care to differentiate the anticoagulant drug labels.

EBP *The Joint Commission has developed a National Patient Safety Goal (03.05.01) that addresses the high risk of patient injury with the use of anticoagulant medications in hospitals. Some of the new standards for the administration of parenteral heparin include the following:*
- *Only prefilled-syringes and premixed IV bags are to be used when these products are available.*
- *Programmable infusion pumps are to be used when heparin is administered intravenously and continuously.*
- *Baseline and ongoing laboratory tests are required for heparin and low molecular weight heparin therapies.*

Other Drugs Measured in Units of Measurement That Require No Conversion

Another drug measured in units is penicillin. With penicillin, like heparin, the unit of measurement in the medication order and on the drug label will always match, and no conversion of units will be needed. Electrolytes (such as potassium) are measured in the unit of measurement "milliequivalent" (mEq). Like the unit of measurement "unit," the mEq is not converted to another unit of measurement when calculating a drug dosage.

Insulin, used to control blood sugar, is another drug that is measured in units. However insulin differs from all other drugs measured in units because it does not require any calculation, and the ordered dose is administered in specially calibrated insulin syringes. Insulin administration is covered in Chapter 13.

APPLY LEARNED KNOWLEDGE 11-2

Calculate the answer to the following drug dosage problems using any method of calculation.

1. The order is for methylprednisolone 60 mg IM now. The following medication is available from the pharmacy:

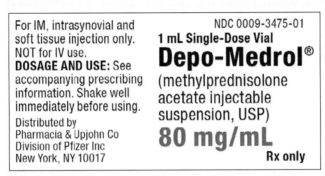

How many mL will the nurse give? _____

Fill in the syringe with the correct amount to administer the ordered dose.

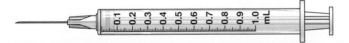

2. The physician orders midazolam 1.25 mg IV now. The following medication is available from the pharmacy:

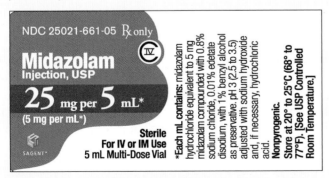

How many mL will the nurse give? _____

Fill in the syringe with the correct amount to administer the ordered dose.

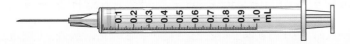

Continued

APPLY LEARNED KNOWLEDGE 11-2—cont'd

3. The order is for amiodarone 125 mg IV now. The following medication is available from the pharmacy:

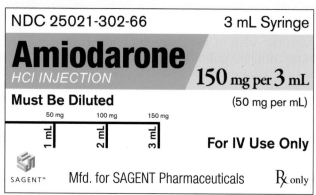

How many mL will the nurse draw up into the syringe? _____

Fill in the syringe with the correct amount to administer the ordered dose.

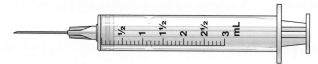

4. The order is for morphine sulfate 9 mg IV now. The following medication is available from the pharmacy:

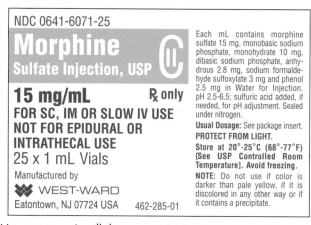

How many mL will the nurse give? _____

Fill in the appropriate syringe with the correct amount to administer the ordered dose.

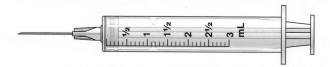

APPLY LEARNED KNOWLEDGE 11-2—cont'd

5. The order is for ondansetron 6 mg IV. Infuse over 15 minutes 30 minutes prior to chemotherapy. The following medication is available from the pharmacy:

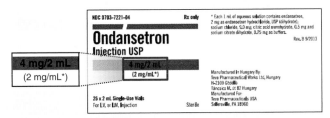

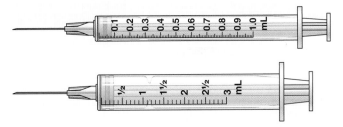

How many mL will the nurse draw up into the syringe? _____

Fill in the appropriate syringe with the correct amount to administer the ordered dose.

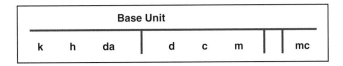

Drug Dosage Calculations Requiring Conversion Within the Metric System

Sometimes the medication that the physician orders is in one unit of measurement, and the drug provided by the pharmacy has a different unit of measurement. In this case, the nurse needs to convert the metric units so that they are the same. Once the units of measurement are the same, the problem can be solved.

Calculations requiring conversion within the metric system can be solved by either working with the metric line to convert from one unit of measurement to another or using a conversion factor. When using the metric line, recall the following steps:

Base Unit							
k	h	da		d	c	m		mc

Step 1: Identify the starting place on the metric line (unit of measurement from the medication order).

Step 2: Identify the desired place on the metric line (unit of measurement from the drug label).

Step 3: Convert to the desired place on the metric line by moving the decimal point.

These steps are applied using the following two examples:

Example 1:

The physician orders desmopressin 0.001 mg subcut BID. The pharmacy sends the following vial of desmopressin. How many mL will the nurse administer to the patient?

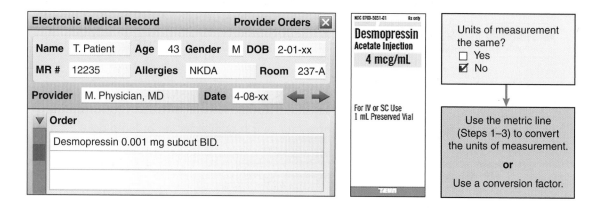

In Example 1, mg is the unit of measurement from the medication order and mcg is the unit of measurement from the drug label. To convert from mg (the starting place) to mcg (the desired place), move the decimal point three places: 0.001 mg equals 1 mcg.

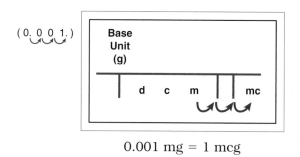

0.001 mg = 1 mcg

If using a conversion factor, the nurse recalls that 1 mg = 1,000 mcg. Now the problem can be solved using one of the methods of calculation.

Linear Ratio & Proportion

Known :: Unknown

4 mcg : 1 mL :: 0.001 mg : x mL

$$4 \text{ mcg} : 1 \text{ mL} :: \underset{1 \text{ mcg}}{\cancel{0.001} \text{ mg}} : x \text{ mL}$$

$$4x = 1 \times 1$$

$$\frac{4x}{4} = \frac{1}{4}$$

$$x = 0.25 \text{ mL}$$

Dimensional Analysis

$$\frac{\text{Ordered}}{\text{Amount}} \times \frac{\text{Dosage}}{\text{Strength}} \times \frac{\text{Conversion}}{\text{Factor}} = \frac{\text{Desired}}{\text{Amount}}$$

$$\frac{0.001 \cancel{\text{ mg}}}{1} \times \frac{1 \text{ mL}}{4 \cancel{\text{ mcg}}} \times \frac{1000 \cancel{\text{ mcg}}}{1 \cancel{\text{ mg}}} = x \text{ mL}$$

$$\frac{0.001 \times 1 \text{ mL} \times 1000}{1 \times 4 \times 1} = \frac{1}{4} = 0.25 \text{ mL}$$

[With dimensional analysis, a conversion factor is used to convert, rather than the metric line.]

Fractional Ratio & Proportion

Known = Unknown

$$\frac{4 \text{ mcg}}{1 \text{ mL}} = \frac{0.001 \text{ mg}}{x \text{ mL}}$$

$$\frac{4 \text{ mcg}}{1 \text{ mL}} \diagup\!\!\!\!\diagdown \frac{\underset{1 \text{ mcg}}{\cancel{0.001} \text{ mg}}}{x \text{ mL}}$$

$$4x = 1 \times 1$$

$$\frac{4x}{4} = \frac{1}{4}$$

$$x = 0.25 \text{ mL}$$

Formula Method

$$\frac{D}{H} \times Q = x$$

$$\frac{0.001 \text{ mg}}{4 \text{ mcg}} \times 1 \text{ mL} = x \text{ mL}$$

$$\frac{\underset{1 \text{ mcg}}{\cancel{0.001} \text{ mg}}}{4 \text{ mcg}} \times 1 \text{ mL} = x \text{ mL}$$

$$\frac{1 \cancel{\text{ mcg}}}{4 \cancel{\text{ mcg}}} \times 1 \text{ mL} = x \text{ mL}$$

$$\frac{1}{4} \times 1 \text{ mL} = 0.25 \text{ mL}$$

The nurse administers 0.25 mL to the patient.

Example 2:

The physician orders amiodarone 0.15 g IV stat. The nurse has the following vial of amiodarone. How many mL will the nurse administer to the patient?

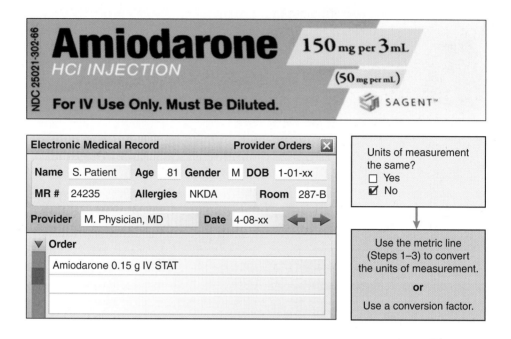

In Example 2, g is the unit of measurement from the MD order and mg is the unit of measurement from the drug label. To convert from g (the starting place) to mg (the desired place), move the decimal point three places: 0.15 g equals 150 mg.

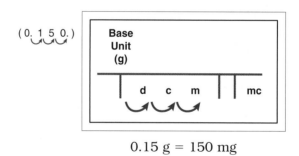

0.15 g = 150 mg

If using a conversion factor, the nurse recalls that 1 g = 1,000 mg. The Amiodarone drug label has two dosage strengths listed. For simplicity, use the smaller numbers. Now the problem can be solved using one of the methods of calculation.

Linear Ratio & Proportion

Known :: Unknown

$50 \text{ mg} : 1 \text{ mL} :: 0.15 \text{ g} : x \text{ mL}$

$$50 \text{ mg} : 1 \text{ mL} :: \underset{150 \text{ mg}}{\cancel{0.15}} \text{ g} : x \text{ mL}$$

$50x = 1 \times 150$

$$\frac{50x}{50} = \frac{150}{50}$$

$x = 3 \text{ mL}$

Dimensional Analysis

$$\underset{\text{Amount}}{\text{Ordered}} \times \underset{\text{Strength}}{\text{Dosage}} \times \underset{\text{Factor}}{\text{Conversion}} = \underset{\text{Amount}}{\text{Desired}}$$

$$\frac{0.15 \ \cancel{g}}{1} \times \frac{1 \text{ mL}}{50 \ \cancel{mg}} \times \frac{1000 \ \cancel{mg}}{1 \ \cancel{g}} = x \text{ mL}$$

$$\frac{0.15 \times 1 \text{ mL} \times 1000}{1 \times 50 \times 1} = \frac{150}{50} = 3 \text{ mL}$$

[With dimensional analysis, a conversion factor is used to convert, rather than the metric line.]

Fractional Ratio & Proportion

Known = Unknown

$$\frac{50 \text{ mg}}{1 \text{ mL}} = \frac{0.15 \text{ g}}{x \text{ mL}}$$

$$\frac{50 \text{ mg}}{1 \text{ mL}} \diagup\!\!\!\!\diagdown \frac{\overset{150 \text{ mg}}{\cancel{0.15}} \text{ g}}{x \text{ mL}}$$

$50x = 1 \times 150$

$$\frac{50x}{50} = \frac{150}{50}$$

$x = 3 \text{ mL}$

Formula Method

$$\frac{D}{H} \times Q = x$$

$$\frac{0.15 \text{ g}}{50 \text{ mg}} \times 1 \text{ mL} = x \text{ mL}$$

$$\frac{\overset{150 \text{ mg}}{\cancel{0.15} \text{ g}}}{50 \text{ mg}} \times 1 \text{ mL} = x \text{ mL}$$

$$\frac{150 \ \cancel{mg}}{50 \ \cancel{mg}} \times 1 \text{ mL} = x \text{ mL}$$

$$\frac{150}{50} \times 1 \text{ mL} = 3 \text{ mL}$$

The nurse administers 3 mL to the patient.

APPLY LEARNED KNOWLEDGE 11-3

Calculate the answer to the following drug dosage problems using any method of calculation.

1. The order is for midazolam 500 mcg IV now. The following medication is available from the pharmacy:

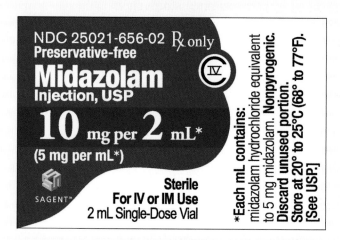

How many mL will the nurse give? _____

Fill in the syringe with the correct amount to administer the ordered dose.

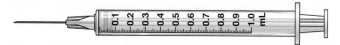

2. The order is for Desmopressin Acetate Injection 0.001 mg IV BID. The following medication is available from the pharmacy:

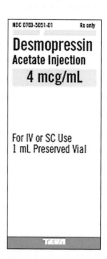

How many mL will the nurse give? _____

Fill in the syringe with the correct amount to administer the ordered dose.

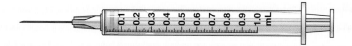

APPLY LEARNED KNOWLEDGE 11-3—cont'd

3. The physician orders propranolol 250 mcg IV now. The following medication is available from the pharmacy:

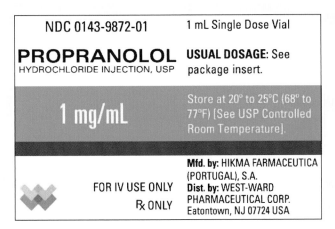

How many mL will the nurse give? _____

Fill in the appropriate syringe with the correct amount to administer the ordered dose.

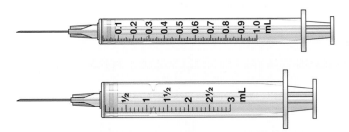

4. The order is for glycopyrrolate 220 mcg IM now.

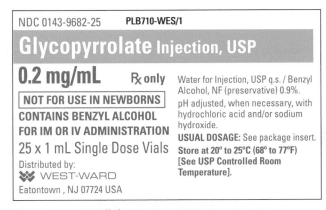

How many mL will the nurse give? _____

Fill in the appropriate syringe with the correct amount to administer the ordered dose.

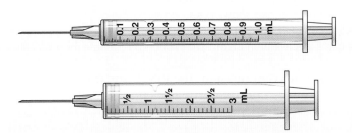

Continued

APPLY LEARNED KNOWLEDGE 11-3—cont'd

5. The physician orders Corvert 100 mcg IV infusion now. The following medication is available from the pharmacy:

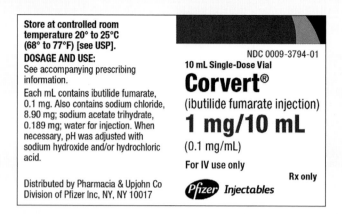

How many mL will the nurse draw up into the syringe? _____

Fill in the appropriate syringe with the correct amount to administer the ordered dose.

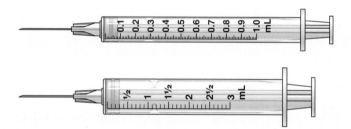

CLINICAL REASONING 11-1

The nurse is preparing a dose of fentanyl 0.1 mg IV to be administered to the patient 30 minutes prior to surgery. The pharmacy has supplied the following vial of fentanyl:

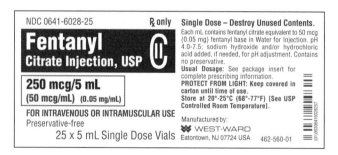

The nurse chooses the dosage strength 250 mcg per 5 mL, calculates the dose, and draws up 2 mL of fentanyl into a syringe. The nurse then shows a second nurse the calculation to verify the dosage. The second nurse uses the 0.05 mg per mL dosage strength, and calculates the dosage as 0.2 mL of medication. Which nurse's calculation is correct? Provide a rationale for your answer.

In summary, agencies such as The Joint Commission, the ISMP, and the CDC have published patient safety standards that promote change in the packaging and handling of parenteral medications. Drug manufacturers now package many parenteral medications in single-use containers that hold only one dose of the drug. This minimizes the number of calculations required before administering a dose of parenteral medication. However, knowledge of how to calculate parenteral doses will always be an essential skill for the nurse to have. Patient safety and patient advocacy demand that every nurse verify the dosage of every medication before the medication is administered.

Developing Competency

Use the drug labels to answer the questions.

1. The order is for phenytoin sodium 80 mg IV now. The following medication is available from the pharmacy. How many mL will the nurse give?

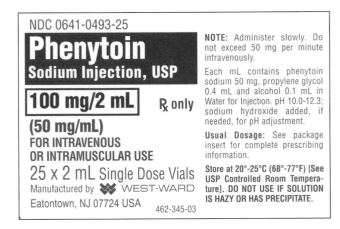

2. The physician orders Granisetron HCl 150 mcg IV now. The nurse has the following vial of medication and the following syringe available. How many mL will the nurse give?

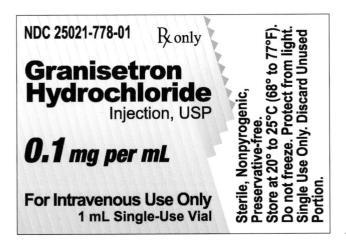

Fill in the syringe with the amount ordered.

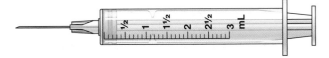

3. The patient is due for a dose of glycopyrrolate 100 mcg IM. The nurse has the following vial of the medication. How many mL will the nurse give?

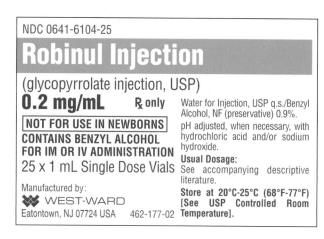

The nurse can draw up the dose in which of the following syringes?
a. 1 mL syringe
b. 3 mL syringe

4. The patient is to receive mesna 210 mg IV now. The pharmacy sends the following vial of mesna, and the nurse has the following syringes available. How many mL will the nurse give?

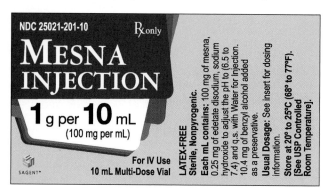

Fill in the appropriate syringe with the ordered dose.

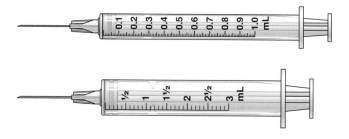

5. The nurse is preparing a 135 mg IV dose of PACLitaxel. The pharmacy sends the following drug and the nurse has a 1 mL, 3 mL, 5 mL, 10 mL, and 30 mL syringe available to use to withdraw the medication from the vial.

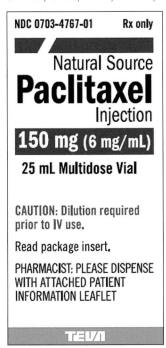

Which of the following applies to the administration of this ordered dose? (Select all that apply.)

a. A conversion is not necessary.
b. 2.25 mL will be administered.
c. All but the 1 mL syringe can be used to measure the ordered dose.
d. The nurse should write date, time, initials, and beyond-use date on the vial after withdrawing the dose.

6. The patient is to receive HYDROmorphone 1.5 mg subcut q.4h prn pain. The following medication is available from the pharmacy. How many mL will the nurse give?

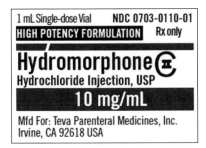

Fill in the appropriate syringe with the amount ordered.

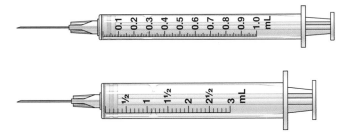

7. The physician orders adenosine 4.5 mg IV STAT. The nurse has available the following prefilled syringe of adenosine:

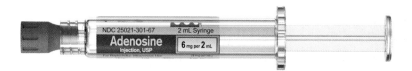

How many mL will the nurse discard from the prefilled syringe? _____

How many mL will the nurse administer? _____

8. The patient is to receive Clindamycin 0.225 g IV q.6h. The nurse has the following vial of Clindamycin. How many mL will the nurse give? Write the appropriate information on the drug label.

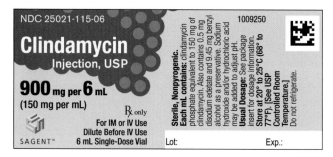

9. The patient complains of incisional pain. The nurse has the following order in the electronic medical record, and the following vial of morphine is available. The nurse checks the medication record and notes that it is time for another pain injection. How many mL will the nurse prepare for the patient?

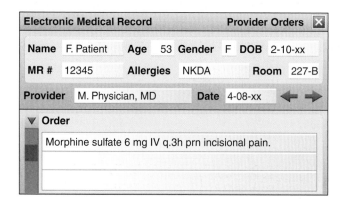
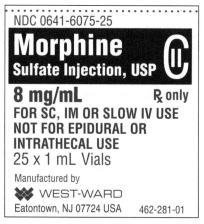

10. The nurse is preparing to administer 0800 medications using the patient's electronic medication administration record. The following vial is in the medication drawer. How many mL will the nurse administer to the patient?

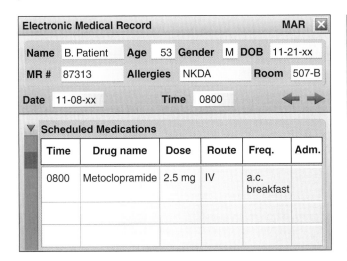

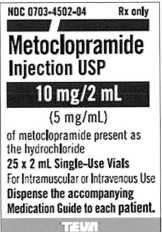

Fill in the syringe with the amount ordered.

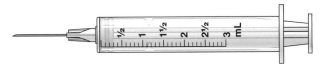

11. The nurse is preparing to administer the 0900 medications to the postoperative patient. The electronic medication administration record lists the scheduled medications, and the following medications are in the patient's medication drawer:

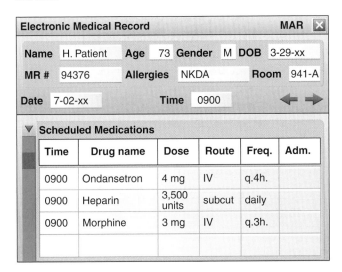

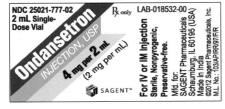

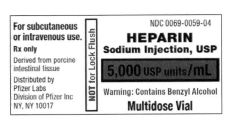

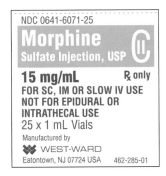

The nurse draws up 2 mL of ondansetron, 0.7 mL of heparin, and 0.2 mL of morphine, and labels the three vials with the date, time, the nurse's initials, and the beyond-use date. Has the nurse calculated the doses and labeled the vials correctly? _____

12. The patient is to have diltiazem 0.012 g IV. The following vial is available. How many mL will the nurse draw up into the syringe?

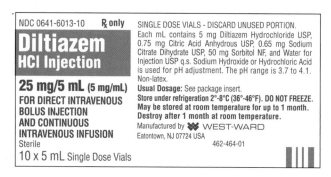

_____

Fill in the syringe with the ordered amount.

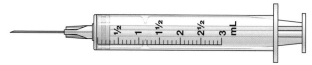

13. The order is for adenosine and the pharmacy sends a disposable syringe of the medication.

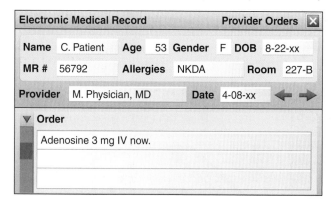

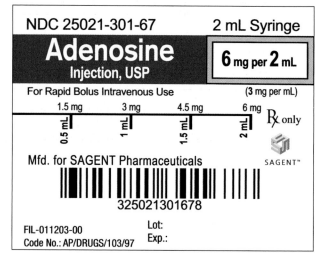

How many mL will the nurse administer?   _____

How many mL will the nurse discard from the prefilled syringe?   _____

14. The physician orders DAUNOrubicin 0.04 g IV daily for 3 days. The pharmacy sends the following drug and the nurse has a 1 mL, 3 mL, 5 mL, and 10 mL syringe available to use to withdraw the medication from the vial.

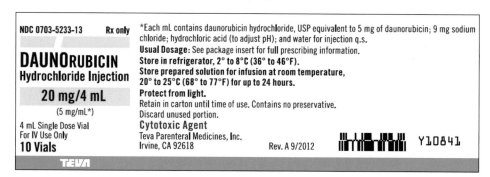

Which of the following applies to the administration of this ordered dose? (Select all that apply.)
a. A conversion is needed.
b. Two dosage strengths are listed on the vial.
c. 2 mL will be administered.
d. The 10 mL syringe is the best choice to measure the ordered dose.

15. The nurse is preparing to administer a dose of pain medication to the patient. The following electronic medication administration record and medication vial is available. How many mL will the nurse administer to the patient? _____

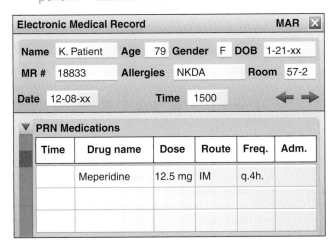

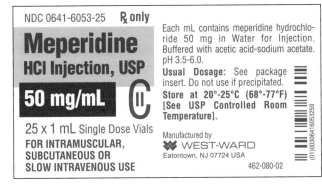

Fill in the syringe with the amount ordered.

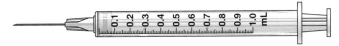

16. The order is for HYDROmorphone 1.5 mg subcut q.4h. The following vial is available. How many mL will the nurse administer to the patient?

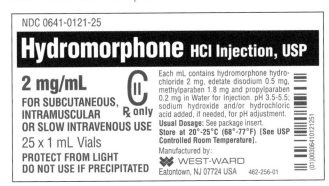

17. The following is the physician's order and available medication:

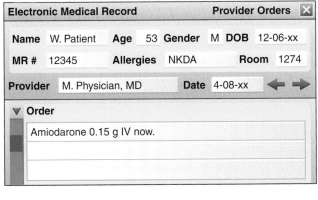

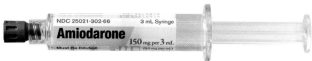

How many mL will the nurse administer? _____

How many mL will the nurse discard from the prefilled syringe? _____

18. The physician orders LORazepam 1,800 mcg IV BID. The pharmacy sends the following drug:

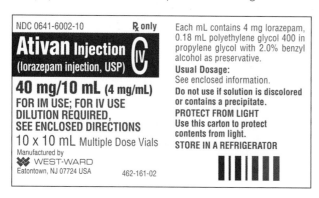

Which of the following applies to the administration of this ordered dose? (Select all that apply.)
a. The nurse has a choice of dosage strengths to use in the calculation.
b. There are two possible routes for this medication.
c. 0.45 mL of lorazepam will be drawn up into the syringe and given directly into the vein.
d. Once opened, the vial can be stored in the refrigerator and used again.

19. The physician orders metoclopramide 8 mg IM now. The nurse has the following vial of metoclopramide. How many mL will the nurse administer?

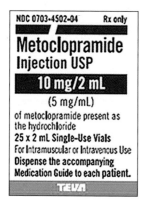

_____

Fill in the appropriate syringe with the ordered amount.

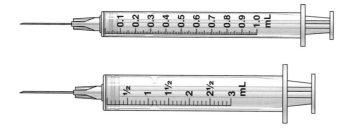

20. The following medication is on the electronic medical record. The nurse withdraws the medication from the automated medication dispensing drawer. How many mL will the nurse administer?

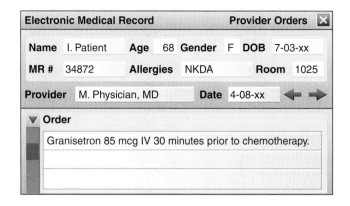

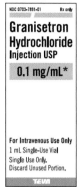

Fill in the syringe with the ordered amount.

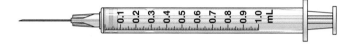

CHAPTER 12

Preparing Powdered Parenteral Medications

LEARNING OUTCOMES

Interpret directions for the reconstitution of powdered medications.

Determine the dosage strength obtained after reconstituting powdered medications.

Calculate doses of single-strength and multiple-strength reconstituted medications.

Sometimes a medication comes in powder rather than in liquid form because it retains its potency for only a short time in solution and must be mixed just before administration. This process, called **reconstitution,** involves adding a liquid (called **diluent**) to the powdered medication, so that it can be used for parenteral injection. The manufacturer prints specific directions for reconstituting the medication.

Current safety standards from the ISMP and American Society of Health System Pharmacists (ASHP) recommend that whenever possible, all drugs should be available in **unit-dose** and in a ready-to-administer form. However, the nurse may occasionally need to reconstitute a powdered medication. The nurse's role in reconstitution is to accurately interpret the directions for reconstitution, choose the appropriate type and amount of diluent, and identify the dosage strength to use in the calculation of the ordered dose.

The Powdered Medication Label

Safe preparation and administration of powdered medication require an understanding of the unique information listed on the label of the powdered medication. The powdered medication label:

- highlights the total amount of drug in the vial, rather than the dosage strength
- identifies the dosage strength on the side of the label or in the package insert
- includes specific directions for reconstitution of the powdered drug

What the nurse will notice first on a reconstitution drug label is the **total amount** of drug in the vial. The total amount, once diluted, provides a specific dosage concentration. The total amount is not a part of the dosage strength and is not used in solving drug dosage problems. To work with drug dosage problems, the nurse must find the **_dosage strength_** listed by the drug manufacturer. The dosage strength is located in the small print on the drug label or in the package insert. Only the dosage strength is used in a dosage calculation. See Figure 12-1.

When some powdered medications are reconstituted, the powder takes up space, causing the volume of the mixed medication to be greater than the amount of diluent added. This is called **_displacement._** For example, in the cefazolin label (Fig. 12-1), 2 mL of diluent is added to the vial and the approximate volume after dilution is 2.2 mL. The displacement volume is 0.2 mL. The displacement volume may not be listed on all drug labels and is not used in dosage calculations.

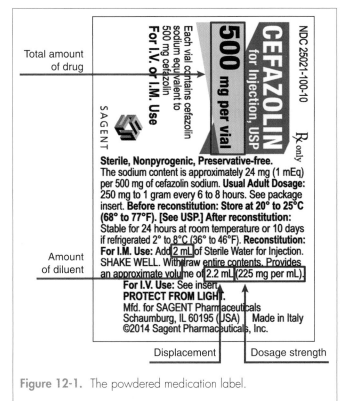

Total amount of drug

NDC 25021-100-10   ℞ only

CEFAZOLIN for Injection, USP

500 mg per vial

Each vial contains cefazolin sodium equivalent to 500 mg cefazolin

For I.V. or I.M. Use

SAGENT

Sterile, Nonpyrogenic, Preservative-free.
The sodium content is approximately 24 mg (1 mEq) per 500 mg of cefazolin sodium. **Usual Adult Dosage:** 250 mg to 1 gram every 6 to 8 hours. See package insert. **Before reconstitution: Store at 20° to 25°C (68° to 77°F). [See USP.] After reconstitution:** Stable for 24 hours at room temperature or 10 days if refrigerated 2° to 8°C (36° to 46°F). **Reconstitution: For I.M. Use:** Add 2 mL of Sterile Water for Injection. SHAKE WELL. Withdraw entire contents. Provides an approximate volume of 2.2 mL (225 mg per mL).
For I.V. Use: See insert.
PROTECT FROM LIGHT.
Mfd. for SAGENT Pharmaceuticals
Schaumburg, IL 60195 (USA)   Made in Italy
©2014 Sagent Pharmaceuticals, Inc.

Amount of diluent

Displacement   Dosage strength

Figure 12-1. The powdered medication label.

 It is not possible to predict the amount of displacement, and sometimes this information is not available on the drug label. For this reason, the nurse must use only the dosage strength given on the drug label or package insert when calculating the drug dosage.

In addition to the total amount and dosage strength, the powdered medication label also has directions for reconstitution of the drug. The type and amount of diluent that can be used are specified by the drug manufacturer. Common diluents for parenteral medications include sterile water for injection and sterile sodium chloride for injection. To obtain the correct dosage strength, reconstitution directions must be followed exactly. It is critical for the nurse to read the directions carefully because the directions may be different based on the parenteral route of administration (i.e., IM or IV).

APPLY LEARNED KNOWLEDGE 12-1

Use the cefazolin label to answer the following questions. Circle T if the statement is true. Circle F if the statement is false and provide a rationale.

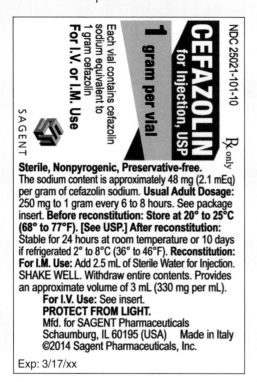

Label text:

NDC 25021-101-10

CEFAZOLIN
for Injection, USP

Rx only

1 gram per vial

Each vial contains cefazolin sodium equivalent to 1 gram cefazolin

For I.V. or I.M. Use

SAGENT

Sterile, Nonpyrogenic, Preservative-free.
The sodium content is approximately 48 mg (2.1 mEq) per gram of cefazolin sodium. **Usual Adult Dosage:** 250 mg to 1 gram every 6 to 8 hours. See package insert. **Before reconstitution:** Store at 20° to 25°C (68° to 77°F). [See USP.] **After reconstitution:** Stable for 24 hours at room temperature or 10 days if refrigerated 2° to 8°C (36° to 46°F). **Reconstitution: For I.M. Use:** Add 2.5 mL of Sterile Water for Injection. SHAKE WELL. Withdraw entire contents. Provides an approximate volume of 3 mL (330 mg per mL).
   For I.V. Use: See insert.
   PROTECT FROM LIGHT.
   Mfd. for SAGENT Pharmaceuticals
   Schaumburg, IL 60195 (USA)   Made in Italy
   ©2014 Sagent Pharmaceuticals, Inc.

Exp: 3/17/xx

1. The order is for cefazolin 0.5 g IM. The amount of diluent to be added to the cefazolin powder is 2.5 mL.

   T   F   _____

2. The nurse may use sterile sodium chloride or sterile water to dilute the powdered medication.

   T   F   _____

3. The dosage strength of the reconstituted medication is 1 g per 2.5 mL.

   T   F   _____

4. If cefazolin 0.5 g IV is ordered, the nurse can use the dosage strength of 330 mg/mL.

   T   F   _____

5. The cefazolin label includes the volume of displacement of the powdered drug.

   T   F   _____

Some powdered drug labels identify the inactive ingredients in addition to the active ingredient, the part of the drug that produces the therapeutic effect. Reading a label with multiple ingredients requires the nurse to distinguish the strength of the active ingredient (the medication) so that the dosage strength of the medication after reconstitution can be identified and used to set up the problem.

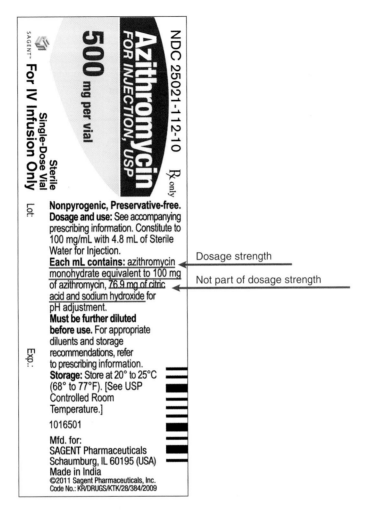

For example, on the Azithromycin label, the dosage strength of the reconstituted medication is expressed as "Each mL contains: azithromycin monohydrate equivalent to 100 mg." This indicates a dosage strength of 100 mg/mL. The other ingredients (76.9 mg of citric acid and sodium hydroxide) are the inactive ingredients and are not part of the dosage strength.

Types of Reconstituted Medications

Many powdered drugs that need to be reconstituted have only one amount of diluent to add, providing only one dosage strength. This is called **single-strength reconstitution.** Other powdered medications allow the nurse to add different amounts of diluent, giving a choice between a more dilute or more concentrated mixed medication. This is called **multiple-strength reconstitution.** Each of these types of reconstitution directions is discussed separately.

SINGLE-STRENGTH RECONSTITUTION

In single-strength reconstitution, the nurse uses the recommended amount of diluent to achieve the dosage strength. For example, in Figure 12-2, the directions state that 3 mL of diluent is to be added to the powdered medication. The dosage strength of the medication after reconstitution is 225 mg/mL.

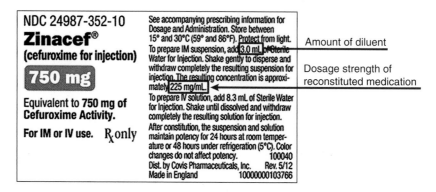

Figure 12-2. Single-strength powdered medication label.

SOLVING SINGLE-STRENGTH RECONSTITUTION PROBLEMS

After the nurse has reconstituted the medication and identified the dosage strength, the problem can be solved. See the following example.

Example:

The order is for 750 mg of cefazolin IM q.8h. The pharmacy sends the following vial of cefazolin (Fig. 12-3). How many mL will the nurse administer to the patient?

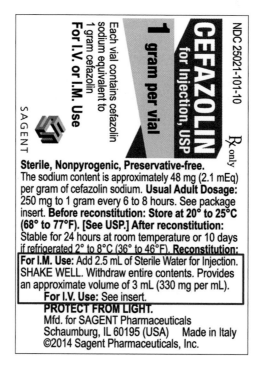

Figure 12-3. Cefazolin for Injection USP.

The nurse adds 2.5 mL of sterile water for injection, and identifies the dosage strength of 330 mg/mL. Then problem can be solved using any one of the following methods of calculation:

Linear Ratio & Proportion

Known :: Unknown

330 mg : 1 mL :: 750 mg : **x** mL

$$330x = 750$$

$$\frac{330x}{330} = \frac{750}{330}$$

$$x = 2.27 \text{ mL}$$

Dimensional Analysis

$$\text{Ordered Amount} \times \text{Dosage Strength} = \text{Desired Amount}$$

$$\frac{750 \cancel{mg}}{1} \times \frac{1 \text{ mL}}{330 \cancel{mg}} = x \text{ mL}$$

$$\frac{750 \times 1 \text{ mL}}{1 \times 330} = \frac{750}{330} = 2.27 \text{ mL}$$

Fractional Ratio & Proportion

Known = Unknown

$$\frac{330 \text{ mg}}{1 \text{ mL}} \quad \frac{750 \text{ mg}}{x \text{ mL}}$$

$$330x = 750$$

$$\frac{330x}{330} = \frac{750}{330}$$

$$x = 2.27 \text{ mL}$$

Formula Method

$$\frac{D}{H} \times Q = x$$

$$\frac{750 \cancel{mg}}{330 \cancel{mg}} \times 1 \text{ mL} = x \text{ mL}$$

$$2.27 \times 1 \text{ mL} = 2.27 \text{ mL}$$

Because there is no syringe that accurately measures 2.27 mL, the answer is rounded to the nearest tenth. The nurse administers 2.3 mL to the patient.

APPLY LEARNED KNOWLEDGE 12-2

Use the medication labels to answer the following questions.

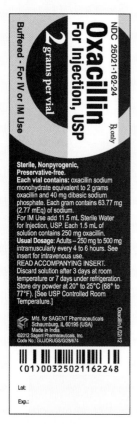

1. The dosage strength of the reconstituted oxacillin is:
   a. 250 mg/1.5 mL
   b. 500 mg/1.5 mL
   c. 2 g/11.5 mL
   d. 2 g/1.5 mL

2. If the physician orders 0.5 g of oxacillin IM q.6h, the nurse will give:
   a. 0.3 mL
   b. 2.8 mL
   c. 2.9 mL
   d. 3 mL

3. If the physician orders 0.4 g of oxacillin IM q.6h, the nurse will give:
   a. 0.24 mL
   b. 0.48 mL
   c. 2.4 mL
   d. 4.8 mL

APPLY LEARNED KNOWLEDGE 12-2—cont'd

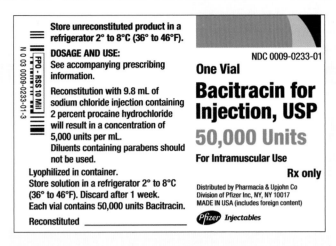

Store unreconstituted product in a refrigerator 2° to 8°C (36° to 46°F).

DOSAGE AND USE:
See accompanying prescribing information.

Reconstitution with 9.8 mL of sodium chloride injection containing 2 percent procaine hydrochloride will result in a concentration of 5,000 units per mL.
Diluents containing parabens should not be used.

Lyophilized in container.
Store solution in a refrigerator 2° to 8°C (36° to 46°F). Discard after 1 week.
Each vial contains 50,000 units Bacitracin.

Reconstituted _____

NDC 0009-0233-01

One Vial

Bacitracin for Injection, USP

50,000 Units

For Intramuscular Use

Rx only

Distributed by Pharmacia & Upjohn Co
Division of Pfizer Inc, NY, NY 10017
MADE IN USA (includes foreign content)

Pfizer *Injectables*

4. The order is for bacitracin 9,000 units IM now. After reconstitution, the nurse will administer:
   a. 0.18 mL
   b. 0.2 mL
   c. 1.8 mL
   d. 2 mL

5. The order is for bacitracin 6,500 units IM now. After reconstitution, the nurse will administer:
   a. 1.2 mL
   b. 0.12 mL
   c. 1.3 mL
   d. 0.13 mL

MULTIPLE-STRENGTH RECONSTITUTION

In multiple-strength reconstitution, the nurse has a choice of making a dilute or a concentrated medication. Different amounts of diluent may be added, as specified by the drug manufacturer. The amount of diluent determines the final concentration. The less diluent added, the stronger the concentration of the medication. The more diluent added, the less concentrated or more dilute the medication.

The nurse decides which concentration is appropriate for the individual patient. Nurses make the decision about the concentration of medication based on several factors:

■ The needs of the patient (For example, a patient with fragile veins may benefit from a more dilute medication.)

■ The route of administration (For example, when reconstituting a medication for IM use, the nurse chooses an amount of diluent that results in a volume small enough to be injected into the muscle.)

■ The medication order (Sometimes the nurse can choose a dosage strength that directly matches the physician's order. This is convenient, as no math is required.)

RELATIONSHIP BETWEEN THE DILUENT AMOUNT AND DOSAGE STRENGTH

Once a certain amount of diluent is added to the powdered medication, the reconstituted medication has a fixed concentration and dosage strength. Look at Figure 12-4. The Pfizerpen label is an example of the manufacturer giving three choices of diluent amounts (75 mL, 33 mL, or 11.5 mL). The dosage strength of the reconstituted medication depends on the amount of diluent that the nurse chooses.

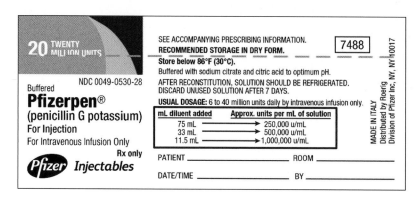

Figure 12-4. Multiple-strength powdered medication.

If the nurse chooses to add 75 mL of diluent, the dosage strength of the mixed medication is 250,000 units/mL. If the nurse adds 33 mL of diluent, the dosage strength is 500,000 units/mL. And if the nurse adds 11.5 mL of diluent, the dosage strength is 1,000,000 units/mL.

SOLVING MULTIPLE-STRENGTH RECONSTITUTION PROBLEMS

Once the nurse has chosen the amount of diluent and identified the dosage strength, the multiple-strength reconstitution problem can be solved.

Example:

The order is for 350,000 units of penicillin G potassium IV q8h. The pharmacy sends the following vial of penicillin G potassium (Fig. 12-5). How many mL will the nurse administer to the patient?

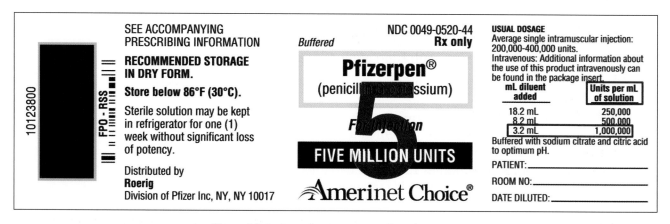

Figure 12-5. Penicillin G potassium for injection.

The nurse reconstitutes the medication using 3.2 mL of diluent, and identifies the dosage strength as 1,000,000 units/mL. The problem can be solved:

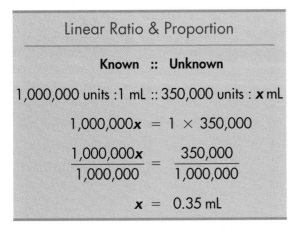

Linear Ratio & Proportion
Known :: Unknown
1,000,000 units : 1 mL :: 350,000 units : **x** mL
1,000,000**x** = 1 × 350,000
$\dfrac{1,000,000x}{1,000,000} = \dfrac{350,000}{1,000,000}$
x = 0.35 mL

Dimensional Analysis
$\dfrac{Ordered}{Amount} \times \dfrac{Dosage}{Strength} = \dfrac{Desired}{Amount}$
$\dfrac{350,000 \ units}{1} \times \dfrac{1 \ mL}{1,000,000 \ units} = x \ mL$
$\dfrac{350,000 \times 1 \ mL}{1 \times 1,000,000} = \dfrac{350,000}{1,000,000} = 0.35 \ mL$

Fractional Ratio & Proportion
Known = Unknown
$\dfrac{1,000,000 \ units}{1 \ mL} \bowtie \dfrac{350,000 \ units}{x \ mL}$
1,000,000**x** = 1 × 350,000
$\dfrac{1,000,000x}{1,000,000} = \dfrac{350,000}{1,000,000}$
x = 0.35 mL

Formula Method
$\dfrac{D}{H} \times Q = x$
$\dfrac{350,000 \ units}{1,000,000 \ units} \times 1 \ mL = x \ mL$
$0.35 \times 1 \ mL = 0.35 \ mL$

The nurse administers 0.35 mL to the patient.

APPLY LEARNED KNOWLEDGE 12-3

Fill in the answers for the following multiple-strength reconstitution problems.

Ampicillin	1 g
Amount of diluent	mg/mL of solution
4.8 mL	125 mg/mL
3.6 mL	250 mg/mL
2.3 mL	500 mg/mL
1.2 mL	1 g/mL

1. The order is for ampicillin 350 mg IV every 6 hours. The pharmacy sends the nurse the above vial of ampicillin.

   If the nurse adds 3.6 mL of diluent, the resulting dosage strength is: _____

   How many mL of the reconstituted medication will the nurse administer? _____

Continued

APPLY LEARNED KNOWLEDGE 12-3—cont'd

2. The physician orders ampicillin 0.6 g IV q.8h. The above vial of ampicillin is available.

If the nurse adds 4.8 mL of diluent, the resulting dosage strength is: _____

How many mL of the reconstituted medication will the nurse administer? _____

Penicillin G	1,000,000 units
Amount of diluent	Units/mL of solution
20 mL	50,000 units/mL
10 mL	100,000 units/mL
4 mL	250,000 units/mL
1.8 mL	500,000 units/mL

3. The order is for penicillin G 200,000 units IM every 8 hours. The pharmacy sends the nurse the above vial of penicillin G.

If the nurse adds 1.8 mL of diluent, the resulting dosage strength is: _____

How many mL of the reconstituted medication will the nurse administer? _____

4. The order is for penicillin G 200,000 units IM every 8 hours. The nurse reconstitutes the vial of penicillin G by adding 4 mL of diluent.

The dosage strength of the medication that the nurse has mixed is: _____

How many mL will the nurse administer? _____

5. The order is for ampicillin 750 mg IV every 8 hours. The pharmacy sends the nurse the following vial of ampicillin:

Ampicillin	2 g
Amount of diluent	mg/mL of solution
3.5 mL	500 mg/mL
6.8 mL	250 mg/mL

If 3.5 mL of diluent is added to the vial, how many mL will the nurse administer? _____

If 6.8 mL of diluent is added to the vial, how many mL will the nurse administer? _____

Variations in Powdered Drug Labels

It is important that the nurse be aware of the variations in the reconstitution directions provided on powdered drug labels. These variations are seen in both single-strength and multiple-strength reconstitution labels.

VARIATIONS IN SINGLE-STRENGTH RECONSTITUTION LABELS

Sometimes drug manufacturers print reconstitution instructions for several different vials all together. Look at the example in Figure 12-6. In this example, reconstitution instructions for 500 mg and 1 g vials of ceFAZolin are included in the same package insert. Sometimes the instructions are different based on the route of administration of the drug. The nurse must be careful to read the correct instructions for reconstitution.

Reconstitution

Preparation of Parenteral Solution

Parental drug products should be SHAKEN WELL when reconstituted, and inspected visually for particulate matter prior to administration. If particulate matter is evident in reconstituted fluids, the drug solutions should be discarded.

When reconstituted or diluted according to the instructions below, Cefazolin for Injection is stable for 24 hours at room temperature or for 10 days if stored under refrigeration (5°C or 41°F).

Reconstituted solutions may range in color from pale yellow to yellow without a change in potency.

Single-Dose Vials

For IM injection, IV direct (bolus) injection or IV infusion, reconstitute with Sterile Water for Injection according to the following table. SHAKE WELL.

Vial Size	Amount of Diluent	Approximate Concentration	Approximate Available Volume
500 mg	2 mL	225 mg/mL	2.2 mL
1 g	2.5 mL	330 mg/mL	3 mL

Excerpt from CeFAZolin package insert.

Figure 12-6. Reconstitution instructions for different sizes of vials.

Figure 12-7 gives another example of a package insert that gives directions for reconstituting vials containing different amounts of the drug (2.25 g, 3.375 g, and 4.5 g vials). These instructions, in a narrative format, are to be read in the order that the vial size and diluent amounts are listed: for a 2.25 g vial, 10 mL of diluent is added; for a 3.375 g vial, 15 mL of diluent is added; and for a 4.5 g vial, 20 mL of diluent is added.

2.5 Reconstitution and Dilution of Powder Formulations

Single-dose vials
Reconstitute piperacillin and tazobactam for injection vials with a compatible reconstitution diluent from the list provided below.

2.25 g, 3.375 g, and 4.5 g piperacillin and tazobactam for injection should be reconstituted with 10 mL, 15 mL, and 20 mL, respectively. Swirl until dissolved.

Compatible Reconstitution Diluents for Single-Dose Vials
0.9% sodium chloride for injection
Sterile water for injection
Dextrose 5%
Bacteriostatic saline/parabens
Bacteriostatic water/parabens
Bacteriorstatic saline/benzyl alcohol
Bacteriostatic water/benzyl alcohol

Excerpt from the piperacillin and tazobactam package insert.

Figure 12-7. Reconstitution instructions for different size vials written in narrative format.

VARIATIONS IN MULTIPLE-STRENGTH RECONSTITUTION LABELS

A multiple-strength drug label can have reconstitution instructions in narrative, table, or combined format. Look at the example in Figure 12-8. In this example, the nurse has to identify the available vial size, and then choose between two amounts of diluent, each yielding a different dosage strength. For example, if the nurse has a 2 g vial of

DIRECTIONS FOR USE:

Intramuscular Administration: Reconstitute ceftriaxone powder with the appropriate diluent (see **COMPATIBILITY AND STABILITY**).

Inject diluent into vial, shake vial thoroughly to form solution. Withdraw entire contents of vial into syringe to equal total labeled dose.

After reconstitution, each 1 mL of solution contains approximately 250 mg or 350 mg equivalent of ceftriaxone according to the amount of diluent indicated below. If required, more dilute solutions could be utilized.

As with all intramuscular preparations, ceftriaxone should be injected well within the body of a relatively large muscle; aspiration helps to avoid unintentional injection into a blood vessel.

Vial Dosage Size	Amount of Diluent to be Added	
	250 mg/mL	350 mg/mL
500 mg	1.8 mL	1.0 mL
1 g	3.6 mL	2.1 mL
2 g	7.2 mL	4.2 mL

Excerpt from CefTRIAXone package insert.

Figure 12-8. Variations in multiple-strength reconstitution instructions.

cefTRIAXone, either 7.2 or 4.2 mL of diluent can be added: if 7.2 mL of diluent is added, the dosage strength is 250 mg/mL, and if 4.2 mL is added, the dosage strength is 350 mg/mL. The nurse must read these instructions very carefully to prevent a medication error.

VARIATIONS IN POWDERED MEDICATION DELIVERY SYSTEMS

Some powdered medications come in a special two-compartment vial (called a **Mix-O-Vial** or **Act-O-Vial**) or attached to an IV bag (called an **ADD-Vantage** system). The Mix-O-Vial contains the powdered medication in one compartment and the diluent in another compartment. The two compartments are separated by a rubber stopper that can be pushed, allowing the diluent and powder to mix together. (See Fig. 12-9.) With the *ADD-Vantage* system, the powdered medication is in a vial that is attached to the IV bag. The plug in the vial is pulled, allowing the medication to mix with the IV fluid prior to administration. The nurse reconstitutes the medication in these systems after verifying the correct drug and dose for the patient. The amount and type of diluent do not need to be verified, as both systems are self-contained (Fig. 12-10).

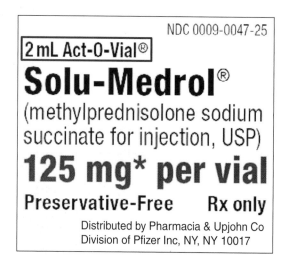

NDC 0009-0047-25

2 mL Act-O-Vial®

Solu-Medrol®

(methylprednisolone sodium succinate for injection, USP)

125 mg* per vial

Preservative-Free   Rx only

Distributed by Pharmacia & Upjohn Co
Division of Pfizer Inc, NY, NY 10017

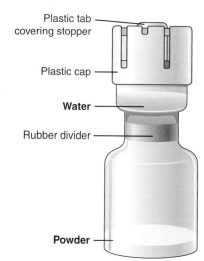

Plastic tab covering stopper

Plastic cap

Water

Rubber divider

Powder

Figure 12-9. Act-O-Vial / Mix-O-Vial.

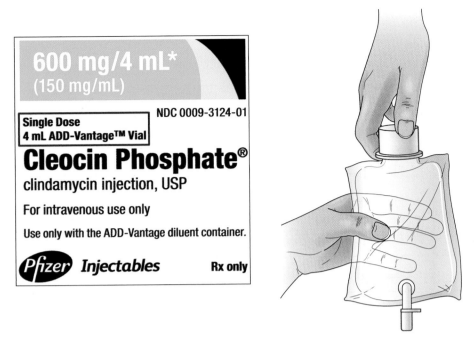

600 mg/4 mL*
(150 mg/mL)

NDC 0009-3124-01

Single Dose
4 mL ADD-Vantage™ Vial

Cleocin Phosphate®

clindamycin injection, USP

For intravenous use only

Use only with the ADD-Vantage diluent container.

Pfizer **Injectables**   **Rx only**

Figure 12-10. ADD-Vantage system.

Other Considerations in Working With Powdered Medications

Best practices recommend that **unit-dose** and ready-to-administer medications be used. But if a multi-dose vial of powdered medication is available, it is imperative that the reconstituted medication be labeled with information regarding how and when the medication was reconstituted. Hospital policy and procedures may have specific information that should be included on the reconstituted medication, including:

■ Dosage strength of the reconstituted drug

■ Type and amount of diluent used

■ Date and time of reconstitution

■ Expiration date and time (beyond-use or discard date of the vial)

■ Initials of the nurse reconstituting the medication

See Figure 12-11 for an example of a label for a reconstituted medication.

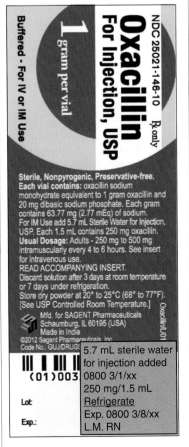

NDC 25021-146-10   Rx only

Oxacillin
For Injection, USP

1 gram per vial

Buffered - For IV or IM Use

Sterile, Nonpyrogenic, Preservative-free.
Each vial contains: oxacillin sodium monohydrate equivalent to 1 gram oxacillin and 20 mg dibasic sodium phosphate. Each gram contains 63.77 mg (2.77 mEq) of sodium.
For IM Use add 5.7 mL Sterile Water for Injection, USP. Each 1.5 mL contains 250 mg oxacillin.
Usual Dosage: Adults - 250 mg to 500 mg intramuscularly every 4 to 6 hours. See insert for intravenous use.
READ ACCOMPANYING INSERT.
Discard solution after 3 days at room temperature or 7 days under refrigeration.
Store dry powder at 20° to 25°C (68° to 77°F).
[See USP Controlled Room Temperature.]
Mfd. for SAGENT Pharmaceuticals
Schaumburg, IL 60195 (USA)
Made in India
©2012 Sagent Pharmaceuticals, Inc.
Code No.: GUJ/DRUG/

(01)003

Lot:

Exp.:

5.7 mL sterile water for injection added
0800 3/1/xx
250 mg/1.5 mL
Refrigerate
Exp. 0800 3/8/xx
L.M. RN

Figure 12-11. Labeling a multi-dose vial of reconstituted medication.

On a multiple-strength reconstitution medication, the nurse should also circle the amount of diluent added and the resulting dosage strength on the medication label. See Figure 12-12.

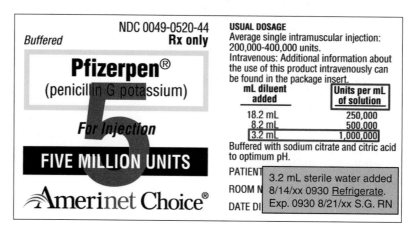

Figure 12-12. Labeling the multiple-strength reconstitution drug label.

 Writing information on the drug label is a form of communication within the healthcare team. This communication ensures that the next nurse knows how and when the powdered medication was reconstituted, and the expiration date. For safe practice, the nurse should never administer a reconstituted medication unless all the appropriate information is written on the drug label.

Storage Information on a Powdered Medication Label

If a vial is to be stored for subsequent doses, recommended storage information is found on the label or package insert. It is the nurse's responsibility to ensure that a reconstituted medication has been prepared and stored according to the manufacturer's instructions. See Figure 12-13.

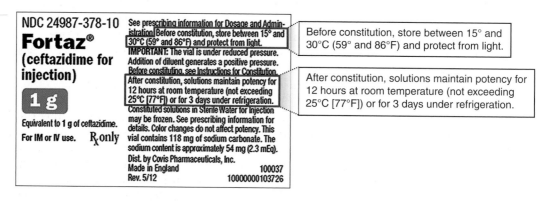

Figure 12-13. Storage information on a powdered medication label.

CLINICAL REASONING 12-1

The nurse is preparing the IV medication for the patient listed on the electronic medical record. The pharmacy sends the following vial of dacarbazine. The nurse prepares by reading the drug label and package insert, adds 19.7 mL of Sterile Water for Injection, and withdraws 1.75 mL into a syringe. After administering the medication and labeling the vial, the nurse puts the vial with the remaining medication into the refrigerator.

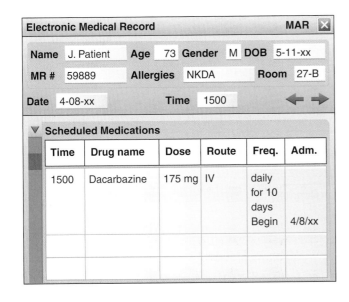

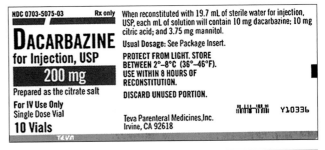

Dacarbazine for injection 200 mg/vial is reconstituted with 19.7 mL of sterile water for injection, USP. Dacarbazine for injection 500 mg/vial is reconstituted with 49.25 mL of sterile water for injection, USP. The resulting solution is drawn into a syringe and administered *only* intravenously.

The reconstituted solution may be further diluted with 5% dextrose injection or sodium chloride injection and administered as an intravenous infusion.

After reconstitution and prior to use, the solution in the vial may be stored at 4°C for up to 72 hours or at normal room conditions (temperature and light) for up to 8 hours. If the reconstituted solution is further diluted in 5% dextrose injection or sodium chloride injection, the resulting solution may be stored at 4°C for up to 24 hours or at normal room conditions for up to 8 hours.

Excerpt from Dacarbazine package insert.

Which of the following are correct regarding the nurse's actions? (Select all that apply.) Provide a rationale for your answer.

A. The nurse added the correct amount and type of diluent to the dacarbazine powder.

B. The dosage strength of the reconstituted dacarbazine is 10 mg per mL.

C. The nurse correctly calculated the dose of reconstituted dacarbazine to administer.

D. If the administration of dacarbazine was delayed until 1600, the reconstituted medication prepared by the nurse could be used.

E. The nurse properly stored the medication remaining in the vial of dacarbazine.

In summary, reconstitution of medications requires the nurse to understand the information on the powdered drug label or to consult the package insert. The nurse must follow the directions for reconstitution of a powdered medication exactly so that he or she may arrive at the correct dosage strength. If a multi-dose vial is used, the nurse must follow the hospital policy about labeling a vial of reconstituted medication. Safe practice requires each nurse to evaluate whether a reconstituted medication can be used for another dose. Most important, the nurse must use the dosage strength identified by the drug manufacturer to solve the drug dosage calculation.

Developing Competency

Use the drug labels or package inserts to answer the questions.

1. The physician orders cefepime 1 g IV q.12h. The nurse has the following vial of cefepime and the package insert for the drug.

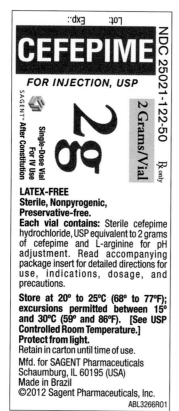

Table 14: Preparation of Solutions of Cefepime for Injection			
Single-Dose Vials for Intravenous/ Intramuscular Administration	Amount of Diluent to be added (mL)	Approximate Available Volume (mL)	Approximate Cefepime Concentration (mg/mL)
cefepime vial content			
1 g (IV)	10	11.3	100
1 g (IM)	2.4	3.6	280
2 g (IV)	10	12.5	160

Excerpt from package insert for Cefepime

Amount of diluent: _____

Dosage strength: _____

Administer: _____

2. The physician orders Vancomycin 0.4 g IV q.8h. The following vial of powdered vancomycin is available.

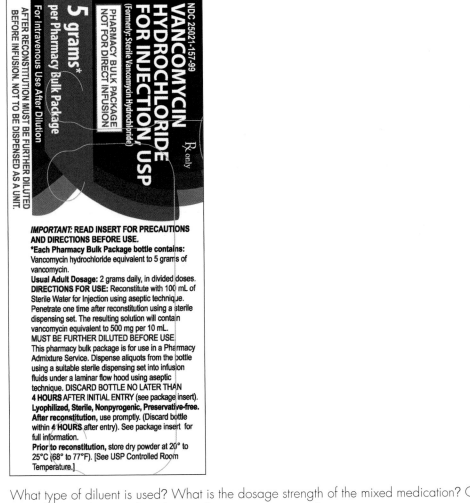

What type of diluent is used? What is the dosage strength of the mixed medication? Once the pharmacy has reconstituted the medication, how long will it retain its potency?

Type of diluent: _____

Dosage strength: _____

Potency: _____

3. The cefTAZIDime vial is reconstituted at 0900 on 2/12/xx and stored in the refrigerator. What is the expiration time and date for the reconstituted medication? _____

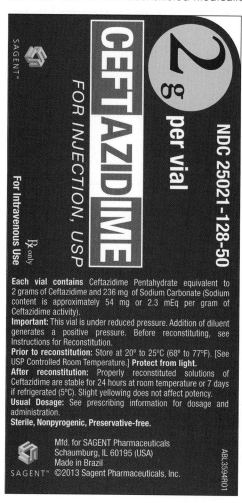

4. The physician orders cefepime 0.75 g IV q.12h. The nurse has the following vial of cefepime and the package insert for the drug.

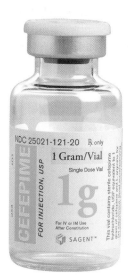

Table 14: Preparation of Solutions of Cefepime for Injection

Single-Dose Vials for Intravenous/ Intramuscular Administration	Amount of Diluent to be Added (mL)	Approximate Available Volume (mL)	Approximate Cefepime Concentration (mg/mL)
cefepime vial content			
1 g (IV)	10	11.3	100
1 g (IM)	2.4	3.6	280
2 g (IV)	10	12.5	160

Excerpt from package insert for Cefepime

Amount of diluent: _____

Dosage strength: _____

Administer: _____

5. The physician orders cefUROXime 500 mg IV q.8hr the nurse has the following vial of cefUROXime and the package insert for the drug.

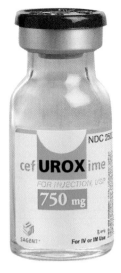

Table 3: Preparation of Solution and Suspension			
Strength	Amount of Diluent to be Added (mL)	Volume to be Withdrawn	Approximate Cefuroxime Concentration (mg/mL)
750 mg Vial	3.0 (IM)	Total*	220
750 mg Vial	8.3 (IV)	Total	90
1.5 gram Vial	16.0 (IV)	Total	90
750 mg Infusion Pack	100 (IV)	---	7.5
1.5 gram Infusion Pack	100 (IV)	---	15

Excerpt from package insert for Cefuroxime

Amount of diluent: _____

Dosage strength: _____

Administer: _____

6. The nurse has the following vial of Solu-Medrol.

For Intramuscular or Intravenous Use Only
Single use vial. Discard unused portion.
Protect from light.
DOSAGE AND USE: See accompanying prescribing information.
*Each 2 mL (when mixed) contains methylprednisolone sodium succinate equivalent to methylprednisolone, 125 mg. Lyophilized in container.

Distributed by Pharmacia & Upjohn Co
Division of Pfizer Inc, NY, NY 10017

LOT/EXP P A A 0 4 5 3 2 3
N 0 03 0009-0047-25 2
FPO GS1 Data Bar Limited (RSS) - 7 mil

NDC 0009-0047-25

2 mL Act-O-Vial®
Solu-Medrol®
(methylprednisolone sodium succinate for injection, USP)
125 mg* per vial
Preservative-Free   Rx only

Once the Act-O-Vial is activated, what is the dosage strength of the medication? _____

If the nurse finds a partial dose of the reconstituted medication stored in the patient's medication drawer, what should the nurse do? _____

7. The physician orders nafcillin 400 mg IM q.6h for the patient. The pharmacy sends the following vial of nafcillin with a package insert.

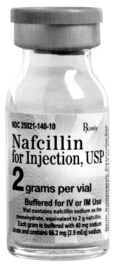

DIRECTIONS FOR USE

For Intramuscular Use
Reconstitute with Sterile Water for Injection, USP, 0.9% Sodium Chloride Injection, USP or Bacteriostatic Water for Injection, USP (with benzyl alcohol or parabens); add 3.4 mL to the 1 g vial for 4 mL resulting solution; 6.6 mL to the 2 g vial for 8 mL resulting solution. All reconstituted vials have a concentration of 250 mg per mL....

For Direct Intravenous Use
The required amount of drug should be diluted in 15 to 30 mL of Sterile Water for Injection, USP or Sodium Chloride Injection, USP and injected over a 5- 10- minute period...

Excerpt from Nafcillin package insert

Identify the amount of diluent to add to the vial. _____

How many mL will the nurse administer to the patient? _____

8. The order is for Fortaz 350 mg IV q.12h. The following vial and package insert are in the patient's medication drawer:

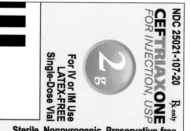

NDC 24987-377-10

Fortaz®
(ceftazidime for injection)

500 mg

Equivalent to **500 mg** of ceftazidime.

For IM or IV use.   R only

See prescribing information for Dosage and Administration. Before constitution, store between 15° and 30°C (59° and 86°F) and protect from light. **IMPORTANT:** The vial is under reduced pressure. Addition of diluent generates a positive pressure. Before constituting, see Instructions for Constitution. After constitution, solutions maintain potency for 12 hours at room temperature (not exceeding 25°C [77°F]) or for 3 days under refrigeration. Constituted solutions in Sterile Water for Injection may be frozen. See prescribing information for details. Color changes do not affect potency. This vial contains 59 mg of sodium carbonate. The sodium content is approximately 27 mg (1.2 mEq). Dist. by Covis Pharmaceuticals, Inc. Made in England
100035   Rev. 5/12   10000000103509

Table 5: Preparation of Solutions of FORTAZ

Size	Amount of Diluent to be Added (mL)	Approximate Available Volume (mL)	Approximate Ceftazidime Concentration (mg/mL)
Intramuscular			
500-mg vial	1.5	1.8	280
1-gram vial	3.0	3.6	280
Intravenous			
500-mg vial	5.3	5.7*	100
1-gram vial	10.0	10.8†	100
2-gram vial	10.0	11.5‡	170
Pharmacy bulk package			
6-gram vial	26	30	200

Excerpt from Fortaz package insert

Amount of diluent: _____

Dosage strength: _____

Administer: _____

9. The nurse uses 0.9% Sodium Chloride Solution to reconstitute a vial of cefTRIAXone for IV use on 5/14/xx and administers a dose to the patient. If the reconstituted medication is stored under refrigeration, when is the last date when the medication can be used for another dose? _____

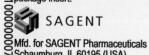

NDC 25021-107-20

CEFTRIAXONE
FOR INJECTION, USP

2 g

For IV or IM Use
LATEX-FREE
Single-Dose Vial

R only

Sterile, Nonpyrogenic, Preservative-free.
Each vial contains ceftriaxone sodium equivalent to 2 grams ceftriaxone.
Usual Dosage: See package insert for Dosage and Administration.
Before reconstitution, store powder at 20° to 25°C (68° to 77°F). [See USP Controlled Room Temperature.]
Protect from light.
Storage after reconstitution: See package insert.

SAGENT

Mfd. for SAGENT Pharmaceuticals Schaumburg, IL 60195 (USA)
Made in Italy
©2009 Sagent Pharmaceuticals, Inc

1000000000072157

Ceftriaxone for injection *intramuscular* solutions remain stable (loss of potency less than 10%) for the following time periods.

Diluent	Concentration mg/mL	Storage	
		Room Temp. (25°C)	Refrigerated (4°C)
Sterile Water for Injection	100	2 days	10 days
	250,350	24 hours	3 days
0.9% Sodium Chloride Solution	100	2 days	10 days
	250,350	24 hours	3 days
5% Dextrose Solution	100	2 days	10 days
	250,350	24 hours	3 days
Bacteriostatic Water + 0.9% Benzyl Alcohol	100	24 hours	10 days
	250,350	24 hours	3 days
1% Lidocaine Solution (without epinephrine)	100	24 hours	10 days
	250,350	24 hours	3 days

Ceftriaxone for injection *intravenous* solutions, at concentrations of 10, 20 and 40 mg/mL, remain stable (loss of potency less than 10%) for the following time periods stored in glass or PVC containers:

Diluent	Storage	
	Room Temp. (25°C)	Refrigerated (4°C)
Sterile Water	2 days	10 days
0.9% Sodium Chloride Solution	2 days	10 days
5% Dextrose Solution	2 days	10 days
10% Dextrose Solution	2 days	10 days
5% Dextrose + 0.9% Sodium Chloride Solution*	2 days	Incompatible
5% Dextrose + 0.45% Sodium Chloride Solution	2 days	Incompatible

*Data available for 10 to 40 mg/mL concentrations in this diluent in PVC containers only.

Excerpt from cefTRIAXone package insert

10. The physician orders penicillin G potassium 400,000 units q.6h. IM. The nurse has the following vial of penicillin G potassium.

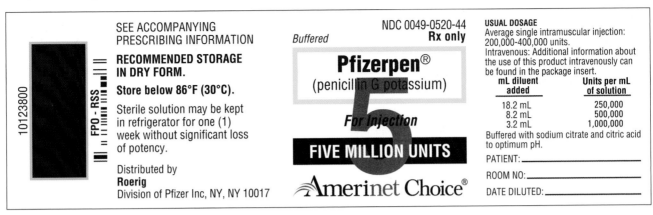

mL diluent added	Units per mL of solution
18.2 mL	250,000
8.2 mL	500,000
3.2 mL	1,000,000

Identify the amount of diluent to add to the vial to make the most concentrated medication.   _____

Dosage strength: _____

Administer: _____

11. The order is for Ampicillin 400 mg IM now. The following vial is in the patient's medication drawer:

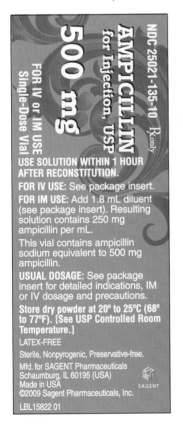

Amount of diluent: _____

Administer: _____

12. The physician orders Gemcitabine 760 mg IV weekly for 7 weeks for the patient with pancreatic cancer. The pharmacy sends four vials of Gemcitabine and a package insert.

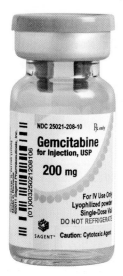

2.7 Preparation for Intravenous Infusion Administration
Reconstitute the vials with 0.9% Sodium Chloride Injection without preservatives.

Add 5 mL to the 200-mg vial or 25 mL to the 1-g vial. These dilutions each yield a Gemcitabine for Injection, USP concentration of 38 mg/mL. Complete withdrawal of the vial contents will provide 200 mg or 1 g of Gemcitabine for Injection, USP. Prior to administration the appropriate amount of drug must be diluted with 0.9% Sodium Chloride Injection. Final concentrations may be as low as 0.1 mg/mL.

Reconstituted Gemcitabine for Injection, USP is a clear, colorless to light straw-colored solution. Inspect visually prior to administration and discard for particulate matter or discoloration. Gemcitabine for Injection, USP solutions are stable for 24 hours at controlled room temperature of 20° to 25°C (68° to 77°F). Do not refrigerate as crystallization can occur.

Excerpt from Gemcitabine package insert.

What amount and type of diluent needs to be added to each vial for reconstitution? What is the resulting dosage strength of the reconstituted medication? How many mL will the nurse administer to the patient each week?

Amount and type of diluent: _____

Dosage strength: _____

Administer: _____

Stable until: _____

13. The following instructions are on a label of powdered medication: "Add 12 mL, 6 mL, or 3 mL of diluent to provide 250 mg, 500 mg, or 1 g per mL, respectively." The nurse adds 6 mL of diluent to the vial. What is the dosage strength of the reconstituted medication? How many mL will the nurse administer to give a 750 mg dose?

Dosage strength: _____

Administer: _____

14. The nurse finds a Mix-O-Vial of Solu-Cortef in the patient's medication cabinet.

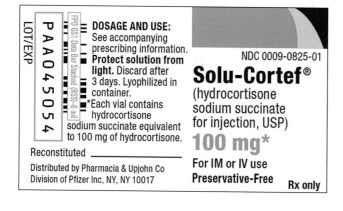

ACT-O-VIAL® System (Single-Dose Vial) in four strengths:	
	100 mg **ACT-O-VIAL** **Each 2 mL** **contains** **(when mixed):**
Hydrocortisone sodium succinate	equiv. to 100 mg Hydrocortisone
Monobasic sodium phosphate anhydrous	0.8 mg
Dibasic sodium phosphate dried	8.73 mg

Excerpt from Solu-Cortef package insert

If the nurse follows the directions for mixing, what is the resulting dosage strength? If the physician orders Solu-Cortef 80 mg IV, how many mL will the nurse administer?

Dosage strength: _____

Administer: _____

15. The nurse has an order to administer Zinacef 1.5 g IV q.6h. The pharmacy sends the following vial of Zinacef.

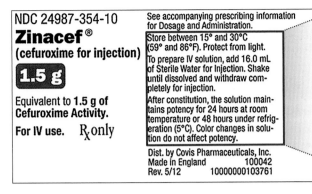

NDC 24987-354-10

Zinacef®
(cefuroxime for injection)

1.5 g

Equivalent to 1.5 g of Cefuroxime Activity.

For IV use.   R only

See accompanying prescribing information for Dosage and Administration.

Store between 15° and 30°C (59° and 86°F). Protect from light. To prepare IV solution, add 16.0 mL of Sterile Water for Injection. Shake until dissolved and withdraw completely for injection.
After constitution, the solution maintains potency for 24 hours at room temperature or 48 hours under refrigeration (5°C). Color changes in solution do not affect potency.

Dist. by Covis Pharmaceuticals, Inc.
Made in England   100042
Rev. 5/12   10000000103761

Store between 15° and 30°C (59° and 86°F). Protect from light. To prepare IV solution, add 16.0 mL of Sterile Water for Injection. Shake until dissolved and withdraw completely for injection.
After constitution, the solution maintains potency for 24 hours at room temperature or 48 hours under refrigeration (5°C). Color changes in solution do not affect potency.

The nurse follows the directions for reconstitution of the powdered medication. How long will the reconstituted medication remain stable? _____

16. The order is for CefTAZidime 500 mg IV q.8h. The following vial is in the patient's medication drawer.

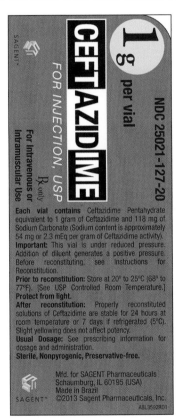

Table 5: Preparation of Solutions of Ceftazidime for Injection

Size	Amount of Diluent to be Added (mL)	Approximate Available Volume (mL)	Approximate Ceftazidime Concentration (mg/mL)
Intramuscular 1 gram vial	3	3.6	280
Intravenous 1 gram vial 2 gram vial	10 10	10.8* 11.5**	100 170

Excerpt from cefTAZidime package insert

What is the dosage strength of the reconstituted medication? How many mL will the nurse administer to the patient? What are the storage directions for the reconstituted medication?

Dosage strength: _____

Administer: _____

Storage directions: _____

17. The physician orders penicillin G potassium 1,200,000 units q.6h. IV. The nurse has the following vial of penicillin G potassium.

20 TWENTY MILLION UNITS	SEE ACCOMPANYING PRESCRIBING INFORMATION.	

SEE ACCOMPANYING PRESCRIBING INFORMATION.
RECOMMENDED STORAGE IN DRY FORM.   7488
Store below 86°F (30°C).
Buffered with sodium citrate and citric acid to optimum pH.
AFTER RECONSTITUTION, SOLUTION SHOULD BE REFRIGERATED.
DISCARD UNUSED SOLUTION AFTER 7 DAYS.
USUAL DOSAGE: 6 to 40 million units daily by intravenous infusion only.

Buffered   NDC 0049-0530-28
Pfizerpen®
(penicillin G potassium)
For Injection
For Intravenous Infusion Only
Rx only
Pfizer Injectables

MADE IN ITALY
Distributed by Roerig
Division of Pfizer Inc, NY, NY 10017

mL diluent added	Approx. units per mL of solution
75 mL	250,000 u/mL
33 mL	500,000 u/mL
11.5 mL	1,000,000 u/mL

PATIENT _____ ROOM _____

DATE/TIME _____ BY _____

Identify the amount of diluent to add to the vial to make the most dilute medication.   _____

Dosage strength: _____

Administer: _____

Storage Instructions: _____

18. The physician orders 450 mg cefazolin IM now. The following medication is available from the pharmacy:

NDC 25021-100-10   **R** only

CEFAZOLIN
for Injection, USP

500 mg per vial

Each vial contains cefazolin
sodium equivalent to
500 mg cefazolin
For I.V. or I.M. Use

SAGENT

Sterile, Nonpyrogenic, Preservative-free.
The sodium content is approximately 24 mg (1 mEq)
per 500 mg of cefazolin sodium. **Usual Adult Dosage:**
250 mg to 1 gram every 6 to 8 hours. See package
insert. **Before reconstitution:** Store at 20° to 25°C
(68° to 77°F). [See USP.] After reconstitution:
Stable for 24 hours at room temperature or 10 days
if refrigerated 2° to 8°C (36° to 46°F). **Reconstitution:**
For I.M. Use: Add 2 mL of Sterile Water for Injection.
SHAKE WELL. Withdraw entire contents. Provides
an approximate volume of 2.2 mL (225 mg per mL).
For I.V. Use: See insert.
PROTECT FROM LIGHT.
Mfd. for SAGENT Pharmaceuticals
Schaumburg, IL 60195 (USA)   Made in Italy
©2014 Sagent Pharmaceuticals, Inc.

Amount of diluent: _____

Volume of displacement: _____

Administer: _____

19. The nurse is preparing to administer IV cefOXItin using the patient's electronic medication administration record. The following vial is in the medication drawer, along with the package insert.

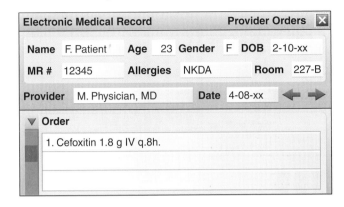

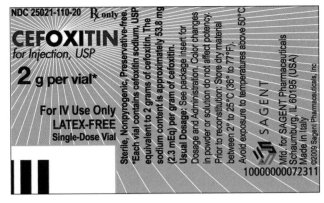

Table 3: Preparation of Solution for Intravenous Administration			
Strength	Amount of Diluent to be Added (mL)++	Approximate Withdrawable Volume (mL)	Approximate Average Concentration (mg/mL)
1 gram Vial	10	10.5	95
2 gram Vial	10 or 20	11.1 or 21	180 or 95

++Shake to dissolve and let stand until clear.

PREPARATION OF SOLUTION
Table 3 is provided for convenience in constituting Cefoxitin for Injection for intravenous administration.

Excerpt from cefOXitin package insert

The nurse adds 10 mL of diluent to the powder in the vial.

Dosage strength: _____

Administer: _____

20. The nurse is preparing to administer 1600 medications using the patient's electronic medication administration record. The pharmacy sends the following vial of powdered medication, along with the package insert.

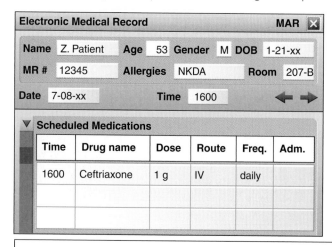

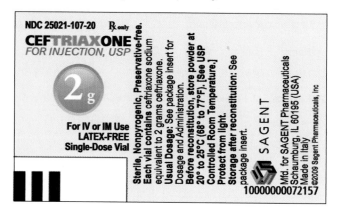

Ceftriaxone
Excerpt from package insert

Directions for Use

Intravenous Administration

Ceftriaxone should be administered intravenously by infusion over a period of 30 minutes. Concentrations between 10 mg/mL and 40 mg/mL are recommended; however, lower concentrations may be used if desired. Reconstitute vials with an appropriate IV diluent (see COMPATIBILITY AND STABILITY).

Vial Dosage Size	Amt. of diluent to be added
500 mg	4.8 mL
1 g	9.6 mL
2 g	19.2 mL

After reconstitution, each 1 mL of solution contains approximately 100 mg equivalent of ceftriaxone. Withdraw entire contents and dilute to the desired concentration with the appropriate IV diluent (sterile water for injection; 0.9% sodium chloride solution).

Excerpt from cefTRIAXone package insert

Amount of diluent: _____

Dosage strength: _____

Administer: _____

CHAPTER 13

Administration of Insulin

LEARNING OUTCOMES

Identify the main types of insulin.

Identify the calibration lines on the U-100 insulin syringes.

Select the appropriate insulin syringe and measure the ordered units of insulin.

Identify safety considerations in working with insulin.

Insulin is a **hormone** produced by the beta cells that are located in the **pancreas** gland. The primary function of the insulin hormone is to assist glucose to enter the cells of the body and to control blood glucose levels. Glucose is released into the blood when food is broken down after a meal. In response to the elevated blood glucose, the pancreas secretes insulin. Insulin functions to lower the glucose level of the blood by assisting the glucose to enter the cells of the body. Glucose is the main source of energy for the cells. If the beta cells of the pancreas do not produce enough insulin, a condition called **diabetes mellitus** develops and a synthetic insulin may be needed to lower and control blood glucose levels.

Synthetically Prepared Insulins

Since the 1980s, recombinant DNA (rDNA) technology has been used to produce the first synthetic insulins called **"human insulin"** and eliminate the need to make insulin from animal sources. Synthetically produced human insulins resemble the structure of the natural insulin made by the beta cells of the pancreas and have decreased the allergic reactions associated with animal insulin sources. Newer forms of synthetic insulins are the insulin **analogs.** Insulin analogs are genetically modified from the synthetic human insulin and improve the action of the insulin once injected into the body. Table 13-1 lists the brand names for the human insulin and the insulin analogs. Human and analog insulins are identified on the drug label with the words "recombinant DNA origin" or "(rDNA origin)" (Fig. 13-1).

Table 13-1. Examples of Human Insulin and Insulin Analogs

HUMAN INSULIN (SYNTHETIC INSULIN)	BRAND NAME
Regular (human insulin)	Humulin R
	Novolin R
NPH (insulin isophane)	Humulin N
	Novolin N
INSULIN ANALOGS (HUMAN INSULIN MODIFIED)	BRAND NAME
Insulin lispro	Humalog
Insulin aspart	Novolog
Insulin glulisine	Apidra
Insulin glargine	Lantus
Insulin detemir	Levemir

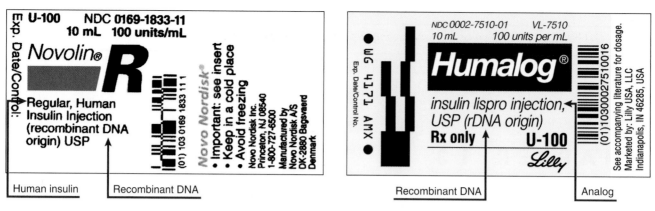

Figure 13-1. Recombinant DNA on insulin drug label.

Types of Insulin and Insulin Characteristics

Drug companies manufacture four main types of insulin: rapid-acting, short-acting, intermediate-acting, and long-acting insulin. Each of these types of insulin is characterized by an onset, peak, and duration of action. **Onset** is the time it takes for the insulin to start lowering blood glucose in the body. **Peak** is the point at which the insulin has the strongest effect on lowering blood glucose, and **duration** is the length of time the insulin continues to lower blood glucose in the body (Table 13-2). Depending on the manufacturer, slight variations in the onset, peak, and duration of insulin may be seen.

Table 13-2. Types of Insulin and Their Onset, Peak, and Duration

| Insulin Type | INSULIN ACTIONS AFTER INJECTION | | |
	Onset	Peak	Duration
Rapid-acting	5 to 10 minutes	1 hour	2 to 4 hours
Short-acting	30 minutes	2 to 3 hours	3 to 6 hours
Intermediate-acting	2 to 4 hours	4 to 12 hours	12 to 18 hours
Long-acting	6 to 10 hours	No peak	20 to 24 hours

Rapid-acting insulin and short-acting insulin are **bolus** types of insulin. These types of insulin are administered a few minutes before a meal and assist the blood glucose to enter into the cells. A patient who uses rapid-acting insulin or short-acting insulin may require multiple injections throughout the day.

Intermediate and long-acting insulin are considered **basal** types of insulin. Basal insulins last longer in the body, provide a steady level of insulin throughout the day, and have the additional benefit of being administered once or twice daily. Depending on the insulin needs, the person with diabetes mellitus may need the administration of a bolus type of insulin, or administration of a basal type of insulin, or a combination of both a bolus and basal insulin.

Insulin Concentration

In the United States, U-100 insulin is the most common **concentration** (strength) available.

U-100 on the insulin drug label indicates a concentration of 100 units of insulin per milliliter of solution. Another concentration available in Europe and Latin America is the U-40 insulin concentration. This concentration indicates 40 units of insulin per milliliter. Insulin is administered with specially calibrated insulin syringes that match the concentration of the insulin being used (U-100 insulin concentration or U-40 insulin concentration).

⚠ *U-500 REGULAR INSULIN*
A U-500 concentration of the short-acting regular insulin is available.

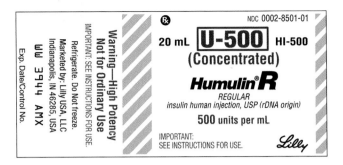

This concentration indicates 500 units of insulin per milliliter and is 5 times more potent than the U-100 concentration of regular insulin. Extreme care must be used when administering U-500 insulin concentration because a specific U-500 insulin syringe is not available. The pharmacist can supply a conversion chart that converts doses of U-500 insulin to be administered with the tuberculin (1 mL) syringe.

Insulin and Dosage Strength

It is important to note that although the U-100 insulin label lists 100 units/mL, indicating a dosage strength, this is not used to determine the amount of insulin that will be administered. When working with insulin, remember the following key points that make the administration of insulin unique:

■ The insulin order identifies the name of the insulin as listed on the drug label.

■ The insulin order identifies the number of units of insulin, not the volume (mL), to be administered per dose.

■ Insulin syringes are made specifically to measure units.

■ The number of units ordered by the physician, such as 17, 26, 45, is the number of units the nurse will draw into the insulin syringe.

The Insulin Drug Label

Safe insulin administration includes an understanding of the information listed on the insulin drug label. The insulin drug label contains the standard components found on a drug label and other important components specific to insulin (Fig. 13-2).

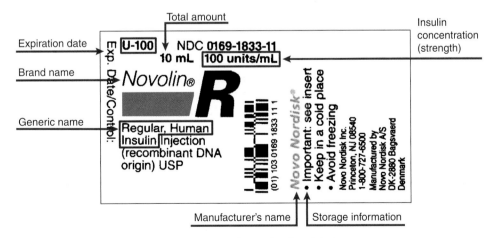

Figure 13-2. The insulin drug label.

Components specific to the insulin drug label include the following:

- *"Unit" as the unit of measurement:* every type of insulin made is measured in units. Recall that a unit expresses the biological activity or potency of a substance that brings about a specific biological response in the body.

- *Brand name:* the brand name followed by a large capital letter has been the standard drug label design for regular insulin and neutral protamine Hagedorn (NPH) insulin. In Figure 13-3, Novolin R is the brand name. The large capital letter R indicates regular insulin. Similarly, Novolin N is the brand name and the large capital letter N indicates NPH insulin.

- *Route of administration:* many of the insulin labels do not list the route of administration. The recommended route of administration for all insulins is the subcutaneous route. In addition to the subcutaneous route, rapid-acting insulin and short-acting insulin are the only insulins that may be administered intravenously.

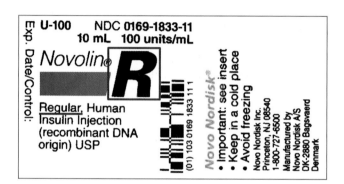

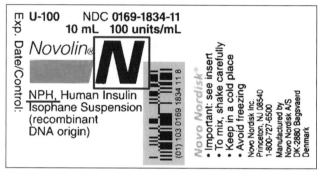

Figure 13-3. Regular human insulin and NPH human insulin drug labels.

 The nurse should always consult a drug reference book or the pharmacist if there is a question about the route of administration.

The Premixed Insulin Drug Label

Drug companies manufacture premixed insulin. Premixed insulin consists of two types of insulin mixed together in fixed proportions. The brand name lists the percentage of the mixed proportions, for example 75/25 and 70/30. The generic name specifies the percentage of each type of insulin (Fig. 13-4). Because insulin needs vary from person to person, the fixed proportions of the premixed insulin may not meet the insulin needs of persons who require changes in the number of units to control blood glucose levels.

Premixed insulin consists of a combination of intermediate-acting insulin with rapid-acting or short-acting insulin in fixed proportions (Table 13-3). Premixed insulin is administered via the subcutaneous injection route and should not to be administered intravenously.

Table 13-3. Premixed Insulin and Insulin Type

PREMIXED HUMAN INSULIN	BRAND NAME	INSULIN TYPE
NPH/Regular	Humulin 70/30	70% Intermediate-acting/30% short-acting
	Novolin 70/30	
Premixed Insulin Analogs		
Insulin lispro protamine suspension/insulin lispro	Humalog Mix 75/25	75% Intermediate-acting/25% rapid-acting
	Humalog Mix 50/50	50% Intermediate-acting/50% rapid-acting
Insulin aspart protamine suspension/insulin aspart	Novolog Mix 70/30	70% Intermediate-acting/30% rapid-acting

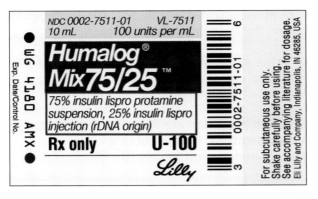
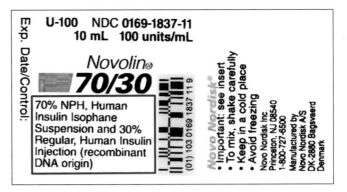

Figure 13-4. Premixed insulin labels.

The Insulin Pen

For ease of administration, various types of insulin are available in prefilled insulin pens. The insulin pen allows the patient to dial the exact insulin dose and administer the insulin by the push of a button. Depending on the manufacturer and the insulin type, the amount of insulin in the pen may vary from 60 units to 300 units. A patient using an insulin pen must be familiar with the specific instructions for proper use and storage as well as the recommended expiration date once the insulin pen is used.

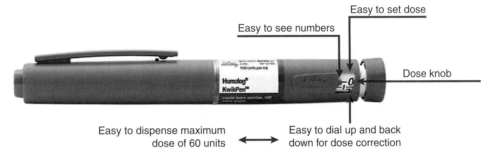

The Insulin Order

The insulin order consists of the name of the insulin, the number of units to administer, the route of administration, and the frequency of administration (Fig. 13-5). The physician considers the actions of insulin (onset, peak, and duration) when ordering the frequency of administration. To ensure that the patient receives the desired effects of the insulin, the nurse must administer the insulin as ordered.

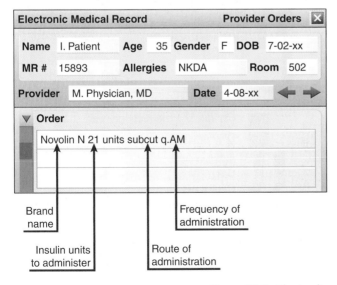
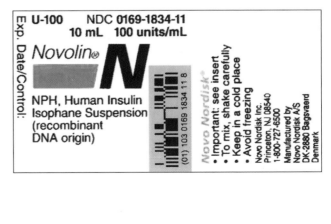

Figure 13-5. The insulin order and insulin drug label.

In carrying out this order, the nurse will select the ordered insulin and the appropriate insulin syringe to accurately measure and draw the ordered number of units.

 A mathematical calculation is not necessary for the administration of insulin. The number of units of insulin that the physician orders is the number of units the nurse will draw in the appropriate insulin syringe.

When a patient is using a premixed insulin, the physician's order will list the name of the insulin identifying the fixed proportions, along with the number of units to administer, the route of administration, and the frequency of administration (Fig. 13-6).

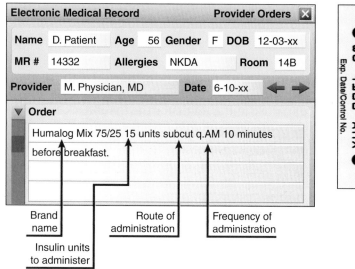

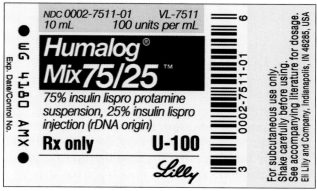

Figure 13-6. The insulin order and premixed insulin drug label.

There are times when the physician orders two insulin types, such as a rapid-acting insulin or short-acting insulin combined with an intermediate-acting insulin, to be mixed in the same insulin syringe. The physician's order will include the name of each insulin, the number of units to be administered for each insulin, the route of administration, and the frequency of administration (Fig. 13-7).

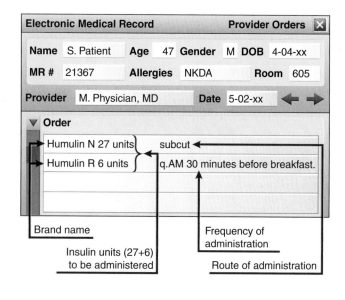

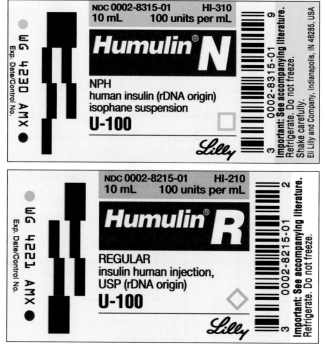

Figure 13-7. The insulin order combining two insulin types and the insulin drug labels.

APPLY LEARNED KNOWLEDGE 13-1

Write the name of the insulin from Column A that corresponds with the statement in Column B. Each insulin name may be used only once.

Column A

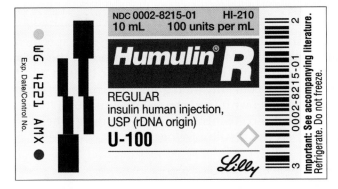

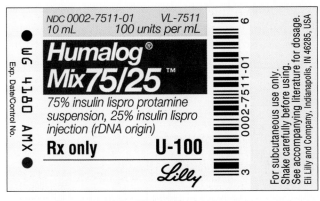

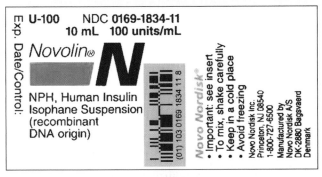

Column B

1. This insulin consists of two insulin types.

_____

2. This insulin may be combined with an intermediate-acting insulin.

_____

3. This insulin lists the route of administration on the label.

_____

4. This insulin is an insulin analog.

_____

Continued

APPLY LEARNED KNOWLEDGE 13-1—cont'd

Column A

Column B

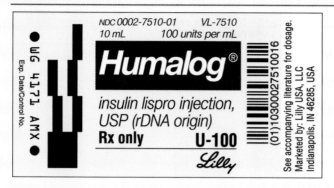

5. This insulin may be combined with a rapid-acting or short-acting insulin.

_____

The Insulin Syringes

The insulin syringe is an integral part of insulin administration because it is specifically made for the administration of insulin. Two distinguishing features found on the insulin syringe include the word "unit," referring to the unit of measurement for insulin and the listing of the insulin concentration. The insulin concentration guides the nurse in matching the insulin concentration from the drug label with the insulin concentration listed on the syringe. Figure 13-8 shows how the insulin concentration from the drug label correlates with the insulin concentration listed on the insulin syringe.

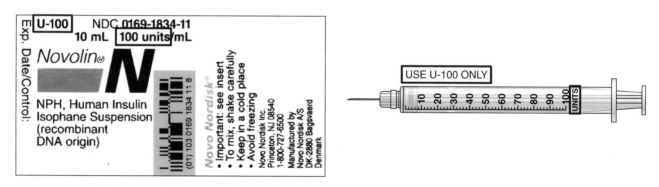

Figure 13-8. The insulin label and the insulin syringe.

The standard insulin syringes include the 100 unit insulin syringe, the 50 unit insulin syringe, and the 30 unit insulin syringe. As indicated by the syringe name, the 100 unit insulin measures a total of 100 units of insulin, the 50 unit insulin measures a total of 50 units of insulin, and the 30 unit syringe measures a total of 30 units of insulin. The volume (mL) the syringe can hold is also identified on the standard insulin syringes (0.3 mL, 0.5 mL, and 1 mL). The syringe volume is not considered when working with the insulin because insulin is ordered by the number of units to administer, not by volume.

Insulin Syringe Calibrations

All insulin syringes are calibrated to measure units. The calibration lines on the 100 unit insulin syringe include the following:

■ A long calibration line identifies every 10 units (i.e., 10, 20, 30, up to 100).
■ Each short calibration line in between equals two units.

The calibration lines on the 50 unit insulin syringe include the following:

■ A long calibration line identifies every five units (i.e., 5, 10, 15, up to 50).

■ Each short calibration line in between equals one unit.

Like the 50 unit insulin syringe, the 30 unit insulin syringe is numbered every five units and each short calibration line equals one unit. The calibration lines on the 30 unit insulin syringe have more spacing between the lines, are easier to read, and are convenient in drawing insulin doses of 30 units or less (Fig. 13-9).

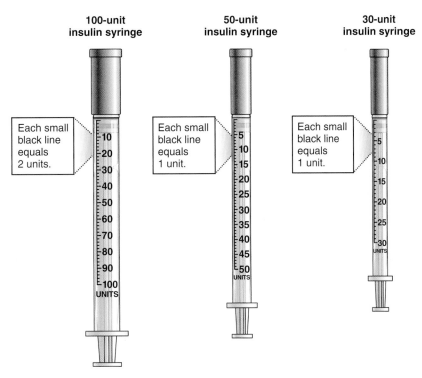

Figure 13-9. Insulin syringes: U-100, U-50, and U-30.

A dual scale insulin syringe is also available and is used to measure even-numbered and odd-numbered insulin doses. For example, the calibration lines on the first scale measure even-numbered doses (2, 4, 6, etc.). The calibration lines on the second scale measure odd-numbered insulin doses (7, 9, 11, etc.) (see Fig. 13-10). In using the dual scale insulin syringe, the nurse must be careful to use the correct scale for the number of units of insulin ordered.

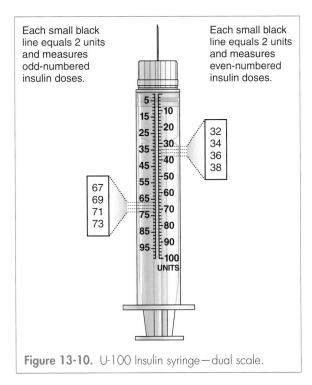

Figure 13-10. U-100 Insulin syringe—dual scale.

Selecting the Most Appropriate Insulin Syringe

The selection of the most appropriate insulin syringe is based on the number of units of insulin that need to be administered. The 100 unit, the 50 unit, and the 30 unit insulin syringes can accurately measure even-numbered insulin doses (i.e., 8, 12, 18, 26). Because of the one unit calibration lines on the 50 unit and the 30 unit insulin syringes, these syringes can also accurately measure odd-numbered insulin doses.

In the following two examples, notice how the number of units of insulin ordered determines the selection of insulin syringe. In Example #1, Novolin 15 units is ordered. The nurse must select the insulin syringe that measures the odd-numbered units of insulin accurately. In Example #2, Humalog 8 units is ordered. The nurse considers all the insulin syringes that accurately measure the even-numbered units of insulin.

Example 1:

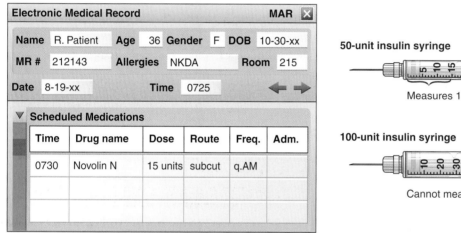

Electronic Medical Record				MAR ☒
Name R. Patient	**Age** 36	**Gender** F	**DOB** 10-30-xx	
MR # 212143	**Allergies** NKDA		**Room** 215	
Date 8-19-xx		**Time** 0725		⬅ ➡

▼ Scheduled Medications

Time	Drug name	Dose	Route	Freq.	Adm.
0730	Novolin N	15 units	subcut	q.AM	

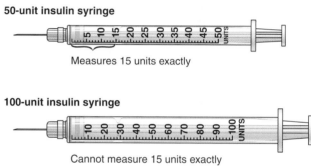

50-unit insulin syringe

Measures 15 units exactly

100-unit insulin syringe

Cannot measure 15 units exactly

The number of units ordered can be measured accurately in the 50 unit insulin syringe. If available, the nurse can also use the 30 unit insulin syringe. The 100 unit insulin syringe can only be used to measure even-numbered doses of insulin.

Example 2:

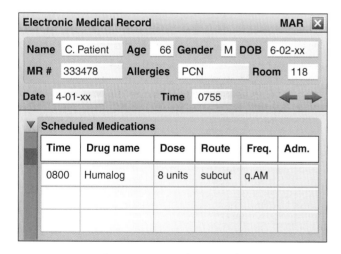

Electronic Medical Record				MAR ☒
Name C. Patient	**Age** 66	**Gender** M	**DOB** 6-02-xx	
MR # 333478	**Allergies** PCN		**Room** 118	
Date 4-01-xx		**Time** 0755		⬅ ➡

▼ Scheduled Medications

Time	Drug name	Dose	Route	Freq.	Adm.
0800	Humalog	8 units	subcut	q.AM	

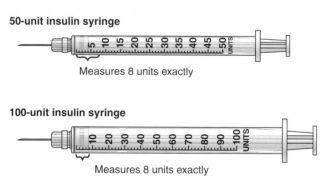

50-unit insulin syringe

Measures 8 units exactly

100-unit insulin syringe

Measures 8 units exactly

The even-numbered of units ordered can be measured accurately in all of the following syringes: the 100 unit insulin syringe, the 50 unit syringe, and the 30 unit insulin syringe.

 For greater accuracy in drawing the number of units of insulin in the insulin syringe, it is recommended to use the smallest insulin syringe that will hold the ordered dose for the patient.

Combining Two Insulins and the Insulin Syringe Selection

Sometimes, the insulin order requires that two insulin doses be combined together in the same syringe. When combining two insulin doses together, the nurse needs to consider the following in the selection of the most appropriate insulin syringe:

■ First, the number of units ordered for each insulin.

■ Second, the total number of units to be administered.

When an insulin order consists of two insulin types to be administered in the same syringe, the nurse needs to first look at the number of units ordered for each insulin type. In the following example, 15 units of Humulin N insulin and 5 units of Humulin R insulin are ordered. Because the insulin orders contain odd-numbered doses of insulin (15 units and 5 units), the nurse begins to consider insulin syringes that measure odd-numbered doses, such as the 30 unit insulin syringe, 50 unit insulin syringe, or the dual scale insulin syringe. Second, the nurse adds the total number of units that will be administered together to ensure that the insulin syringe can hold the total number of units (15 units + 5 units = 20 units total). For the administration of this insulin order, the nurse may use the 30 unit insulin syringe, the 50 unit insulin syringe, or the dual scale insulin syringe. Any time the insulin order contains an odd-numbered dose, the nurse needs to select the insulin syringe that measures odd-numbered doses accurately.

Example:

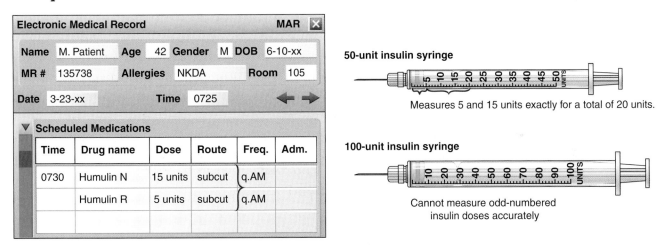

50-unit insulin syringe

Measures 5 and 15 units exactly for a total of 20 units.

100-unit insulin syringe

Cannot measure odd-numbered insulin doses accurately

Electronic Medical Record — MAR ☒

| Name | M. Patient | Age | 42 | Gender | M | DOB | 6-10-xx |

| MR # | 135738 | Allergies | NKDA | Room | 105 |

| Date | 3-23-xx | Time | 0725 |

▼ **Scheduled Medications**

	Time	Drug name	Dose	Route	Freq.	Adm.
	0730	Humulin N	15 units	subcut	q.AM	
		Humulin R	5 units	subcut	q.AM	

Combining two insulins in the same insulin syringe requires the nurse to adhere to a specific procedure that helps maintain the action of each insulin. Nurses need to consult the manufacturer's guidelines, the agency's policy and procedure for combining insulins, the pharmacist, or other reliable reference sources if unsure of the recommended procedure for combining two insulin doses.

APPLY LEARNED KNOWLEDGE 13-2

Read the Medication Administration Record from Column A and fill in the number of units of insulin that will be administered in the most appropriate syringe from Column B.

Column A   **Column B**

1.

Electronic Medical Record — MAR ☒

Name	V. Patient	Age	52	Gender	F	DOB	11-20-xx
MR #	822245		Allergies	NKDA		Room	110
Date	11-06-xx			Time	0720		← →

▼ Scheduled Medications

Time	Drug name	Dose	Route	Freq.	Adm.
0730	Novolin R	7 units	subcut	q.AM	

50-unit insulin syringe

100-unit insulin syringe

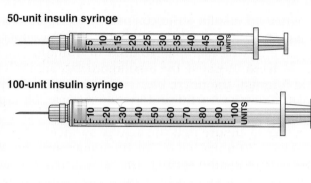

2.

Electronic Medical Record — MAR ☒

Name	S. Patient	Age	54	Gender	M	DOB	10-10-xx
MR #	453790		Allergies	NKDA		Room	214
Date	9-11-xx			Time	1650		← →

▼ Scheduled Medications

Time	Drug name	Dose	Route	Freq.	Adm.
0700	Lantus	26 units	subcut	q.PM	

50-unit insulin syringe

100-unit insulin syringe

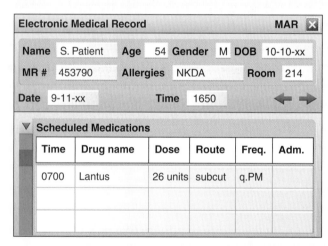
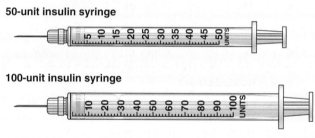

3.

Electronic Medical Record — MAR ☒

Name	NS. Patient	Age	66	Gender	M	DOB	8-17-xx
MR #	61287		Allergies	NKDA		Room	404
Date	10-03-xx			Time	1125		← →

▼ Scheduled Medications

Time	Drug name	Dose	Route	Freq.	Adm.
1130	Novolog	4 units	subcut	stat	

30-unit insulin syringe

100-unit insulin syringe

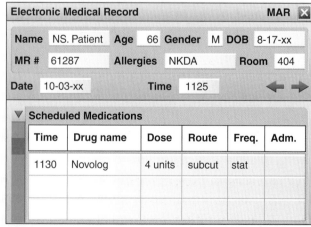
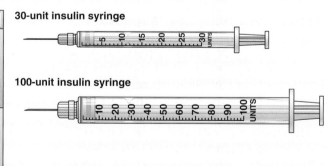
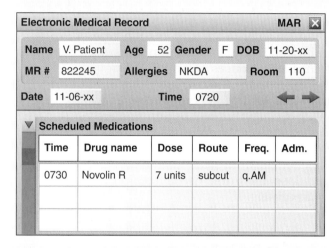

APPLY LEARNED KNOWLEDGE 13-2—cont'd

Column A	Column B

4.

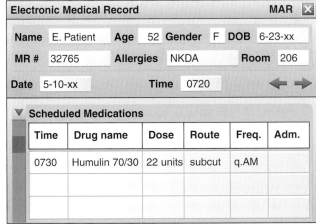

Electronic Medical Record **MAR** ✕

| Name | E. Patient | Age | 52 | Gender | F | DOB | 6-23-xx |

| MR # | 32765 | Allergies | NKDA | Room | 206 |

| Date | 5-10-xx | | Time | 0720 | ← → |

▼ Scheduled Medications

Time	Drug name	Dose	Route	Freq.	Adm.
0730	Humulin 70/30	22 units	subcut	q.AM	

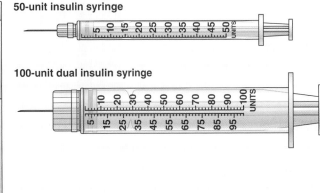

50-unit insulin syringe

100-unit dual insulin syringe

5.

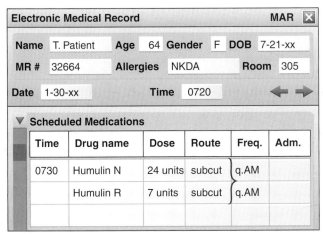

Electronic Medical Record **MAR** ✕

| Name | T. Patient | Age | 64 | Gender | F | DOB | 7-21-xx |

| MR # | 32664 | Allergies | NKDA | Room | 305 |

| Date | 1-30-xx | | Time | 0720 | ← → |

▼ Scheduled Medications

Time	Drug name	Dose	Route	Freq.	Adm.
0730	Humulin N	24 units	subcut	q.AM	
	Humulin R	7 units	subcut	q.AM	

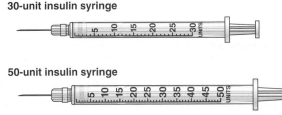

30-unit insulin syringe

50-unit insulin syringe

Safety in the Administration of Insulin

Insulin is identified as a ***"High Alert"*** medication by the Institute for Safe Medication Practices. High alert medications are known to have an increased risk of causing serious injury or harm to patients when an error occurs. Every effort must be made to reduce the risk of potential errors in the administration of insulin. Nurses have a significant role in medication administration, because in applying the Six Rights of Medication Administration the nurse is the final person to review the ordered medication, the ordered dose, and the route of administration prior to administering the medication to the right patient.

In the administration of insulin, it is important to note that the brand names of synthetic insulins may sound alike or look alike, for example, Novolog Mix 70/30 and Novolin 70/30, but the action of each insulin is different (Table 13-4).

Table 13-4. Insulin Brand Names

DO NOT CONFUSE		
Humalog	⟷	Novolog
Humulin 70/30	⟷	Novolin 70/30
Humulin N	⟷	Novolin N
Humulin R	⟷	Novolin R
ALSO		
Novolin 70/30	⟷	Novolog Mix 70/30

CLINICAL REASONING 13-1

The nurse has an order to administer 12 units of Novolin 70/30 subcut now. The nurse finds the following insulin vial in the refrigerator.

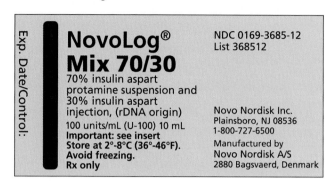

Which action by the nurse is most appropriate? Provide a rationale for your answer.

A. Draw up the 12 units of insulin in a 50 unit insulin syringe.
B. Use a 30 unit insulin syringe to administer the ordered dose.
C. Obtain a vial of Novolin 70/30 insulin from the pharmacy.
D. Clarify the insulin order with the physician.

Organizations such as the Institute for Safe Medication Practices recommend that the word "unit" be spelled out and never abbreviated because it may be misinterpreted for a zero, contributing to an increased risk for medication errors.

In summary, as a patient advocate, the nurse must administer the insulin exactly as it is prescribed, question insulin orders that are unclear, and double-check all insulin doses with another licensed nurse prior to administration.

Developing Competency

Circle "Correct" or "Incorrect" for the following 10 questions. For problems with incorrect answers, provide a rationale to support your answer.

1. In administering insulin, the nurse will use the 100 units/mL listed on the drug label to calculate the dose.
Correct   Incorrect
Rationale: _____

2. U-100 on the insulin label refers to the insulin concentration.
Correct   Incorrect
Rationale: _____

3. The physician orders Humalog 6 units subcut now. The nurse has a vial of Novolog insulin. The nurse may use Novolog insulin to administer the 6 units of insulin.
Correct   Incorrect
Rationale: _____

4. Humulin 70/30 insulin may be mixed with a rapid-acting insulin in the same syringe.
Correct   Incorrect
Rationale: _____

5. The nurse selects the 100 unit insulin syringe to combine 7 units of Humulin R and 23 units of Humulin N.
Correct   Incorrect
Rationale: _____

6. Levemir is a synthetic insulin.
Correct   Incorrect

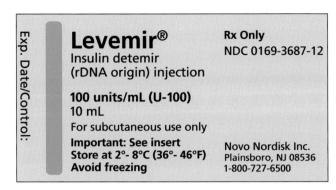

Rationale: _____

7. 25 units of insulin have been drawn into the insulin syringe.
Correct   Incorrect

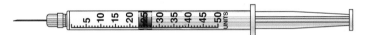

Rationale: _____

8. 13 units of insulin have been drawn into the insulin syringe.
Correct   Incorrect

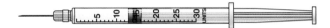

Rationale: _____

9. 35 units of insulin have been drawn into the insulin syringe.
Correct   Incorrect

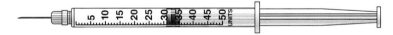

Rationale: _____

10. 42 units of insulin have been drawn into the insulin syringe.
Correct   Incorrect

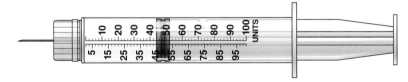

Rationale: _____

Shade in the ordered number of units of insulin in the appropriate syringe for following five questions.

11.

Electronic Medical Record				MAR ☒
Name V. Patient	**Age** 49	**Gender** M	**DOB** 4-12-xx	
MR # 67533	**Allergies** NKDA		**Room** 412	
Date 4-12-xx		**Time** 0720		← →

	Scheduled Medications					
	Time	**Drug name**	**Dose**	**Route**	**Freq.**	**Adm.**
	0730	Humulin N	13 units	subcut	q.AM	
		Humulin R	5 units	subcut	q.AM	

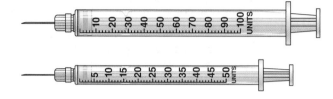

12.

Electronic Medical Record				MAR ☒
Name M. Patient	**Age** 62	**Gender** F	**DOB** 11-01-xx	
MR # 93658	**Allergies** NKDA		**Room** 106	
Date 1-22-xx		**Time** 0800		← →

	Scheduled Medications					
	Time	**Drug name**	**Dose**	**Route**	**Freq.**	**Adm.**
	0800	Novolog	10 units	subcut	q.AM	

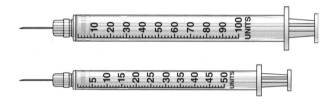

13.

Electronic Medical Record				MAR ☒
Name C. Patient	**Age** 48	**Gender** F	**DOB** 3-17-xx	
MR # 035786	**Allergies** NKDA		**Room** 235	
Date 6-02-xx		**Time** 0800		← →

	Scheduled Medications					
	Time	**Drug name**	**Dose**	**Route**	**Freq.**	**Adm.**
	0800	Humulin 70/30	15 units	subcut	q.AM	

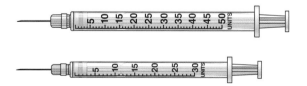

14.

Electronic Medical Record					MAR ✕
Name A. Patient	**Age** 55	**Gender** M	**DOB** 6-20-xx		
MR # 28653	**Allergies** NKDA		**Room** 317		
Date 10-03-xx		**Time** 0720		← →	

▼ **Scheduled Medications**

Time	Drug name	Dose	Route	Freq.	Adm.
0730	Humulin N	27 units	subcut	q.AM	

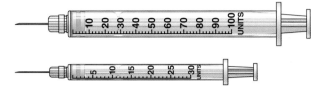

15.

Electronic Medical Record					MAR ✕
Name S. Patient	**Age** 47	**Gender** M	**DOB** 7-15-xx		
MR # 15490	**Allergies** NKDA		**Room** 601		
Date 2-28-xx		**Time** 0720		← →	

▼ **Scheduled Medications**

Time	Drug name	Dose	Route	Freq.	Adm.
0730	Humulin N	21 units	subcut	q.AM	
	Humulin R	7 units	subcut	q.AM	

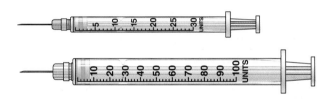

Administration of Medications

Unit Review—Evaluate for Clinical Decision Making

*For each question, use your clinical judgment to determine whether the nurse's decision is **Correct** or **Incorrect**. For incorrect problems, write the correct answer.*

1. MD order: Prenisolone oral solution 75 mg every other day for 2 weeks.
Pharmacy sends:

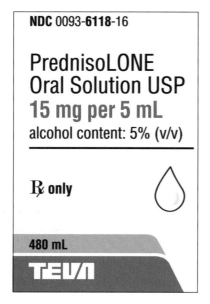

NDC 0093-**6118**-16

PrednisoLONE
Oral Solution USP
15 mg per 5 mL
alcohol content: 5% (v/v)

℞ only

480 mL

TEVA

The nurse measures the ordered dose in the medicine cup.

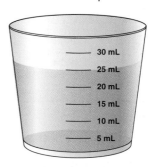

The amount of prednisolone measured is:

Correct	Incorrect	Answer: _____

2. MD order: Digoxin elixir 250 mcg PO q.AM.
Pharmacy sends: Digoxin elixir 0.05 mg per mL
The nurse measures the ordered dose in the medicine cup.

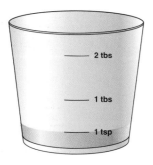

The amount of digoxin measured is:

Correct	Incorrect	Answer: _____

3. MD order: Warfarin Sodium 3 mg tab PO q.AM.
Pharmacy sends:

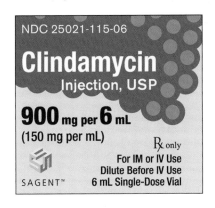

Usual Dosage: See package brochure.

Pharmacist: Dispense one Medication Guide with each prescription.

Dispense with a child-resistant closure in a tight, light-resistant container.

Protect from light.

Store at 20° to 25°C (68° to 77°F) [See USP Controlled Room Temperature].

BARR LABORATORIES, INC.
Pomona, NY 10970
R10-06 (v.4)
10001187

barr.
Laboratories, Inc.

Warfarin Sodium
Tablets, USP
6 mg

HIGHLY POTENT ANTICOAGULANT
WARNING: Serious bleeding results from overdosage. Do not use or dispense before reading directions and warnings in package brochure.

℞ only   **100 Tablets**

The nurse decides to administer 0.5 tab.

Correct	Incorrect	Answer: _____

4. MD order: Clindamycin 815 mg IVPB. Infuse over 30 minutes.
Pharmacy sends:

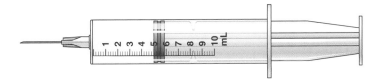

NDC 25021-115-06

Clindamycin
Injection, USP

900 mg per **6** mL
(150 mg per mL)

℞ only
For IM or IV Use
Dilute Before IV Use
6 mL Single-Dose Vial

SAGENT™

The nurse draws up the ordered dose in the syringe.

The nurse's decision is:

Correct	Incorrect	Answer: _____

5. MD order: Midazolam 8 mg IVP before meals.
Pharmacy sends:

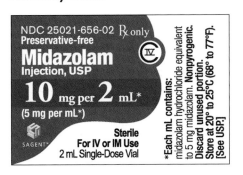

NDC 25021-656-02 ℞ only
Preservative-free
Midazolam
Injection, USP
10 mg per **2** mL*
(5 mg per mL*)

SAGENT™
Sterile
For IV or IM Use
2 mL Single-Dose Vial

*Each mL contains: midazolam hydrochloride equivalent to 5 mg midazolam. Nonpyrogenic. Discard unused portion. Store at 20° to 25°C (68° to 77°F). [See USP.]

℞ only   IV

The nurse draws up the following amount of Midazolam in the syringe.

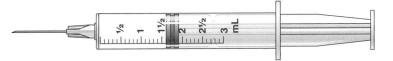

The nurse's decision is:

Correct	Incorrect	Answer: _____

6. MD order: Oxacillin 300 mg IM now.
Pharmacy sends:

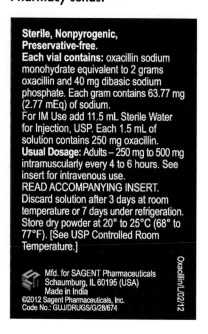

Sterile, Nonpyrogenic, Preservative-free.
Each vial contains: oxacillin sodium monohydrate equivalent to 2 grams oxacillin and 40 mg dibasic sodium phosphate. Each gram contains 63.77 mg (2.77 mEq) of sodium.
For IM Use add 11.5 mL Sterile Water for Injection, USP. Each 1.5 mL of solution contains 250 mg oxacillin.
Usual Dosage: Adults – 250 mg to 500 mg intramuscularly every 4 to 6 hours. See insert for intravenous use.
READ ACCOMPANYING INSERT.
Discard solution after 3 days at room temperature or 7 days under refrigeration. Store dry powder at 20° to 25°C (68° to 77°F). [See USP Controlled Room Temperature.]

Mfd. for SAGENT Pharmaceuticals
Schaumburg, IL 60195 (USA)
Made in India
©2012 Sagent Pharmaceuticals, Inc.
Code No.: GUJ/DRUGS/G/28/674

Oxacillin/L/02/12

The nurse adds 11.5 mL of sterile water to the vial of powdered Oxacillin, shakes the vial, and draws up 1.7 mL into a syringe. After administering the dose, the nurse labels the vial and puts it in the refrigerator.

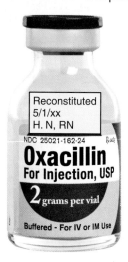

The nurse's calculation of the dose (1.7 mL) and labeling of the vial of reconstituted medication is:

Correct	Incorrect	Answer: _____

7. MD order: Ceftriaxone 400 mg IM now.
Pharmacy sends:

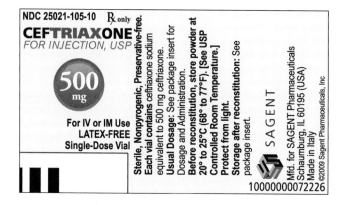

NDC 25021-105-10   ℞ only
CEFTRIAXONE
FOR INJECTION, USP
500 mg
For IV or IM Use
LATEX-FREE
Single-Dose Vial

Sterile, Nonpyrogenic, Preservative-free.
Each vial contains ceftriaxone sodium equivalent to 500 mg ceftriaxone.
Usual Dosage: See package insert for Dosage and Administration.
Before reconstitution, store powder at 20° to 25°C (68° to 77°F). [See USP Controlled Room Temperature.]
Protect from light.
Storage after reconstitution: See package insert.

SAGENT

Mfd. for SAGENT Pharmaceuticals
Schaumburg, IL 60195 (USA)
Made in Italy
©2009 Sagent Pharmaceuticals, Inc
10000000072226

Vial Dosage Size	Amount of Diluent to be Added	
	250 mg/mL	350 mg/mL
500 mg	1.8 mL	1.0 mL
1 g	3.6 mL	2.1 mL
2 g	7.2 mL	4.2 mL

Excerpt from CefTRIAXone package insert.

The nurse adds 1 mL of diluent to the vial of powdered CefTRIAXone, shakes the vial, and draws up 1.1 mL into a syringe. The nurse's decision is:

Correct	Incorrect	Answer: _____

8. MD order: Humalog insulin 7 units subcut now.
   Fill in the most appropriate syringe with the ordered dose.

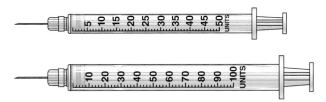

9. MD order: Novolin 70/30 insulin 36 units subcut q.AM
   30 minutes before breakfast.
   Fill in the most appropriate syringe with the ordered dose.

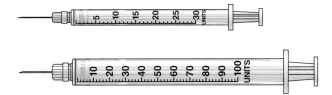

10. MD order: Humulin N insulin 21 units with Humulin R insulin
   5 units subcut q.AM 30 minutes before breakfast.
   Fill in the most appropriate syringe with the ordered dose.

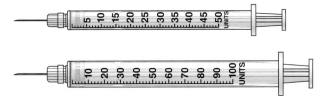

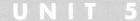

UNIT 5

IV Therapy and Administration of Intravenous Medications

Intravenous fluids and IV medications infuse directly into the circulatory system and have an immediate effect on the patient. Accuracy and vigilance in the preparation, calculation, and monitoring of the patient are essential when administering IV fluids and medications. This unit teaches you how to calculate IV infusion rates, determine the infusion and completion time of an IV, label an IV bag, and calculate the rate of administration for direct IV medications.

 APPLICATION TO NURSING PRACTICE

The nurse learns in the morning handoff report that the patient's IV was started at 0330 and is to infuse over 8 hours. The nurse assesses the patient at 0730 and observes the IV is infusing via an IV pump at 125 mL/hr.

To validate that the IV is infusing as ordered, the nurse must review the IV order and use clinical reasoning to determine whether:

■ the correct rate is set on the IV pump

■ the correct volume of IV fluid has infused

■ the IV is labeled correctly

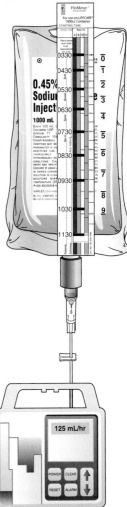

275

Intravenous Infusion and Infusion Rates

Discuss IV infusion therapy, including the components of the physician's order, line markings on the IV bag, and infusion sets used to administer primary IVs and IV piggybacks.

Discuss IV infusion by infusion pump and by gravity.

Determine the flow rate of an IV infusing by pump (mL/hr).

Determine the flow rate of an IV infusing by gravity (gtt/min).

Fluids, electrolytes, and medications can be administered directly into the vascular system by the intravenous route. Intravenous (IV) therapy is very common in the clinical setting, and most patients have IV fluids or IV medications ordered as part of their medical treatment. With the IV route, fluids and medications are given directly into a vein and are absorbed immediately. The nurse must take great care to calculate all IV flow rates correctly to promote patient safety and prevent potentially serious adverse reactions in the patient.

The nurse's role in IV therapy is to take the information contained in the physician's order and implement it safely and accurately at the **point of care.** This includes selecting the correct IV solution and administration equipment and calculating the correct rate of infusion or **flow rate** for the IV. Once the infusion has started, the nurse monitors it to prevent complications and ensure that the IV continues to flow at the correct rate.

Common Clinical Terminology for IV Infusion Therapy

When learning about IV infusion therapy, it is important to know the terminology used by the nurse in the clinical setting. Here are some common terms that refer to IV infusion therapy:

- **IV catheter:** An IV catheter is a small plastic tube that is inserted into a vein for the administration of fluids and medications directly into the circulatory system.
- **Primary IV:** A primary IV is a large volume IV used to administer fluids and electrolytes to the patient on a continuous basis.
- **IV piggyback:** An IV piggyback (IVPB) is a small volume IV used to administer IV medications. An IVPB (also called a **secondary IV**) is superimposed or "piggybacked" on a primary IV line to administer the medication on an intermittent basis, such as q.8h.

■ **Peripheral IV:** A peripheral IV or peripheral **line** is an IV that is inserted into a vein in the hand or arm. Most primary IVs or IVPBs can be infused through a peripheral line.

■ **Central IV:** A central IV or central line is an IV that is inserted into a large vein near the heart, such as the subclavian or jugular vein. A central IV can be inserted directly through the chest wall, or through a peripheral vein and threaded into the large vein (called a peripherally inserted central catheter, or **PICC** line). Any type of IV (primary or IVPB) can be infused through a central line.

■ **IV lock:** An IV lock is a short IV line that is attached to an IV catheter. The IV lock has an end cap that can be accessed by a needle or a needleless system to administer IV medications intermittently. The IV lock can be flushed with saline **("saline lock")** or with heparin **("heparin lock")** to keep the IV line **patent.**

IV Solutions

IV solutions contain water and electrolytes, and may contain dextrose or other nutrients. The name of the IV solution is often abbreviated, and the nurse must carefully read the label to ensure that the correct solution is infusing. See Table 14-1 for the names and abbreviations of common IV solutions.

Table 14-1. Common IV Solutions

COMPONENT	ABBREVIATION	COMMENTS	EXAMPLES
Saline	NS (normal saline)	Normal saline (0.9% sodium chloride solution) has the same concentration as that of body fluids.	• NS (0.9% NaCl) • 0.9% NaCl
	NaCl (sodium chloride) or saline solutions	Sodium chloride solutions with less than 0.9% NaCl are less concentrated than body fluids.	• ½ NS (0.45% NaCl) • ¼ NS (0.225% NaCl)
		A few sodium chloride solutions have more than 0.9% NaCl. These IV solutions are more concentrated than body fluids.	• 3% sodium chloride
Dextrose	D	Dextrose is a common component of IV fluids used to restore blood glucose levels and provide calories.	• D_5W (5% Dextrose in Water) • $D_{10}W$ (10% Dextrose in Water)
Lactated Ringer's	LR RL	Lactated Ringer's is an IV solution that contains electrolytes, such as potassium, magnesium, and calcium chloride. LR has the same concentration as body fluids.	
Combined solutions		Some IV solutions combine dextrose with saline or LR.	• D_5NS (D_5/0.9% NaCl) • D_5½ NS (D_5/0.45% NaCl) • D_5¼ NS (D_5/0.225% NaCl) • D_5LR
		KCl is a common additive to IV solutions. It is measured in milliequivalents (mEq).	• 20 mEq KCl in D_5NS • 30 mEq KCl in D_5½ NS

The Primary IV

A primary IV is a large volume IV, usually 1,000 mL for the adult. The physician's order for a primary IV includes the following:

■ type of IV solution

■ volume to be infused (liters or mL)

■ time for the IV to infuse (total number of hours, or mL/hr)

Figure 14-1 shows examples of how a primary IV order may be written.

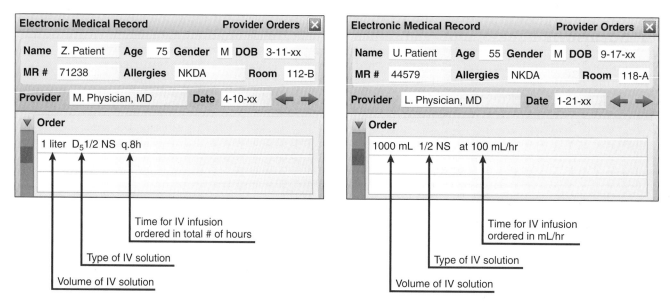

Figure 14-1. The primary IV order.

THE PRIMARY IV BAG

Most primary IV solutions come in plastic bags with detailed information on the label about the components of the IV solution, the volume in the IV bag, safe storage and handling of the IV bag, and the expiration date.

Primary IV bags have numbered line markings on the right side of the bag. There may or may not be a starting or zero line at the top of the IV bag, and the last number (10 for a 1,000 mL bag) is not written on the IV (see Fig. 14-2). The single-digit numbers (each of which represents one hundred mL) increase in value down the side of the bag, representing the volume of fluid that has infused into the patient. For example, if the IV fluid is at the level of the number 2, this indicates that 200 mL has infused into the patient.

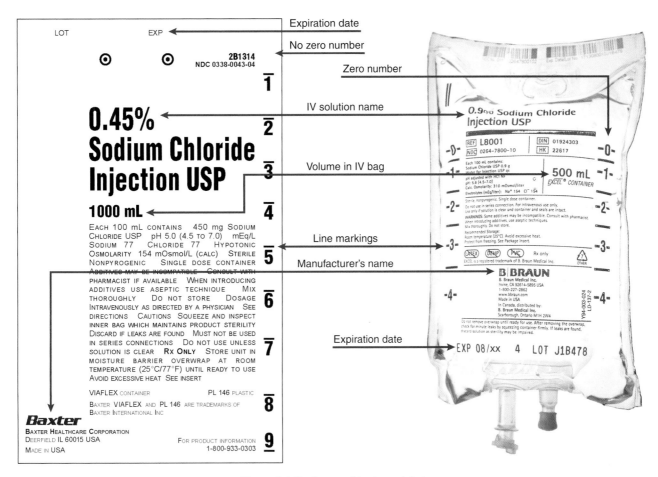

Figure 14-2. Primary IV solution labels.

THE PRIMARY IV INFUSION SET

A primary IV has several parts including the IV bag and an IV infusion set that allows the IV fluid to flow from the IV bag to the IV catheter in the patient's vein (see Fig. 14-3).

The **primary IV infusion set** is a long plastic tubing with an enlarged section at the top, called the **drip chamber.** The nurse can observe the drops of IV fluid through the drip chamber and the clear plastic tubing allows the nurse to assess the IV fluid as it flows into the patient. **Injection ports** provide access into the tubing so that the nurse can attach an IV piggyback or a syringe to administer medication. Most injection ports allow for needleless entry into the IV tubing.

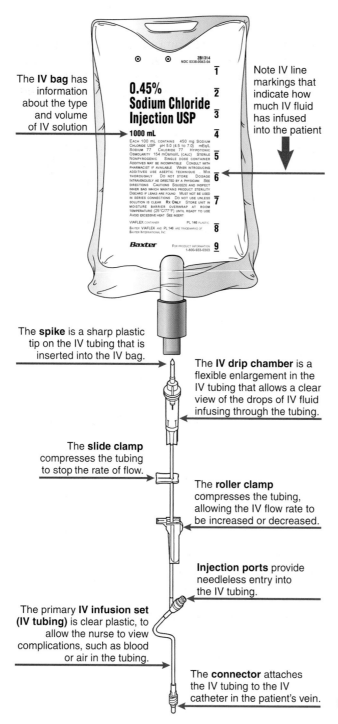

The **IV bag** has information about the type and volume of IV solution

Note IV line markings that indicate how much IV fluid has infused into the patient

0.45% Sodium Chloride Injection USP

1000 mL

The **spike** is a sharp plastic tip on the IV tubing that is inserted into the IV bag.

The **IV drip chamber** is a flexible enlargement in the IV tubing that allows a clear view of the drops of IV fluid infusing through the tubing.

The **slide clamp** compresses the tubing to stop the rate of flow.

The **roller clamp** compresses the tubing, allowing the IV flow rate to be increased or decreased.

Injection ports provide needleless entry into the IV tubing.

The primary **IV infusion set (IV tubing)** is clear plastic, to allow the nurse to view complications, such as blood or air in the tubing.

The **connector** attaches the IV tubing to the IV catheter in the patient's vein.

Figure 14-3. The primary IV and infusion set.

OTHER PRIMARY INTRAVENOUS INFUSIONS

In addition to IV fluids and IV medications, the nurse also administers other solutions intravenously, such as blood products or **parenteral nutrition.** Blood products are administered using blood administration sets (see Fig. 14-4). Calculating the infusion rate of blood products and parenteral nutrition is the same as is done for any IV fluid. These calculations are discussed at the end of this chapter.

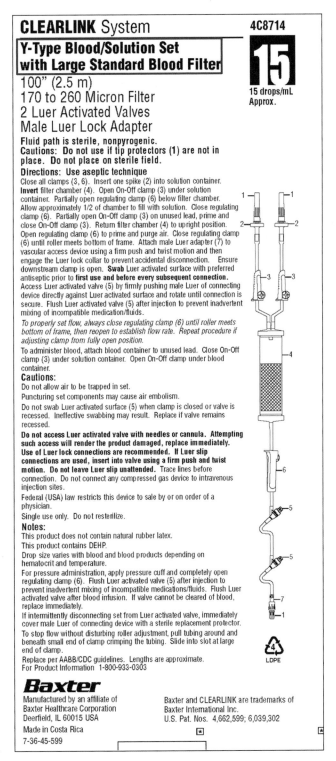

Figure 14-4. Blood administration set.

The IV Piggyback

An IV piggyback (IVPB), also referred to as a secondary IV, is a small volume IV (usually 50 or 100 mL) that contains a medication diluted in an IV solution such as normal saline or D_5W. The order for an IVPB is similar to an order for any medication. It includes the medication's name, dose, route, and time or frequency of administration (see Fig. 14-5). The amount and type of IV solution used to dilute the medication is not specified in the order, but is determined by the drug manufacturer.

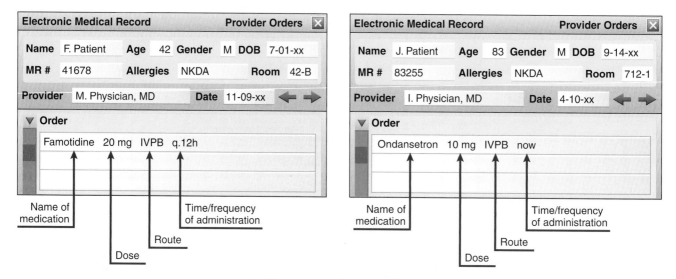

Figure 14-5. The IVPB order.

Like a primary IV, IV piggybacks come in plastic bags labeled with information about the type of IV solution, the volume in the IV bag, storage, and the expiration date. Unlike the primary IV bag, IV piggyback bags do not have numbered line markings.

Premixed IVPBs

Many IVPBs come premixed from the drug manufacturer. The label of the premixed IVPB contains information including the name of the medication, the dosage strength, and information about the IV solution in which the medication is diluted. In Figure 14-6 below, note how the Fluconazole IVPB clearly states the dosage strength of the medication (200 mg/ 100 mL). The Famotidine IVPB has the strength of the medication (20 mg) listed separately from the form of the drug (50 mL). The most important number for the nurse to locate when calculating the infusion rate for an IVPB is the volume of solution in the IV bag.

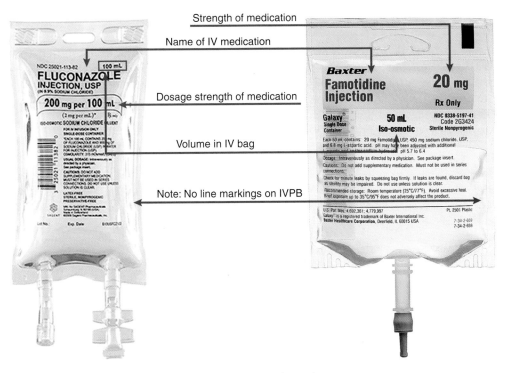

Figure 14-6. Premixed IVPB bags.

When a commercially prepared pre-mixed IVPB is not available, the pharmacist will add the IV medication to a small volume IV bag. In this case, the pharmacist will label the IV bag with the appropriate information, using a label such as the following:

MEDICATION ADDED

PATIENT _____ RM. _____

DRUG_____

AMOUNT_____

ADDED BY_____ BASE SOL'N _____

DATE _____ TIME _____

START TIME _____ DATE_____ FLOW RATE _____

EXP. DATE_____

THIS LABEL MUST BE AFFIXED TO ALL INFUSION FLUIDS CONTAINING ADDITIONAL MEDICATION.

In some instances, the nurse may need to add IV medication into a small-volume IV bag through the injection port on the IV bag. Best practices dictate that pre-mixed IVPB medications or IVPBs prepared in the pharmacy be used.

The Secondary IV Infusion Set

A **secondary IV infusion set** is a short IV tubing, specifically designed to facilitate the IVPB to "piggyback" into the primary line through an injection port (see Fig. 14-7). A secondary infusion set has a drip chamber, clamp, and needleless connector.

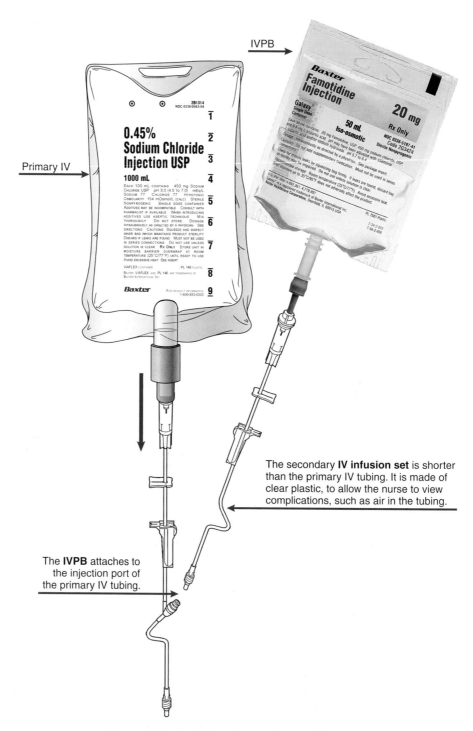

IVPB

Primary IV

The secondary **IV infusion set** is shorter than the primary IV tubing. It is made of clear plastic, to allow the nurse to view complications, such as air in the tubing.

The **IVPB** attaches to the injection port of the primary IV tubing.

Figure 14-7. The IVPB and secondary IV infusion set.

APPLY LEARNED KNOWLEDGE 14-1

For each of the IV orders below, decide whether the nurse has correctly carried out the order. Provide a rationale for your answer.

1. Order: 1 L D$_5$½ NS every 10 hours. The nurse chooses a primary IV infusion set to administer this IV.

   Correct   Incorrect

   Rationale: _____

2. Order: 1,000 mL ½ NS q.12h. The liter IV bag was hung by the nurse on the previous shift. When the 12 hour IV infusion has completed, the nurse discontinues the IV.

   Correct   Incorrect

   Rationale: _____

3. Order: Ampicillin 500 mg IVPB q.6h. The nurse calls the physician to clarify the IV solution that should be used to administer the ampicillin.

   Correct   Incorrect

   Rationale: _____

4. Order: 1 L D$_5$/0.9% NaCl with 20 mEq KCl @ 75 mL/hr. The nurse chooses a secondary IV infusion set to administer this IV.

   Correct   Incorrect

   Rationale: _____

5. Order: 1,000 mL D$_5$/0.45 NaCl @ 10:00 AM. The nurse calls the physician to question the IV order before starting this IV.

   Correct   Incorrect

   Rationale: _____

Methods of Administering IV Fluids

There are two methods by which IV fluids and IVPBs can be infused into the patient: by IV infusion pump or by gravity.

- An **IV infusion pump** allows the nurse to set a precise flow rate (mL/hr) for the IV. A pump is used for administration of potent IV medications or as indicated by the patient's age or health condition.
- An **IV infusion by gravity** allows the nurse to regulate the flow rate (gtt/min) of an IV by means of the roller clamp on the IV tubing. It is used for infusion of IV fluids and some IVPBs.

IV INFUSION PUMPS

IV infusion pumps are very common in the clinical setting. These are electronic devices that are programmed to deliver IV fluids and medications at precisely controlled rates. IV pumps have a control panel that allows the nurse to set the flow rate, the volume to be infused, and other parameters pertinent to the IV infusion.

There are many types of IV pumps, including **volumetric pumps, syringe pumps, patient-controlled analgesia (PCA) pumps,** and **peristaltic pumps** (Table 14-2). Newer "smart" infusion pumps contain software that includes information on IV medications and dosing guidelines for drugs given intravenously. This helps prevent errors with the amount or rate of medication administered to patients. The alarms on IV pumps alert the nurse to potential errors and guide the nurse's assessment of the IV pump and IV infusion.

Table 14-2. IV Infusion Pumps

TYPE OF PUMP	ACTION	CLINICAL EXAMPLE
Volumetric pump 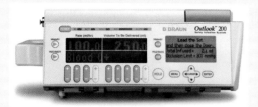	A volumetric pump is an electronic infusion device that pumps a set volume of IV fluid. A special IV tubing is required for this pump. The rate on a volumetric pump is set at mL/hr.	A patient has a primary IV infusing at 125 mL/hr. The patient has IVPBs ordered q.6h. Both the primary IV and the IVPBs are infused via a volumetric pump.
Syringe pump 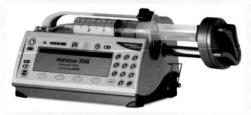	A syringe pump is a motor-driven system that pushes the plunger of a syringe to deliver a small volume of fluid or high-potency medication at a precise rate of infusion. The rate on a syringe pump is set at mL/hr.	A pediatric patient requires an infusion of a small volume of a cardiac medication. The medication is diluted in saline and administered at the precise rate of 12 mL/hr.
Patient-controlled analgesia (PCA) pump 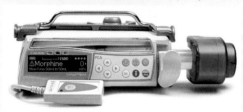	A PCA pump is a specialized type of syringe pump. It has a feature that allows the patient to self-administer medication by pushing a button on the pump. Limits on the amount and frequency of medication administration are programmed into the PCA pump.	A postoperative patient has a PCA pump for pain management during the first 2 days after surgery. The patient self-administers a dose of the medication to control postoperative pain.
Ambulatory pump 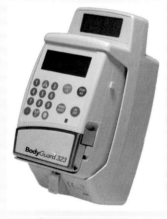	Ambulatory pumps are small, lightweight pumps that are powered by a battery and allow mobility for the patient. Battery-powered ambulatory pumps are set in mL/hr.	An oncology patient receives a chemotherapeutic drug at home via an ambulatory pump.
Peristaltic pump	A peristaltic pump has a set of rollers that intermittently squeeze the IV tubing and push fluid downward into the tubing. The rate on a peristaltic pump is set at mL/hr.	A patient has a primary IV infusing at 125 mL/hr. The IV is infusing via a peristaltic pump.
Nonelectric pump	Nonelectric disposable pumps, such as elastomeric balloon pumps, are also available for ambulatory use. These pumps work by positive pressure inherent in the balloon. No infusion rate is set on an elastomeric balloon pump.	A home-care patient receives intermittent antibiotics at home via an elastomeric balloon pump.

*Despite the convenience of IV pumps and the improvements in design, IV pumps have been associated with medication errors and **sentinel events** affecting patient safety. Both the FDA and the ISMP have published recommendations for best practices including:*

- *having a second clinician perform an independent double check of infusion pump settings with all high-risk medications and infusions.*
- *monitoring the patient and infusion according to nursing best practices rather than just relying on the pump settings and alarms.*

Additional recommendations related to IV pump safety can be found at http://www.fda.gov/infusionpumps.

Calculating the Flow Rate in mL/hr

With IV infusion pumps, the flow rate is set in mL/hr. Recall that the physician's order for an IV can include either the mL/hr or the total number of hours that the IV will infuse. Here are two examples of how the flow rate is written in an IV order:

Example 1:

The physician's order includes the number of mL per hour for the infusion:

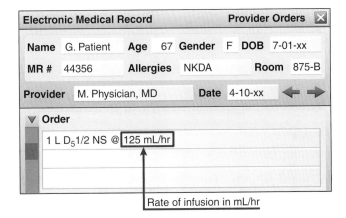

Electronic Medical Record		Provider Orders ☒
Name G. Patient **Age** 67 **Gender** F **DOB** 7-01-xx		
MR # 44356 **Allergies** NKDA **Room** 875-B		
Provider M. Physician, MD **Date** 4-10-xx ← →		
▼ **Order**		
1 L D₅1/2 NS @ 125 mL/hr		

Rate of infusion in mL/hr

In this case, there is no math to do. The nurse programs the number of mL/hr into the IV pump.

Example 2:

The physician's order includes the total number of hours for the IV infusion:

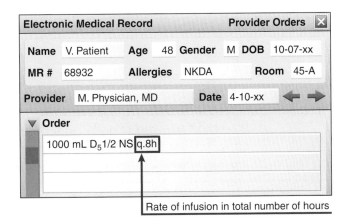

Electronic Medical Record		Provider Orders ☒
Name V. Patient **Age** 48 **Gender** M **DOB** 10-07-xx		
MR # 68932 **Allergies** NKDA **Room** 45-A		
Provider M. Physician, MD **Date** 4-10-xx ← →		
▼ **Order**		
1000 mL D₅1/2 NS q.8h		

Rate of infusion in total number of hours

When the total number of hours for the infusion is ordered, the nurse will need to calculate the number of mL/hr to set on the IV pump. The information needed for this calculation includes

■ the volume of IV fluid.

■ the amount of time it is to infuse.

Many methods of calculation can be used to find the flow rate in mL/hr. The formula method used to solve most drug dosage calculations, $\frac{D}{H} \times Q = x$ cannot be applied to IV flow rate calculations. Instead, an alternate simple formula is used:

> ### Formula: mL/hr
>
> $$\frac{\text{volume (mL)}}{\text{#hr}} = x \text{ mL/hr}$$

This formula is the simplest method to use, although ratio and proportion and dimensional analysis can also be used to solve for the mL/hr flow rate.

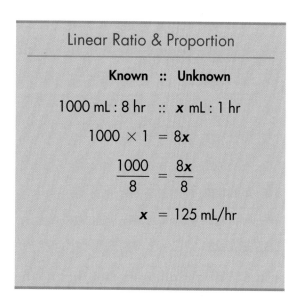

Linear Ratio & Proportion

Known :: Unknown

1000 mL : 8 hr :: *x* mL : 1 hr

1000 × 1 = 8*x*

$$\frac{1000}{8} = \frac{8x}{8}$$

x = 125 mL/hr

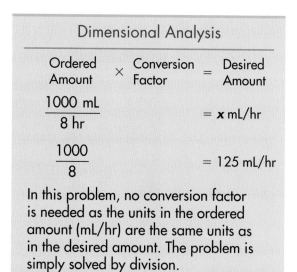

Dimensional Analysis

$$\underset{\text{Amount}}{\text{Ordered}} \times \underset{\text{Factor}}{\text{Conversion}} = \underset{\text{Amount}}{\text{Desired}}$$

$$\frac{1000 \text{ mL}}{8 \text{ hr}} = x \text{ mL/hr}$$

$$\frac{1000}{8} = 125 \text{ mL/hr}$$

In this problem, no conversion factor is needed as the units in the ordered amount (mL/hr) are the same units as in the desired amount. The problem is simply solved by division.

Fractional Ratio & Proportion

Known = Unknown

$$\frac{1000 \text{ mL}}{8 \text{ hr}} \quad \frac{x \text{ mL}}{1 \text{ hr}}$$

1000 × 1 = 8*x*

$$\frac{1000}{8} = \frac{8x}{8}$$

x = 125 mL/hr

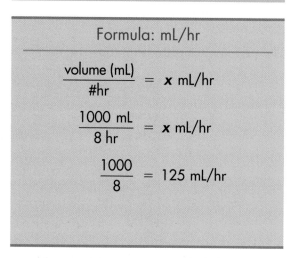

Formula: mL/hr

$$\frac{\text{volume (mL)}}{\text{#hr}} = x \text{ mL/hr}$$

$$\frac{1000 \text{ mL}}{8 \text{ hr}} = x \text{ mL/hr}$$

$$\frac{1000}{8} = 125 \text{ mL/hr}$$

The nurse sets the flow rate on the IV pump at 125 mL/hr.

Sometimes a conversion is needed before the problem can be solved. Look at the following example of a calculation for flow rate in mL/hr where a conversion is needed.

The nurse recalls that 1 L = 1,000 mL and uses this conversion to change the unit L to mL so that the units of measurement in the problem match. The problem can be solved using one of the methods of calculation.

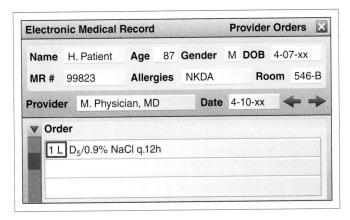

Electronic Medical Record			Provider Orders ☒
Name H. Patient	**Age** 87	**Gender** M **DOB** 4-07-xx	
MR # 99823	**Allergies** NKDA		**Room** 546-B
Provider M. Physician, MD		**Date** 4-10-xx ← →	

▼ **Order**

1 L D$_5$/0.9% NaCl q.12h

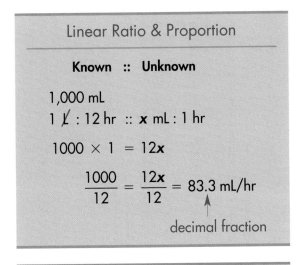

Linear Ratio & Proportion

Known :: Unknown

1,000 mL

$1 \cancel{L} : 12 \, hr :: x \, mL : 1 \, hr$

$1000 \times 1 = 12x$

$\dfrac{1000}{12} = \dfrac{12x}{12} = 83.3 \, mL/hr$

↑ decimal fraction

Dimensional Analysis

$$\underset{\text{Amount}}{\text{Ordered}} \times \underset{\text{Factor}}{\text{Conversion}} = \underset{\text{Amount}}{\text{Desired}}$$

$$\dfrac{1 \cancel{L}}{12 \, hr} \times \dfrac{1000 \, mL}{1 \cancel{L}} = x \, mL/hr$$

$$\dfrac{1 \times 1000 \, mL}{12 \, hr \times 1} = \dfrac{1000}{12} = 83.3 \, mL/hr$$

↑ decimal fraction

Fractional Ratio & Proportion

Known = Unknown

1,000 mL

$$\dfrac{1 \cancel{L}}{12 \, hr} \; ⤪ \; \dfrac{x \, mL}{1 \, hr}$$

$1000 \times 1 = 12x$

$\dfrac{1000}{12} = \dfrac{12x}{12} = 83.3 \, mL/hr$

↑ decimal fraction

Formula: mL/hr

$$\dfrac{\text{volume (mL)}}{\#hr} = x \, mL/hr$$

1000 mL

$$\dfrac{1 \cancel{L}}{12 \, hr} = x \, mL/hr$$

$$\dfrac{1000}{12} = 83.3 \, mL/hr$$

↑ decimal fraction

When the answer is not a whole number, work the problem to the tenths place to determine the decimal fraction. Because IV pumps are set in mL/hr, the answer must be rounded to the nearest whole number. The nurse sets the flow rate on the IV pump to 83 mL/hr.

APPLY LEARNED KNOWLEDGE 14-2

For each of the following IV orders, calculate the flow rate in mL/hr, and enter the answer on the IV pump.

1.

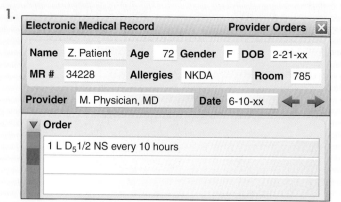

Electronic Medical Record   **Provider Orders** ☒

Name Z. Patient   **Age** 72 **Gender** F **DOB** 2-21-xx

MR # 34228   **Allergies** NKDA   **Room** 785

Provider M. Physician, MD   **Date** 6-10-xx ← →

▼ **Order**

1 L D$_5$1/2 NS every 10 hours

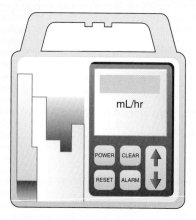

mL/hr

POWER CLEAR ↑
RESET ALARM ↓

2.

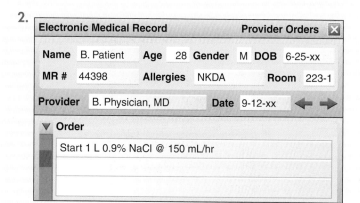

Electronic Medical Record   **Provider Orders** ☒

Name B. Patient   **Age** 28 **Gender** M **DOB** 6-25-xx

MR # 44398   **Allergies** NKDA   **Room** 223-1

Provider B. Physician, MD   **Date** 9-12-xx ← →

▼ **Order**

Start 1 L 0.9% NaCl @ 150 mL/hr

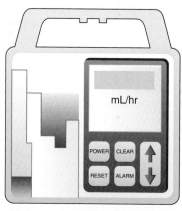

mL/hr

POWER CLEAR ↑
RESET ALARM ↓

3.

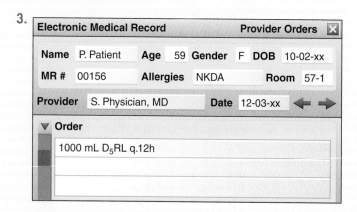

Electronic Medical Record   **Provider Orders** ☒

Name P. Patient   **Age** 59 **Gender** F **DOB** 10-02-xx

MR # 00156   **Allergies** NKDA   **Room** 57-1

Provider S. Physician, MD   **Date** 12-03-xx ← →

▼ **Order**

1000 mL D$_5$RL q.12h

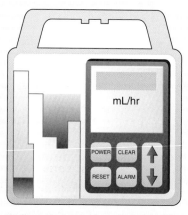

mL/hr

POWER CLEAR ↑
RESET ALARM ↓

APPLY LEARNED KNOWLEDGE 14-2—cont'd

4.

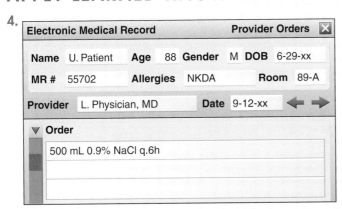

Electronic Medical Record		Provider Orders ☒
Name U. Patient	**Age** 88 **Gender** M **DOB** 6-29-xx	
MR # 55702	**Allergies** NKDA	**Room** 89-A
Provider L. Physician, MD	**Date** 9-12-xx ⬅ ➡	
▼ **Order**		
500 mL 0.9% NaCl q.6h		

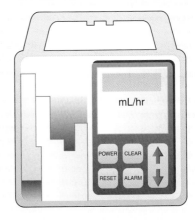

5.

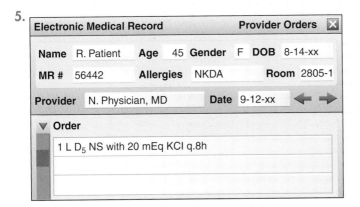

Electronic Medical Record		Provider Orders ☒
Name R. Patient	**Age** 45 **Gender** F **DOB** 8-14-xx	
MR # 56442	**Allergies** NKDA	**Room** 2805-1
Provider N. Physician, MD	**Date** 9-12-xx ⬅ ➡	
▼ **Order**		
1 L D_5 NS with 20 mEq KCl q.8h		

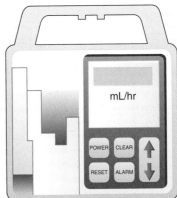

IV Infusions by Gravity

When an IV is infused by gravity, the flow rate is measured in drops (gtt) per minute. Recall that the enlarged section at the top of the IV tubing, called the **drip chamber,** allows the nurse to observe and count the number of drops infusing into the patient.

THE DROP FACTOR

IV infusion sets, or IV tubings, come in a variety of lengths and sizes. The size of each drop varies with the type of IV tubing. Therefore, the number of drops in a mL (called the **drop factor**) will vary. For example, in an IV tubing with a drop factor of 60 gtt/mL, the drops are very small: 1 mL of IV fluid is made up of 60 drops. An IV tubing with a drop factor of 15 gtt/mL has larger drops: 15 drops make up 1 mL of IV fluid.

There are two main types of IV tubing:

- **macrodrip**
- **microdrip**

Each type of IV infusion set has a specific size of drop that flows into the drip chamber.

Macrodrip IV Infusion Sets

A macrodrip IV infusion set has a relatively large plastic opening through which the drops are formed. With macrodrip tubing, the size of the drop varies according to the manufacturer. Macrodrip IV infusion sets are available with the following drop factors:

- 10 gtt = 1 mL
- 15 gtt = 1 mL
- 20 gtt = 1 mL

As there are several available sizes of macrodrip tubing, the nurse needs to read the package of the infusion set carefully to determine the drop factor. The drop factor is usually displayed in large numbers on the package labeling (Fig. 14-8), but is not found on the tubing itself, so the nurse needs to read the package before discarding it.

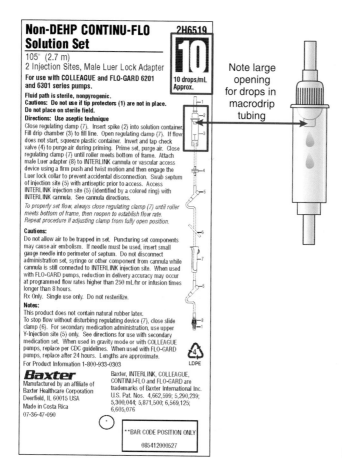

Figure 14-8. Macrodrip tubing set.

Microdrip IV Infusion Sets

A microdrip IV infusion set has a small needlelike projection through which the drops are formed. Microdrip tubing produces very small drops of IV fluid. Regardless of the manufacturer, microdrip IV infusion sets are available with only one drop factor:

- 60 gtt = 1 mL

Microdrip sets are also called pediatric (pedidrip) or minidrip infusion sets (Fig. 14-9).

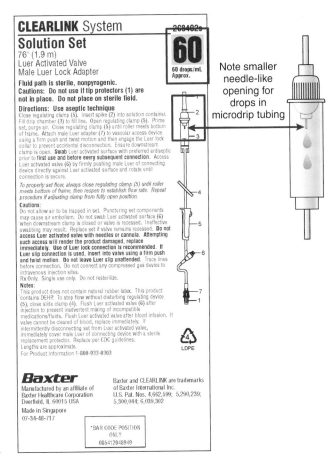

Figure 14-9. Microdrip tubing set.

 *It is easy to get confused between the drop factor (gtt/**mL**) and the gravity flow rate (gtt/**min**). It is important to know the difference between the two when working IV flow rate problems.*

- The **drop factor** indicates the number of drops per **mL** of the IV tubing. A certain number of drops make up a mL: for example, 15 gtt/mL or 60 gtt/mL. This information is written on the infusion set package.
- The gravity **flow rate** is the number of drops per **minute** of the IV. The flow rate is calculated, and used by the nurse to set up and monitor the gtt/min of the IV infusion.

CALCULATING THE FLOW RATE IN GTT/MIN

When an IV is to infuse by gravity, the nurse needs to count the number of drops of IV fluid that fall into the IV drip chamber each minute. As this information is not included in the IV order, a calculation is always required to find the flow rate in gtt/min. To calculate the number of gtt/min for the IV infusion, the nurse needs the following:

■ the drop factor of the IV tubing

■ the volume (mL) to be infused

■ the time the IV is to infuse (in minutes)

The easiest method to use to solve for the number of gtt/min is a formula:

$$\frac{\text{volume (mL)} \times \text{drop factor}}{\text{time (min)}} = \textbf{x} \text{ gtt/min}$$

In many gravity flow rate calculations, the nurse will need to convert so that the units of measurement match. Common conversions used in gravity flow rate problems include 1 L = 1,000 mL, and 1 hr = 60 minutes. In addition, if the answer to the flow rate problem contains a decimal fraction, the problem is worked to the tenths place and the answer is rounded to the nearest whole number, as the nurse only counts whole drops. Look at the following four examples showing how to use the formula to calculate gravity flow rate in gtt/min.

Example 1:

An IV is ordered to infuse at 100 mL/hr. The nurse has an IV infusion set with a drop factor of 15 gtt/mL. What is the flow rate?

   Notice how the numbers are placed in the formula setup: the ordered mL is put in the numerator of the fraction, and the hr is used in the denominator of the fraction. Because the formula solves for the gtt/min, the 1 hr is changed to 60 minutes when it is placed in the formula.

$$\text{Formula: gtt/min}$$

$$\frac{\text{volume (mL)} \times \text{drop factor}}{\text{time (min)}} = x \text{ gtt/min}$$

$$\frac{100 \text{ mL} \times 15 \text{ gtt/mL}}{1 \text{ hr (convert to min)}} = x \text{ gtt/min}$$

$$\frac{100 \text{ mL} \times 15 \text{ gtt/mL}}{60 \text{ min}} = x \text{ gtt/min}$$

$$\frac{100 \times 15 \text{ gtt}}{60 \text{ min}} = x \ \frac{1500}{60} = 25 \text{ gtt/min}$$

   The flow rate for this gravity IV infusion is 25 gtt/min.

Example 2:

The physician's order reads: Infuse 1 unit of packed cells (250 mL) over 3 hours. The nurse has a blood administration set with a drop factor of 10 gtt/mL. What is the flow rate for this transfusion?

   In this problem, the order includes the total number of hours for the infusion, rather than the mL/hr. The ordered mL is put in the numerator of the fraction in the formula. The 3 hr is used in the denominator of the fraction, but because the formula requires the time in minutes, notice how the 3 hr is multiplied by 60 minutes to arrive at the total number of minutes for the formula.

$$\text{Formula: gtt/min}$$

$$\frac{\text{volume (mL)} \times \text{drop factor}}{\text{time (min)}} = x \text{ gtt/min}$$

$$\frac{250 \text{ mL} \times 10 \text{ gtt/mL}}{3 \text{ hr (convert to min)}} = x \text{ gtt/min}$$

$$\frac{250 \text{ mL} \times 10 \text{ gtt/mL}}{3 \times 60 \text{ min}} = x \text{ gtt/min}$$

$$\frac{250 \times 10 \text{ gtt}}{180 \text{ min}} = x \ \frac{2500}{180} = 13.8 \text{ gtt/min}$$

$$x = 14 \text{ gtt/min}$$

   The answer is worked to the tenths place and rounded to the nearest whole number. The flow rate for this IV fluid infusing by gravity is 14 gtt/min.

Example 3:

The IV order is written as follows: Start 1 L 0.9% NaCl to infuse in 6 hr. The IV tubing has a drop factor of 15 gtt/mL. What is the flow rate in gtt/min?

This example requires two conversions before the problem can be solved: the unit L needs to be converted to mL, and the hours must be converted to minutes in order to set up and solve the problem.

$$\text{Formula: gtt/min}$$

$$\frac{\text{volume (mL)} \times \text{drop factor}}{\text{time (min)}} = x \text{ gtt/min}$$

$$\frac{1 \text{ L} \times 15 \text{ gtt/mL}}{6 \text{ hr (convert to min)}} = x \text{ gtt/min}$$

$$\frac{1000 \text{ mL} \times 15 \text{ gtt/mL}}{6 \times 60 \text{ min}} = x \text{ gtt/min}$$

$$\frac{1000 \times 15 \text{ gtt}}{360 \text{ min}} = x = \frac{15{,}000}{360} = 41.6 \text{ gtt/min}$$

$$x = 42 \text{ gtt/min}$$

The answer is worked to the tenths place and rounded to the nearest whole number. The flow rate for this IV fluid infusing by gravity is 42 gtt/min.

Example 4:

The order is to infuse an IVPB of 50 mL of D_5W with 500 mg ampicillin over 15 minutes. The nurse chooses a macrodrip IV tubing with a drop factor of 10 gtt/mL. What is the flow rate for this IVPB?

With this example the other methods of calculation will be used to solve for flow rate in gtt/min. The ratio and proportion method requires two steps: first to solve for the mL/min, then to solve for the gtt/min.

Linear Ratio & Proportion

Solve for mL / min :

Known :: Unknown

(ordered amount)

50 mL : 15 min :: x mL : 1 min

$50 \times 1 = 15x$

$\dfrac{50}{15} = \dfrac{15x}{15} = 3.3$ mL/min

Solve for mL/min:

Known :: Unknown

(drop factor)

10 gtt : 1 mL :: x gtt/min : 3.3 mL/min

$10 \times 3.3 = 1x$

$\dfrac{33}{1} = \dfrac{1x}{1} = 33$ gtt/min

Dimensional Analysis

$\dfrac{\text{Ordered}}{\text{Amount}} \times \dfrac{\text{Conversion}}{\text{Factor}} = \dfrac{\text{Desired}}{\text{Amount}}$

$\dfrac{50 \;\cancel{mL}}{15 \;min} \times \dfrac{10 \;gtt}{1 \;\cancel{mL}} = x$ gtt/min

$\dfrac{50 \times 10 \;gtt}{15 \times 1} = \dfrac{500}{15} = 33.3$ gtt/min

$x = 33$ gtt/min

Fractional Ratio & Proportion

Solve for mL/min:

Known :: Unknown

(ordered amount)

$\dfrac{50 \;mL}{15 \;min} \diagup\kern-1.2em\diagdown \dfrac{x \;mL}{1 \;min}$

$50 \times 1 = 15x$

$\dfrac{50}{15} = \dfrac{15x}{15} = 3.3$ mL/min

Solve for mL/min:

Known :: Unknown

(drop factor)

10 gtt : 1 mL :: x gtt/min : 3.3 mL/min

$10 \times 3.3 = 1x$

$\dfrac{33}{1} = \dfrac{1x}{1} = 33$ gtt/min

Formula: gtt/min

$\dfrac{\text{volume (mL)} \times \text{drop factor}}{\text{time (min)}} = x$ gtt/min

$\dfrac{50 \;mL \times 10 \;gtt/mL}{15 \;min} = x$ gtt/min

$\dfrac{50 \;\cancel{mL} \times 10 \;gtt/\cancel{mL}}{15 \;min} = x$ gtt/min

$\dfrac{50 \times 10 \;gtt}{15 \;min} = \dfrac{500}{15} = 33.3$ gtt/min

$x = 33$ gtt/min

The flow rate for this IVPB infusing by gravity is 33 gtt/min.

Here is a useful shortcut: When the drop factor of an IV infusion set is 60 gtt/mL, the number of mL/hr is equal to the number of gtt/min.

For example, the IV order is to infuse 500 mL D₅½NS @ 40 mL/hr. The nurse chooses a microdrip IV infusion set (60 gtt/mL). The gravity flow rate of this IV will be 40 gtt/min (the same as the ordered mL/hr).

APPLY LEARNED KNOWLEDGE 14-3

Calculate the flow rate in gtt/min for each of the following IV orders. Fill in the clock with the correct flow rate.

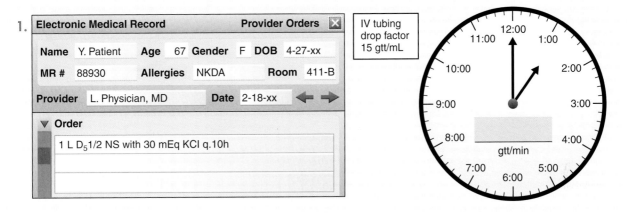

1. **Electronic Medical Record**   **Provider Orders** ☒

   Name Y. Patient   **Age** 67 **Gender** F **DOB** 4-27-xx

   MR # 88930   **Allergies** NKDA   **Room** 411-B

   Provider L. Physician, MD   **Date** 2-18-xx ⬅ ➡

   ▼ **Order**

   1 L D₅1/2 NS with 30 mEq KCl q.10h

   IV tubing drop factor 15 gtt/mL

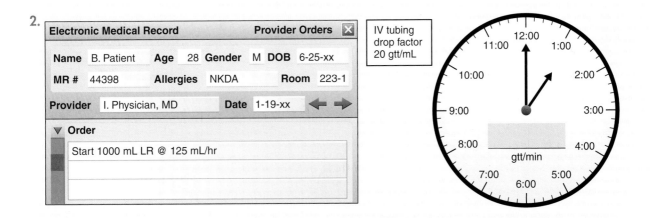

2. **Electronic Medical Record**   **Provider Orders** ☒

   Name B. Patient   **Age** 28 **Gender** M **DOB** 6-25-xx

   MR # 44398   **Allergies** NKDA   **Room** 223-1

   Provider I. Physician, MD   **Date** 1-19-xx ⬅ ➡

   ▼ **Order**

   Start 1000 mL LR @ 125 mL/hr

   IV tubing drop factor 20 gtt/mL

Continued

APPLY LEARNED KNOWLEDGE 14-3—cont'd

3.

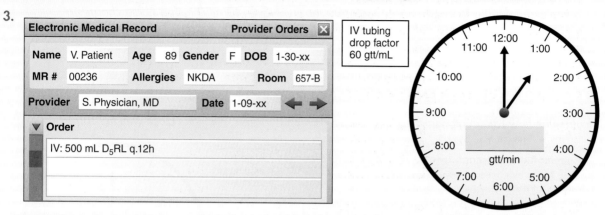

Electronic Medical Record   Provider Orders   ☒

Name V. Patient   **Age** 89 **Gender** F **DOB** 1-30-xx

MR # 00236   **Allergies** NKDA   **Room** 657-B

Provider S. Physician, MD   **Date** 1-09-xx ⬅ ➡

▼ **Order**

IV: 500 mL D$_5$RL q.12h

IV tubing drop factor 60 gtt/mL

gtt/min

4.

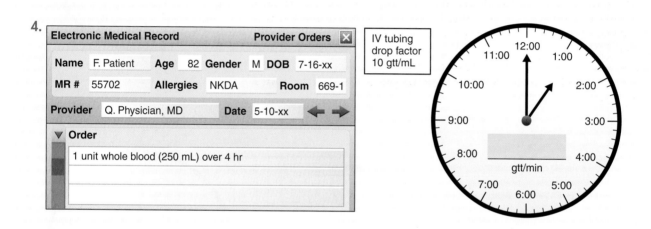

Electronic Medical Record   Provider Orders   ☒

Name F. Patient   **Age** 82 **Gender** M **DOB** 7-16-xx

MR # 55702   **Allergies** NKDA   **Room** 669-1

Provider Q. Physician, MD   **Date** 5-10-xx ⬅ ➡

▼ **Order**

1 unit whole blood (250 mL) over 4 hr

IV tubing drop factor 10 gtt/mL

gtt/min

5.

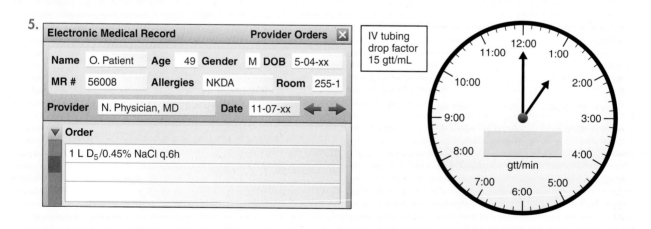

Electronic Medical Record   Provider Orders   ☒

Name O. Patient   **Age** 49 **Gender** M **DOB** 5-04-xx

MR # 56008   **Allergies** NKDA   **Room** 255-1

Provider N. Physician, MD   **Date** 11-07-xx ⬅ ➡

▼ **Order**

1 L D$_5$/0.45% NaCl q.6h

IV tubing drop factor 15 gtt/mL

gtt/min

CLINICAL REASONING 14-1
The doctor's order for the primary IV is for 1 L D₅W to infuse over
8 hours by gravity. The night nurse begins the IV at 0645 using
the tubing shown. The day-shift nurse assesses the IV at 0700 and
counts the flow rate as 31 drops per minute. The nurse decides
to continue to monitor the IV. At 1100, the physician decreases
the IV to 75 mL/hr, and the nurse adjusts the gravity IV flow rate
to 19 gtt/min. The nurse's decisions are (choose all that apply):

A. 0700; correct in validating the flow rate of 31 gtt/min.
B. 0700; incorrect; the flow rate should be 25 gtt/minute.
C. 1100; correct; the flow rate should be changed to 19 gtt/min.
D. 1100; incorrect; the flow rate should be changed to 18 gtt/minute
E. incorrect; the IV tubing should be changed to a pedidrip set.

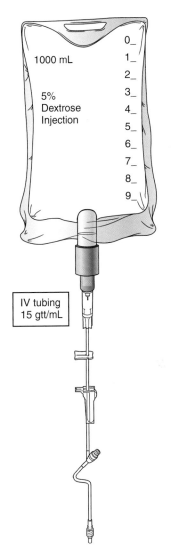

IV tubing
15 gtt/mL

Careful calculation and monitoring of IV flow rates is essential to patient safety. IV solutions that infuse too rapidly can overload the cardiac and respiratory systems of the patient. IV solutions that infuse too slowly will fail to meet the fluid and electrolyte needs of the patient. If the IV contains medication, the correct flow rate is essential to ensuring the therapeutic effect of the medication and preventing potential adverse reactions. To reduce medication errors and prevent patient injury, careful calculation and vigilant patient monitoring are a necessity.

Developing Competency

Work the problems and answer the questions below.

1. The IV order is as follows:

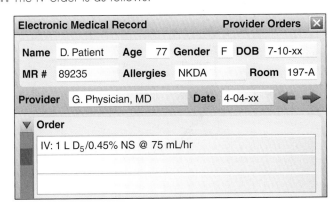

Which of the following applies to this IV?
a. This IV can be infused by gravity or by an IV pump.
b. A conversion is needed if the nurse chooses an IV pump.
c. If the nurse chooses to run the IV by gravity with a tubing that has a drop factor of 10 gtt/mL, the flow rate is 75 gtt/min.

2. The doctor orders ciprofloxacin 200 mg IVPB q.12h. The pharmacy sent the following premixed IVPB of ciprofloxacin. The drug reference states that IV ciprofloxacin is to be administered over 60 min. What rate will the nurse set on the IV pump (mL/hr)? _____

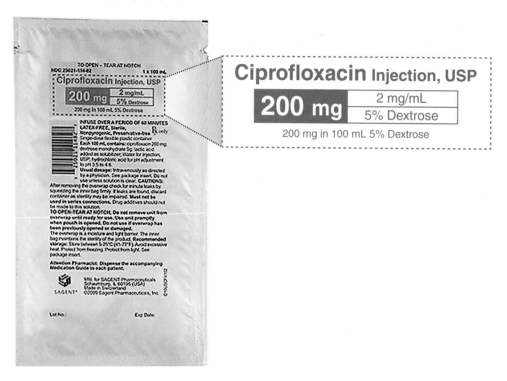

3. The IV order is as follows: 1,000 mL D$_5$/0.9% NaCl over 12 hr. How many mL/hr will the nurse set on the IV pump? _____

4. The IV order is to infuse 1 L 0.9% NaCl over 6 hr. Calculate the flow rate in mL/hr. _____

5. The nurse is preparing to hang a unit of blood on the patient. The unit contains 235 mL and the order is to infuse the blood over 4 hours. The nurse has the following blood tubing administration set. Calculate the flow rate in gtt/min for this infusion. _____

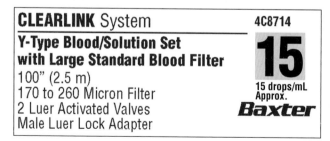

6. The physician orders an IV of 0.9% NaCl 250 mL to infuse over 2½ hours. Calculate the mL/hr. _____

7. The physician orders vancomycin 1 g IVPB q.12h. The pharmacy sends the following IVPB. The vancomycin is to infuse over 90 min. How many mL/hr will the nurse set on the IV pump? _____

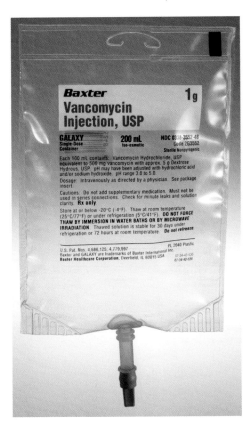

8. The nurse is to infuse 1 L lactated Ringer's over 10 hours. The IV tubing set has a drop factor of 20 gtt/min. Calculate the flow rate in gtt/min. _____

9. The order is to infuse 500 mL D5/0.225% NaCl over 10 hr. The nurse has the following IV tubing. Calculate flow rate in gtt/min. _____

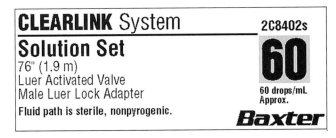

10. The physician orders an IV to infuse at 30 mL/hr. The nurse chooses a microdrip IV infusion set. Calculate the gravity flow rate for this IV. _____

11. The nurse is preparing to administer 0900 medications using the patient's electronic medication administration record. The following IVPB is in the medication drawer:

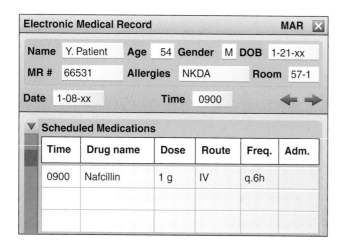

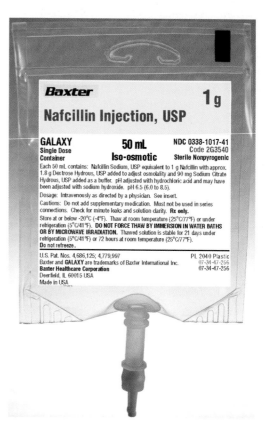

The IVPB is to be infused over 60 minutes. The nurse has an IV solution set with a drop factor of 15 gtt/mL. Calculate the flow rate in gtt/min. _____

12. The 1,000 mL IV is to infuse over 6 hours. The nurse has an infusion set with a drop factor of 15 gtt/mL. Calculate the flow rate in gtt/min. _____

13. A 1 L IV is to infuse over 8 hours. The nurse has an infusion set with a drop factor of 15 gtt/mL. Calculate the flow rate in gtt/min. _____

14. 500 mL D$_5$/0.225% NaCl is to infuse over 8 hr. Calculate the mL/hr. _____

15. The physician writes the following order on the electronic medical record. The nurse has a tubing administration set with a drop factor of 15 gtt/mL. Calculate the gtt/min for this gravity IV. _____

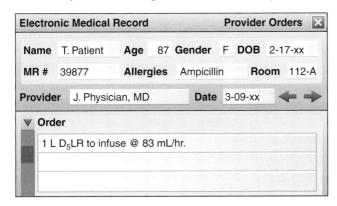

Electronic Medical Record	Provider Orders ☒

Name T. Patient	**Age** 87	**Gender** F	**DOB** 2-17-xx
MR # 39877	**Allergies** Ampicillin		**Room** 112-A
Provider J. Physician, MD		**Date** 3-09-xx ⬅ ➡	

▼ **Order**

1 L D$_5$LR to infuse @ 83 mL/hr.

16. The IV order is to infuse 250 mL 0.9% NaCl with 10 mEq KCl over 4 hours. How many mL/hr will the nurse set on the IV pump? _____

17. The patient is to receive one unit of packed cells (280 mL) over 3 hours. The blood administration set has a drop factor of 10 gtt/mL. Calculate the gravity flow rate in gtt/min. _____

18. The nurse is to infuse 500 mL D$_5$/0.45% NaCl over 4 hours. Calculate the mL/hr for this IV infusion. _____

19. The physician writes the following order for IV therapy:

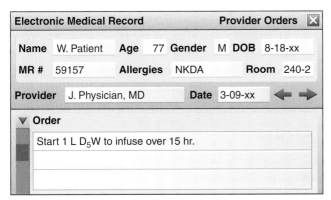

Electronic Medical Record	Provider Orders ☒

Name W. Patient	**Age** 77	**Gender** M	**DOB** 8-18-xx
MR # 59157	**Allergies** NKDA		**Room** 240-2
Provider J. Physician, MD		**Date** 3-09-xx ⬅ ➡	

▼ **Order**

Start 1 L D$_5$W to infuse over 15 hr.

The nurse sets up the IV to infuse vial a volumetric pump. How many mL/hr will the nurse set on the pump? _____

20. The physician orders 3 L D$_5$/0.45% NaCl with 20 mEq KCl to infuse over 24 hours. How many mL will the patient receive per hour? _____

CHAPTER 15

Calculating Infusion and Completion Time

LEARNING OUTCOMES

Calculate the infusion time of an IV in hours and minutes.

Calculate the completion time of an IV.

Use a flow meter to label the IV bag using military time.

Use the flow meter to identify the infused and the remaining amount of IV fluid.

A patient who is receiving intravenous therapy requires careful monitoring so that the amount of intravenous fluid infuses as ordered. The nurse calculates the infusion and completion time of the IV fluid to ensure that the patient receives the amount of IV fluid ordered by the physician. Knowing the infusion time helps the nurse to know how long the ordered IV fluid will take to infuse into the patient. Calculation of the completion time helps the nurse maintain continuous IV therapy by preparing and hanging the next IV bag or discontinuing the IV therapy in a timely manner.

Infusion Time and the IV Order

Infusion time is the amount of time (hours and minutes) that it will take to infuse the ordered amount of IV fluid. The nurse uses the IV order to calculate the infusion time. An IV order (Fig. 15-1) is written so that it identifies either

- the total amount of IV fluid over a specific number of hours, or
- the total amount of IV fluid and the specific hourly rate (mL/hr).

When the IV order includes the specific number of hours, the nurse does not need to calculate the infusion time because the IV order already specifies the length of time the IV fluid needs to be infused. In the IV order example, 1 L D_5W q.8h, the infusion time is 8 hours.

However, when the IV order includes a specific rate (mL/hr), the nurse needs to calculate the infusion time.

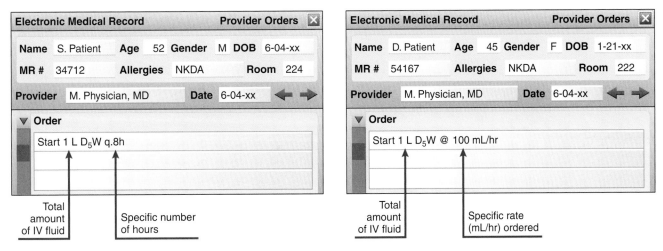

Figure 15-1. Intravenous therapy orders and infusion time.

Many methods of calculation can be used to calculate the infusion time. The formula method used to solve drug dosage calculations, $\dfrac{D}{H} \times Q = x$ cannot be applied to infusion time calculations. Instead, an alternate simple formula is used:

> **Formula : Infusion Time**
>
> $$\dfrac{\text{Total volume (mL)}}{\text{Ordered hourly (mL)}} \times 1\ \text{hr} = x\ \text{hr}$$

Example 1:

The IV order states: Start 1,000 mL of Lactated Ringer's at 125 mL/hr. What is the infusion time for this IV?

Linear Ratio & Proportion

Known :: Unknown

$$125\ \text{mL} : 1\ \text{hr} :: 1000\ \text{mL} : x\ \text{hr}$$

$$125x = 1000$$

$$\frac{125x}{125} = \frac{1000}{125}$$

$$x = 8\ \text{hr}$$

Dimensional Analysis

$$\frac{\text{Ordered}}{\text{Amount}} \times \frac{\text{Conversion}}{\text{Factor}} = \frac{\text{Desired}}{\text{Amount}}$$

$$\frac{1000\ \cancel{mL}}{1} \times \frac{1\ \text{hr}}{125\ \cancel{mL}} = x\ \text{hr}$$

$$\frac{1000 \times 1\ \text{hr}}{1 \times 125} = \frac{1000}{125} = 8\ \text{hr}$$

In dimensional analysis, the ordered IV rate (mL / hr) is the conversion factor used in the problem.

Fractional Ratio & Proportion	Formula: Infusion Time
Known = Unknown	$\dfrac{\text{Total volume (mL)}}{\text{Ordered hourly (mL)}} \times \textbf{1 hr} = \textbf{x hr}$
$\dfrac{125 \text{ mL}}{1 \text{ hr}} \diagup\!\!\!\diagdown \dfrac{1000 \text{ mL}}{\textbf{x hr}}$	$\dfrac{1000 \text{ mL}}{125 \text{ mL}} \times 1 \text{ hr} = \textbf{x hr}$
$125\textbf{x} = 1000$	$\dfrac{1000}{125} \times 1 \text{ hr} = 8 \text{ hr}$
$\dfrac{125\textbf{x}}{125} = \dfrac{1000}{125}$	
$\textbf{x} = 8 \text{ hr}$	

The infusion time for this IV is 8 hours.

Example 2:

The IV order states: Start 500 mL of 0.9% Sodium Chloride at 50 mL/hr. What is the infusion time for this IV?

Linear Ratio & Proportion	Dimensional Analysis
Known :: Unknown	$\begin{array}{ccc}\text{Ordered} \\ \text{Amount}\end{array} \times \begin{array}{ccc}\text{Conversion} \\ \text{Factor}\end{array} = \begin{array}{ccc}\text{Desired} \\ \text{Amount}\end{array}$
$50 \text{ mL} : 1 \text{ hr} :: 500 \text{ mL} : \textbf{x hr}$	$\dfrac{500 \text{ mL}}{1} \times \dfrac{1 \text{ hr}}{50 \text{ mL}} = \textbf{x hr}$
$50\textbf{x} = 500$	$\dfrac{500 \times 1 \text{ hr}}{1 \times 50} = \dfrac{500}{50} = 10 \text{ hr}$
$\dfrac{50\textbf{x}}{50} = \dfrac{500}{50}$	In dimensional analysis, the ordered IV rate (mL/hr) is the conversion factor used in the problem.
$\textbf{x} = 10 \text{ hr}$	

Fractional Ratio & Proportion	Formula: Infusion Time
Known = Unknown	$\dfrac{\text{Total volume (mL)}}{\text{Ordered hourly (mL)}} \times \textbf{1 hr} = \textbf{x hr}$
$\dfrac{50 \text{ mL}}{1 \text{ hr}} \diagup\!\!\!\diagdown \dfrac{500 \text{ mL}}{\textbf{x mL}}$	$\dfrac{500 \text{ mL}}{50 \text{ mL}} \times 1 \text{ hr} = \textbf{x hr}$
$50\textbf{x} = 500$	$\dfrac{500}{50} \times 1 \text{ hr} = 10 \text{ hr}$
$\dfrac{50\textbf{x}}{50} = \dfrac{500}{50}$	
$\textbf{x} = 10 \text{ hr}$	

The infusion time for this IV is 10 hours.

Calculation of Minutes

Not all infusion time problems end evenly in a whole number (8 hours, 10 hours, etc.). Some infusion time problems include a decimal fraction. This decimal fraction represents part of an hour and needs to be converted to minutes. Converting the part of an hour to minutes requires working the problem as follows:

■ First, work the problem to two places to the right of the decimal point.

■ Second, calculate the minutes, using one of the four methods of calculation.

■ Third, use the rounding rules to convert the minutes to a whole number.

For example, the nurse starts 1,000 mL of 0.9% Sodium Chloride at 75 mL/hr. What is the infusion time for this IV?

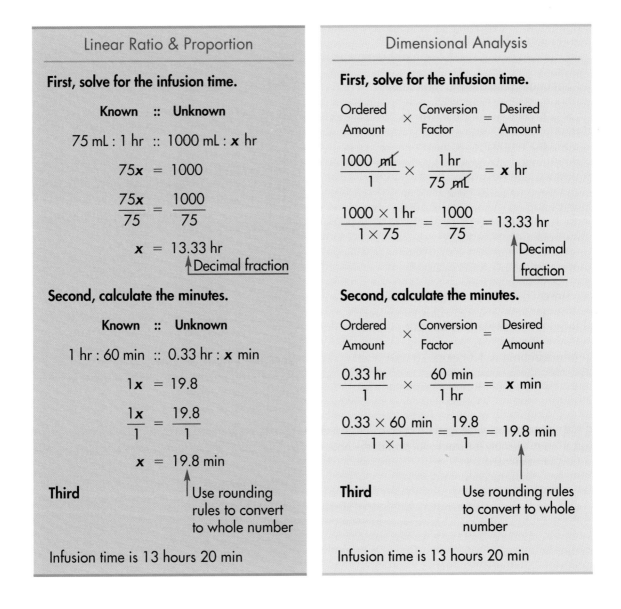

Linear Ratio & Proportion

First, solve for the infusion time.

Known   ::   Unknown

75 mL : 1 hr :: 1000 mL : **x** hr

$$75x = 1000$$

$$\frac{75x}{75} = \frac{1000}{75}$$

$$x = 13.33 \text{ hr}$$
↑Decimal fraction

Second, calculate the minutes.

Known   ::   Unknown

1 hr : 60 min :: 0.33 hr : **x** min

$$1x = 19.8$$

$$\frac{1x}{1} = \frac{19.8}{1}$$

$$x = 19.8 \text{ min}$$

Third   ↑Use rounding rules to convert to whole number

Infusion time is 13 hours 20 min

Dimensional Analysis

First, solve for the infusion time.

$$\frac{\text{Ordered}}{\text{Amount}} \times \frac{\text{Conversion}}{\text{Factor}} = \frac{\text{Desired}}{\text{Amount}}$$

$$\frac{1000 \text{ mL}}{1} \times \frac{1 \text{ hr}}{75 \text{ mL}} = x \text{ hr}$$

$$\frac{1000 \times 1 \text{ hr}}{1 \times 75} = \frac{1000}{75} = 13.33 \text{ hr}$$
↑Decimal fraction

Second, calculate the minutes.

$$\frac{\text{Ordered}}{\text{Amount}} \times \frac{\text{Conversion}}{\text{Factor}} = \frac{\text{Desired}}{\text{Amount}}$$

$$\frac{0.33 \text{ hr}}{1} \times \frac{60 \text{ min}}{1 \text{ hr}} = x \text{ min}$$

$$\frac{0.33 \times 60 \text{ min}}{1 \times 1} = \frac{19.8}{1} = 19.8 \text{ min}$$
↑

Third   Use rounding rules to convert to whole number

Infusion time is 13 hours 20 min

Fractional Ratio & Proportion

First, solve for infusion time.

Known   =   Unknown

$$\frac{75 \text{ mL}}{1 \text{ hr}} \quad \frac{1000 \text{ mL}}{x \text{ hr}}$$

$$75x = 1000$$

$$\frac{75x}{75} = \frac{1000}{75}$$

$$x = 13.33 \text{ hr}$$
↑ Decimal fraction

Second, calculate the minutes.

Known   =   Unknown

$$\frac{60 \text{ min}}{1 \text{ hr}} \quad \frac{x \text{ min}}{0.33 \text{ hr}}$$

$$1x = 19.8$$

$$\frac{1x}{1} = \frac{19.8}{1}$$

$$x = 19.8 \text{ min}$$

Third   ↑ Use rounding rules to convert to whole number

Infusion time is 13 hours 20 min

Formula: Infusion Time

First, solve for infusion time.

$$\frac{\text{Total volume (mL)}}{\text{Ordered hourly (mL)}} \times 1 \text{ hr} = x \text{ hr}$$

$$\frac{1000 \text{ mL}}{75 \text{ mL}} \times 1 \text{ hr} = x \text{ hr}$$

$$\frac{1000}{75} \times 1 \text{ hr} = 13.33 \text{ hr}$$
↑ Decimal fraction

Second, calculate the minutes.

$$\frac{0.33 \text{ hr}}{1 \text{ hr}} \times 60 \text{ min} = x \text{ min}$$

$$\frac{0.33}{1} \times 60 \text{ min} = 19.8 \text{ min}$$
↑ Use rounding rules to convert to whole number

Third

Infusion time is 13 hours 20 min

 Regardless of the method of calculation used, a simple mathematical way to solve for the minutes is to multiply the fractional part of the hour by 60. Then apply the rounding rules once the answer is calculated.

APPLY LEARNED KNOWLEDGE 15-1

Calculate the infusion time for the following IV orders.

1.
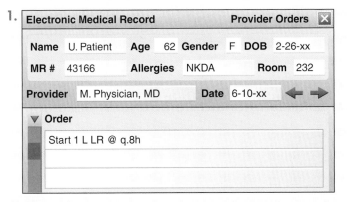

Electronic Medical Record   **Provider Orders** ☒

| **Name** U. Patient | **Age** 62 | **Gender** F | **DOB** 2-26-xx |
| **MR #** 43166 | **Allergies** NKDA | | **Room** 232 |

Provider M. Physician, MD   **Date** 6-10-xx ← →

▼ **Order**

Start 1 L LR @ q.8h

What is the infusion time for this IV order? _____

2.
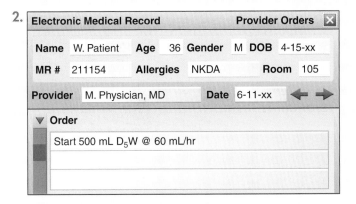

Electronic Medical Record   **Provider Orders** ☒

| **Name** W. Patient | **Age** 36 | **Gender** M | **DOB** 4-15-xx |
| **MR #** 211154 | **Allergies** NKDA | | **Room** 105 |

Provider M. Physician, MD   **Date** 6-11-xx ← →

▼ **Order**

Start 500 mL D_5W @ 60 mL/hr

What is the infusion time for this IV order? _____

3.

Electronic Medical Record   **Provider Orders** ☒

| **Name** B. Patient | **Age** 47 | **Gender** F | **DOB** 10-23-xx |
| **MR #** 5719 | **Allergies** NKDA | | **Room** 422 |

Provider M. Physician, MD   **Date** 2-12-xx ← →

▼ **Order**

Start 1 L 0.9% NaCL @ 80 mL/hr

What is the infusion time for this IV order? _____

Continued

APPLY LEARNED KNOWLEDGE 15-1—cont'd

4.

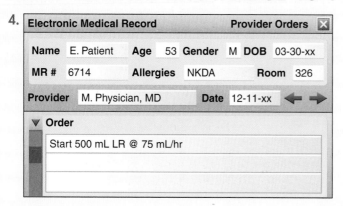

Electronic Medical Record   **Provider Orders** ☒

Name E. Patient	**Age** 53	**Gender** M	**DOB** 03-30-xx
MR # 6714	**Allergies** NKDA		**Room** 326
Provider M. Physician, MD		**Date** 12-11-xx ← →

▼ **Order**

Start 500 mL LR @ 75 mL/hr

What is the infusion time for this IV order? _____

5.

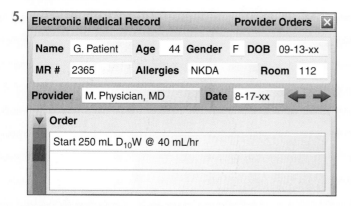

Electronic Medical Record   **Provider Orders** ☒

Name G. Patient	**Age** 44	**Gender** F	**DOB** 09-13-xx
MR # 2365	**Allergies** NKDA		**Room** 112
Provider M. Physician, MD		**Date** 8-17-xx ← →

▼ **Order**

Start 250 mL $D_{10}W$ @ 40 mL/hr

What is the infusion time for this IV order? _____

Military Time

After the nurse calculates the infusion time, the nurse can use military time to solve for the completion time. Military time is used frequently; therefore, it is important to understand how to read and write military time (Table 15-1).

Table 15-1. Comparison of the 24-Hour Clock and the 12-Hour AM–PM Clock

24-HOUR CLOCK—MILITARY TIME	12-HOUR AM–PM CLOCK TIME
Features:	**Features:**
• The use of 0 to 24 to represent the hours of the day	• The use of 12 numbers (1 to 12) to represent morning and evening hours
• The use of 4 digits (i.e., 1230)	• The use of the colon (:) to separate the hours from the minutes (i.e., 12:30)
• The first two digits represent the hours; the last two digits represent the minutes. (i.e., 1230) hours ↑ ↑minutes	hours↑ ↑minutes
• No colon is used to separate the hours and minutes.	• The use of AM to identify before noon. The use of PM to identify after noon
• 2400 represents the end of the day or midnight.	• Day starts at 12:00 AM
• 0000 represents the start of the new day.	• Day ends at 11:59 PM

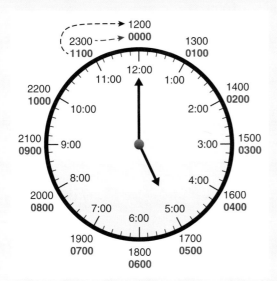

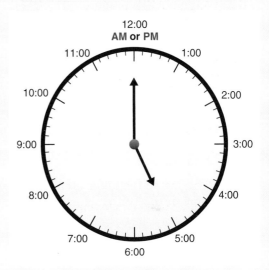

APPLY LEARNED KNOWLEDGE 15-2

Write in the answers to the following problems.

1. Write 3:15 p.m. using military time. _____

2. Write 8:25 a.m. using military time. _____

3. Write 11:30 p.m. using military time. _____

4. Write 1845 using clock time. _____

5. Write 0248 using clock time. _____

Completion Time

Completion time is the clock time (hours and minutes) when the ordered amount of IV fluid is completely infused into the patient. Calculating the completion time is easiest when military time is used to set up and work the problem. To calculate the completion time requires:

■ Identifying the start time of the IV using military time.

■ Adding the infusion time (hours and minutes) to the start time.

For example, the nurse begins a liter of D_5W at 0900 to infuse over 8 hours. What is the completion time of the IV?

Start time: 0900
Add the infusion time: +0800
Completion time: 1700 or 5:00 p.m.

ONLY 24 HOURS IN A DAY

There are only 24 hours in a day. When calculating the completion time, if the answer is equal to or greater than 2400 hours, it is necessary to subtract 2400 from the answer to arrive at the correct completion time. This will identify the hours after midnight or the completion time on the next day.

Example 1:

The nurse begins a liter of 0.9% NS at 2300 to infuse over 10 hours. What is the completion time of the IV?

Start time: 2300
Add the infusion time: +1000
3300 ◄——

Because there are only 24 hours in a day, this time needs to be changed to identify the completion time, which will be on the next day.

> To work the problem when the hours are greater than 24 hours, set up the answer from the problem: 3300
> subtract: −2400
> Completion time: 0900 or 9:00 AM (the next day)

Example 2:

The nurse begins a liter of D_5W at 2200 to infuse over 8 hours. What is the completion time of the IV?

Start time: 2200
Add the infusion time: +0800
3000 ◄——

Because there are only 24 hours in a day, this time needs to be changed to identify the completion time, which will be on the next day.

> To work the problem when the hours are greater than 24 hours, set up the answer from the problem: 3000
> subtract −2400
> **Completion time:** 0600 or 6:00 AM (the next day)

CALCULATING THE COMPLETION TIME

In the previous examples, the infusion time of the IV was identified as " over 10 hours," over "5 hours," and so on. There are times when the IV order identifies the mL/hr (Fig. 15-2). To solve for the completion time, the nurse must first begin by calculating the infusion time.

For example, using the IV order in Figure 15-2, the nurse starts the 500 mL of $D_{10}W$ at 1400. What is the completion time of the IV?

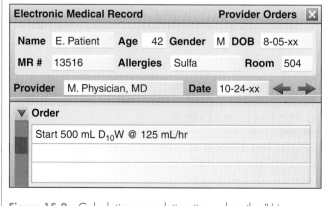

Figure 15-2. Calculating completion time when the IV is ordered in mL/hr.

Linear Ratio & Proportion

First, solve for infusion time.

Known   ::   Unknown

$125 \text{ mL} : 1 \text{ hr} :: 500 \text{ mL} : x \text{ hr}$

$125x = 500$

$$\frac{125x}{125} = \frac{500}{125}$$

$x = 4 \text{ hr}$

Second, calculate the completion time.

Start time: 1400

Add the infusion time: +0400

Completion time: 1800

Dimensional Analysis

First, solve for infusion time.

$$\frac{\text{Ordered}}{\text{Amount}} \times \frac{\text{Conversion}}{\text{Factor}} = \frac{\text{Desired}}{\text{Amount}}$$

$$\frac{500 \text{ mL}}{1} \times \frac{1 \text{ hr}}{125 \text{ mL}} = x \text{ hr}$$

$$\frac{500 \times 1 \text{ hr}}{1 \times 125} = \frac{500}{125} = 4 \text{ hr}$$

Second, calculate the completion time.

Start time: 1400

Add the infusion time: +0400

Completion time: 1800

Fractional Ratio & Proportion

First, solve for infusion time.

Known   =   Unknown

$$\frac{125 \text{ mL}}{1 \text{ hr}} \quad \frac{500 \text{ mL}}{x \text{ hr}}$$

$125x = 500$

$$\frac{125x}{125} = \frac{500}{125}$$

$x = 4 \text{ hr}$

Second, calculate the completion time.

Start time: 1400

Add the infusion time: +0400

Completion time: 1800

Formula: Infusion Time

First, solve for infusion time.

$$\frac{\text{Total volume (mL)}}{\text{Ordered hourly (mL)}} \times 1 \text{ hr} = x \text{ hr}$$

$$\frac{500 \text{ mL}}{125 \text{ mL}} \times 1 \text{ hr} = x \text{ hr}$$

$$\frac{500}{125} \times 1 \text{ hr} = 4 \text{ hr}$$

Second, calculate the completion time.

Start time: 1400

Add the infusion time: +0400

Completion time: 1800

THE COMPLETION TIME INCLUDES THE MINUTES

The start time of an IV includes both hours and minutes, because an IV can be started at any time during the shift. Recall that in writing and reading military time, the last two digits represent the minutes: 1230.

hours ↑ ↑minutes

Look at how the minutes are identified in this example: The nurse begins a liter of lactated Ringer's at 0245 to infuse over 12 hours. What is the completion time of the IV?

Start time: 0245
Add the infusion time: +1200
Completion time: 1445 or 2:45 PM
hours ↑ ↑minutes

ONLY 60 MINUTES IN AN HOUR

There are only 60 minutes in an hour. In calculating the minutes in the completion time, if the answer is equal to or greater than 60 minutes, it is necessary to subtract 60 from the number of minutes and then add the equivalent 1 hour to arrive at the correct completion time.

Example 1:

The nurse begins 500 mL of D_5W at 0345 to infuse over 5 hours 30 minutes. What is the completion time of the IV?

Start time: 0345
Add the infusion time: +0530
Completion time: 0875 ◄——— The minutes are greater than 60.
hours ↑ ↑minutes

To work the problem when the minutes are equal to or greater than 60, set up the:
Answer from the problem: 0875
subtract   −0060 minutes (1 hour)
0815
+0100 (now **add** the **1 hour** obtained from the 60 minutes subtracted)
Completion time: 0915

Example 2:

The nurse begins a liter of 0.45% NS at 1355 to infuse over 8.5 hours. What is the completion time of the IV?

Start time: 1355
Add the infusion time: +0830
Completion time: 2185 ◄——— The minutes are greater than 60.
hours ↑ ↑minutes

To work the problem when the minutes are equal to or greater than 60, set up the:
Answer from the problem: 2185
subtract   −0060 minutes (1 hour)
2125
+0100 (now **add** the **1 hour** obtained from the 60 minutes subtracted)
Completion time: 2225

APPLY LEARNED KNOWLEDGE 15-3

Calculate the completion time for the following problems. Write the answer in military time.

1. The nurse begins 250 mL of 0.9% NS at 0815 to infuse over 3 hours. What is the completion time of the IV?

   _____

2. The IV of 1,000 mL of 0.45% NS is started at 2045 to infuse at 125 mL/hr. What is the completion time of the IV?

   _____

3. A liter of 0.45% NS is started at 0215 to infuse at 75 mL/hr. What is the completion time of the IV?

   _____

4. The nurse begins 500 mL of D_5/0.9% NS at 1145 to infuse over 8.5 hours. What is the completion time of the IV?

   _____

5. The nurse begins 500 mL 0.9% NS at 1515 to infuse over 5 hours. What is the completion time of the IV?

   _____

The Flow Meter Label for Monitoring IV Therapy

Any patient who is receiving intravenous therapy needs to be monitored frequently to ensure that the IV fluid is infusing as ordered. Intravenous fluid may be infused using an infusion pump or by gravity. The infusion pump allows the nurse to set the hourly rate (mL/hr) of the IV, thereby facilitating the exact amount of fluid infused every hour. Information about the use of infusion pumps in IV fluid therapy is found in Chapter 14, IV Therapy and Infusion Rates.

When a patient's IV is infused by gravity, the nurse uses a flow meter to monitor the hourly fluid intake. The flow meter is a long narrow strip of paper that is applied to the IV bag and is used to communicate three important points related to the infusion of an IV:

■ The **start time** of the IV.
■ The **hourly fluid level** based on the mL/hr.
■ The **completion time** or end time of the IV.

In clinical practice, these three points guide the nurse in communicating the status of an IV. For example: 1,000 mL D_5W is started at 1200 (start time) to infuse at 125 mL/hr. At 1400, the IV has 750 mL left (fluid level based on hourly rate). The completion time is calculated as 2000 (based on the start time + infusion time).

COMMERCIAL IV FLOW METERS

Commercial flow meters are available for 500 mL and 1,000 mL IV bags. In working with commercial flow meters, notice how the start time and the end time are identified on the flow meter (Fig. 15-3). On the right outer edge of these flow meters, the line markings identify every 50 mL of fluid. Every 100 mL of fluid is marked with a number (100, 200, 300, etc.). These line markings help the nurse to identify the fluid level based on the mL/hr.

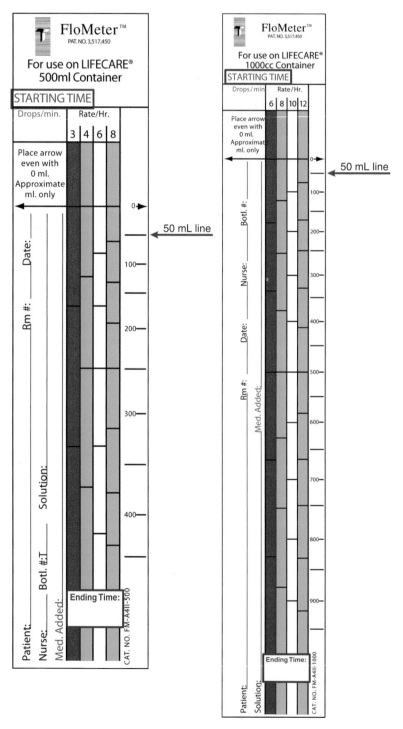

Figure 15-3. Commercial IV flow meters.

THE IV BAG

Intravenous solutions come in a variety sizes. The IV bag provides information about the type and amount of IV solution, expiration date, and numbered line markings that identify every 50 mL or 100 mL depending on the IV bag size (Fig. 15-4).

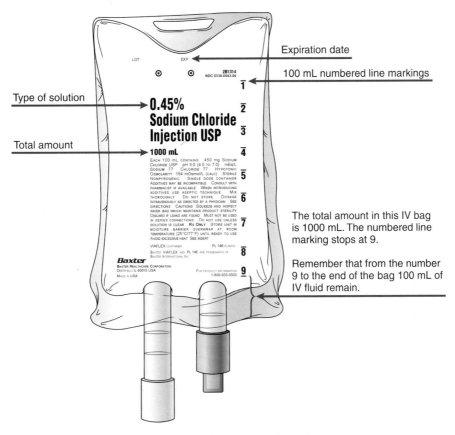

Figure 15-4. Information on the IV bag.

Labeling the Flow Meter Using the mL/hr

To label the flow meter correctly, the nurse must

■ write in the start time of the IV.

■ draw lines from the numbered line markings and enter the military time to identify the fluid level based on the mL/hr.

■ write in the completion/end time of the IV.

The flow meter is then applied to the IV bag so that the numbered line markings on the IV bag (1, 2, 3, etc.) match the numbered line markings from the flow meter (100, 200, 300, etc.) (Fig. 15-5). For example, the nurse starts 500 mL of 0.9% sodium chloride at 1500 to infuse at 100 mL/hr.

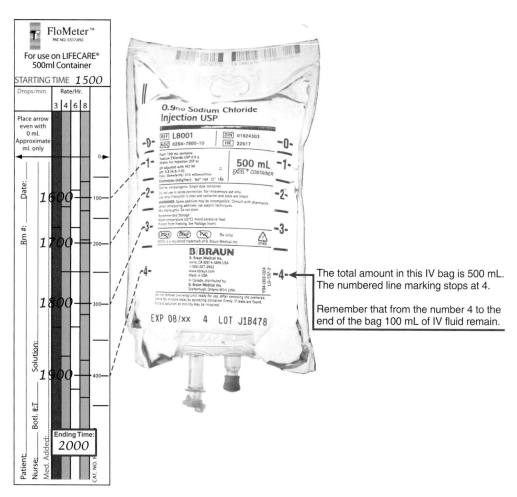

The total amount in this IV bag is 500 mL. The numbered line marking stops at 4.

Remember that from the number 4 to the end of the bag 100 mL of IV fluid remain.

Figure 15-5. 500 mL flow meter labeled and applied to IV bag.

Estimating the Fluid Level

There are times when the ordered mL/hr cannot be measured accurately using the numbered line markings. To effectively complete the flow meter, the nurse will need to estimate the hourly fluid level on the flow meter and then calculate the completion time (Fig. 15-6).

Look at how the flow meter is labeled using this example: The nurse starts 500 mL 0.9% sodium chloride at 0900 to infuse at 75 mL/hr.

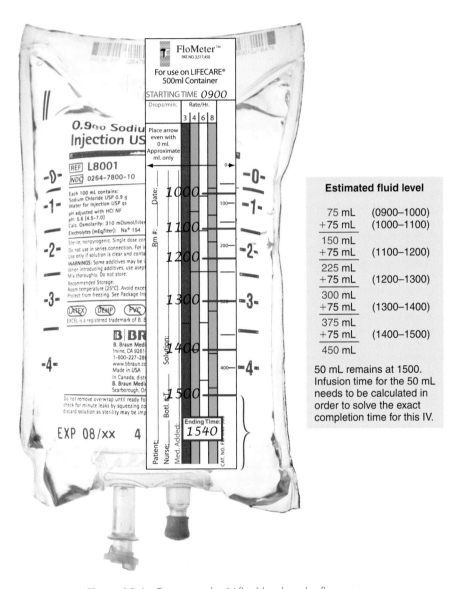

Estimated fluid level

75 mL	(0900–1000)
+75 mL	(1000–1100)
150 mL	
+75 mL	(1100–1200)
225 mL	
+75 mL	(1200–1300)
300 mL	
+75 mL	(1300–1400)
375 mL	
+75 mL	(1400–1500)
450 mL	

50 mL remains at 1500. Infusion time for the 50 mL needs to be calculated in order to solve the exact completion time for this IV.

Figure 15-6. Estimating the IV fluid level on the flow meter.

To solve for the exact completion time, use the ordered mL/hr to calculate the amount of time (in minutes) it will take to infuse the 50 mL that remain in the IV bag.

Linear Ratio & Proportion

First, solve for the time (hr).

Known :: Unknown

75 mL : 1 hr :: 50 mL : x hr

$$75x = 50$$

$$\frac{75x}{75} = \frac{50}{75}$$

$$x = 0.66 \text{ hr}$$

↑ Decimal fraction

Second, convert to minutes.

Known :: Unknown

1 hr : 60 min :: 0.66 hr : x min

$$1x = 39.6$$

$$\frac{1x}{1} = \frac{39.6}{1}$$

$$x = 39.6 \text{ min}$$

Third   Use rounding rules
                    to convert to
                    whole number

Infusion time for the remaining amount
of IV fluid is 40 minutes.

Dimensional Analysis

First

$$\frac{\text{Remaining}}{\text{Amount}} \times \frac{\text{Conversion}}{\text{Factor}} \times \frac{\text{Conversion}}{\text{Factor}} = \frac{\text{Desired}}{\text{Amount}}$$

$$\frac{50 \text{ mL}}{1} \times \frac{1 \text{ hr}}{75 \text{ mL}} \times \frac{60 \text{ min}}{1 \text{ hr}} = x \text{ min}$$

$$\frac{50 \times 1 \times 60 \text{ min}}{1 \times 75 \times 1} = \frac{3000}{75} = 40 \text{ min}$$

Infusion time for the remaining amount
of IV fluid is 40 minutes.

In dimensional analysis, the ordered IV
rate (mL / hr) is one of the conversion
factors used in the problem.

Fractional Ratio & Proportion

First, solve for the time (hr).

Known = Unknown

$$\frac{75 \text{ mL}}{1 \text{ hr}} \bowtie \frac{50 \text{ mL}}{x \text{ hr}}$$

$$75x = 50$$

$$\frac{75x}{75} = \frac{50}{75}$$

$$x = 0.66 \text{ hr}$$
↑Decimal fraction

Second, convert to minutes.

Known = Unknown

$$\frac{60 \text{ min}}{1 \text{ hr}} \bowtie \frac{x \text{ min}}{0.66 \text{ hr}}$$

$$1x = 39.6$$

$$\frac{1x}{1} = \frac{39.6}{1}$$

$$x = 39.6 \text{ min}$$

Third ↑ Use rounding rules to convert to whole number

Infusion time for the remaining amount of IV fluid is 40 minutes.

Formula: Infusion Time

First, solve for the time (hr).

$$\frac{\text{Total volume (mL)}}{\text{Ordered hourly (mL)}} \times 1 \text{ hr} = x \text{ hr}$$

$$\frac{50 \text{ mL}}{75 \text{ mL}} \times 1 \text{ hr} = x \text{ hr}$$

$$\frac{50}{75} \times 1 \text{ hr} = 0.66 \text{ hr}$$
↑ Decimal fraction

Second, convert to minutes.

$$\frac{0.66 \text{ hr}}{1 \text{ hr}} \times 60 \text{ min} = x \text{ min}$$

$$\frac{0.66}{1} \times 60 \text{ min} = 39.6 \text{ min}$$

Third ↑ Use rounding rules to convert to whole number

Infusion time for the remaining amount of IV fluid is 40 minutes.

Additional Numbered Line Markings on the Flow Meter

Both the 1000 mL and the 500 mL flow meters have additional line markings to guide in identifying the hourly fluid level for commonly ordered infusion times. Notice the line markings under the numbers of 6, 8, 10, and 12 hours in the 1000 mL flow meter. These line markings can be used to readily mark the hourly fluid level based on the infusion times of 6 hours, 8 hours, 10 hours, and 12 hours (Fig. 15-7).

An IV 1000 mL of D₅W was started at 1200 to infuse over 8 hours.

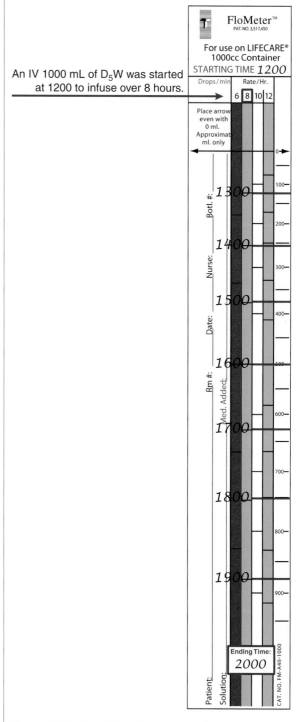

Figure 15-7. Use of the 8-hour line marking on the 1000 mL.

There may be times when a commercial flow meter is not available. The nurse may use a piece of tape and write the same information as found on a commercial flow meter. The tape is then attached to the IV bag (Fig. 15-8).

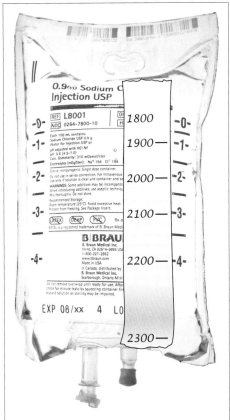

Figure 15-8. Use of tape as a flow meter: start time, 100 mL hourly markings, end time.

The flow meter, whether a commercial flow meter or the use of tape as a flow meter, serves as a communication tool that assists all licensed health-care providers to monitor and maintain the IV fluid therapy for the patient.

APPLY LEARNED KNOWLEDGE 15-4

Complete the flow meter with the start time, the hourly fluid level time based on the mL/hr, and the completion time for the following three flow meter problems.

1. 1 liter D$_5$W is started at 100 mL/hr at 1000.

2. 500 mL 0.9% NS is started at 125 mL/hr at 1400.

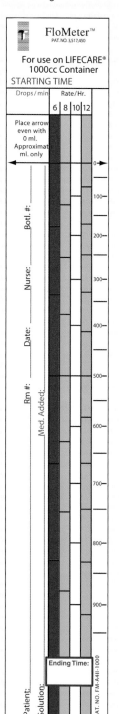

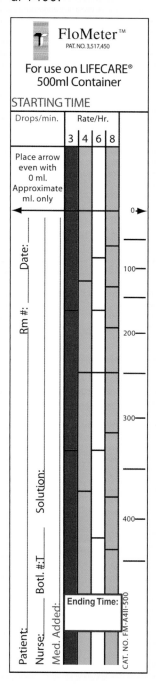

APPLY LEARNED KNOWLEDGE 15-4—cont'd

3. 1 L LR is started at 150 mL/hr at 2000.

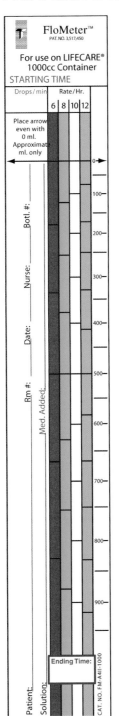

4. A 1 liter IV is to infuse at 75 mL/hr. What is the infusion time?

_____

5. A 1 liter IV is started at 2200 to infuse at 75 mL/hr. What is the completion time?

_____

Reading the Amount of IV Fluid Infused

As IV fluid infuses into a patient, the line markings on the IV bag provide information (Fig. 15-9) that show:

- how much fluid has infused.
- how much fluid remains **(remaining amount)** in the bag.

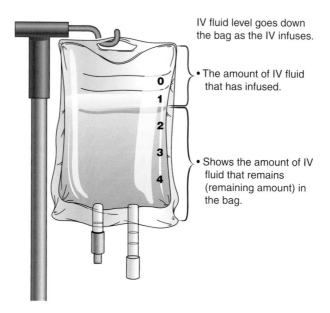

Figure 15-9. IV bag showing infused amount and remaining amount of IV fluid.

Reading the flow meter provides the same information and helps the nurse to determine how much IV fluid has infused into the patient during the shift and how much IV fluid remains at a specific time. Look at the following two examples (Fig. 15-10). The IV order is to infuse 500 mL at 125 mL/hr.

The infused amount will be recorded as part of the parenteral intake for the shift and the remaining amount will be used to inform the next nurse how much fluid is left in the IV bag.

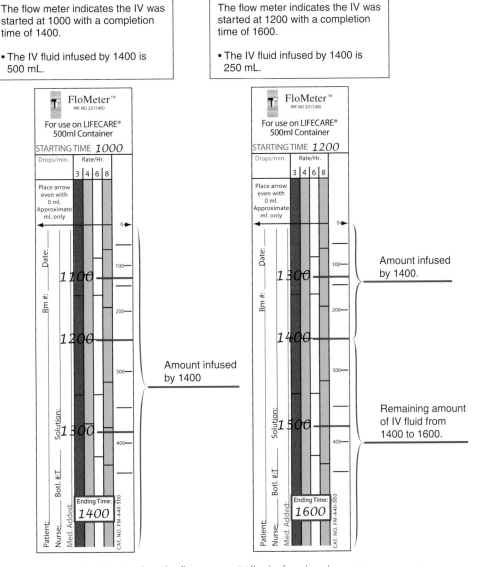

Figure 15-10. Reading the flow meter: IV fluid infused and remaining amount.

 CLINICAL REASONING 15-1
The physician orders 1 liter lactated Ringer's to infuse at 80 mL/hr. The night nurse starts the IV at 0100 and completes the flow meter. On checking the IV at 0800, the day nurse notices a completion time of 1230 on the flow meter. The day nurse decides to continue monitoring the IV as indicated on the flow meter. Is the nurse's decision correct?

The care of patients who are receiving intravenous therapy is common practice in the acute care setting. Every nurse must know how to calculate infusion and completion times of an IV, read a flow meter, and evaluate the accuracy of the information on a flow meter. This will help to ensure the timely delivery of IV fluids and assist in communicating the IV fluid needs of each patient.

Developing Competency

Answer the following IV problems using the Provider Orders.

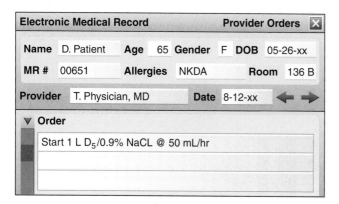

Electronic Medical Record   **Provider Orders** ☒

Name D. Patient   **Age** 65 **Gender** F **DOB** 05-26-xx

MR # 00651   **Allergies** NKDA   **Room** 136 B

Provider T. Physician, MD   **Date** 8-12-xx ⬅ ➡

▼ **Order**

Start 1 L D$_5$/0.9% NaCL @ 50 mL/hr

1. What is the infusion time for this IV order? _____

2. The nurse starts this IV at 2300. What is the completion time? _____

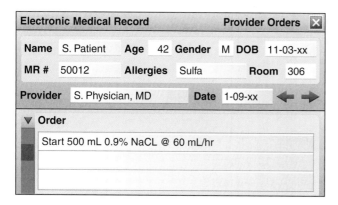

Electronic Medical Record   **Provider Orders** ☒

Name S. Patient   **Age** 42 **Gender** M **DOB** 11-03-xx

MR # 50012   **Allergies** Sulfa   **Room** 306

Provider S. Physician, MD   **Date** 1-09-xx ⬅ ➡

▼ **Order**

Start 500 mL 0.9% NaCL @ 60 mL/hr

3. What is the infusion time for this IV order? _____

4. The nurse starts this IV at 0700. What is the completion time? _____

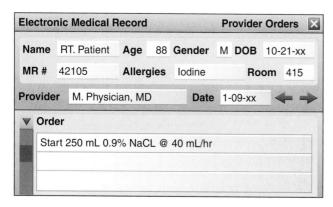

Electronic Medical Record   **Provider Orders** ☒

Name RT. Patient   **Age** 88 **Gender** M **DOB** 10-21-xx

MR # 42105   **Allergies** Iodine   **Room** 415

Provider M. Physician, MD   **Date** 1-09-xx ⬅ ➡

▼ **Order**

Start 250 mL 0.9% NaCL @ 40 mL/hr

5. What is the infusion time for this IV order? _____

6. The nurse starts this IV at 0230. What is the completion time? _____

Determine the correct answer.

7. 5:30 p.m. written in military time is _____

8. 2145 written in clock time is _____

Circle the correct answer.

9. The nurse begins 1 liter of D$_5$W at 0900 at 125 mL/hr. By 1400, the nurse is correct to report that <u>575 mL,</u> <u>625 mL,</u> or <u>700 mL</u> has infused into the patient.

10. The nurse hangs 1 liter of D5/0.9% NS at 1800 to infuse at 75 mL/hr. By 2200, the nurse is correct to report that <u>300 mL,</u> <u>375 mL,</u> or <u>425 mL</u> of IV fluid has infused.

11. The nurse hangs 500 mL of D5/0.45% NS at 1500 to infuse at 50 mL/hr. By 2200, the nurse is correct to report that <u>250 mL,</u> <u>350 mL,</u> or <u>400 mL</u> of IV fluid has infused.

12. The nurse starts 1 liter of lactated Ringer's at 2300 at 75 mL/hr. By 0600, the nurse expects the remaining amount of IV fluid to be <u>400 mL,</u> <u>475 mL,</u> or <u>525 mL.</u>

13. The nurse hangs 1 liter of lactated Ringer's at 0000 at 85 mL/hr. By 0500, the nurse expects the remaining amount of IV fluid to be <u>425 mL,</u> <u>500 mL,</u> or <u>575 mL.</u>

14. The physician orders 1 liter of 0.9% NS q.10h. The nurse starts the first liter at 0700. If the IV infuses as ordered, the nurse can expect the remaining amount of IV fluid at 1400 to be <u>300 mL,</u> <u>500 mL,</u> or <u>700 mL.</u>

Evaluate the following flow meters. Select the answer that correctly identifies the error in the flow meter.

15.

Order: Infuse 500 mL at 125 mL/hr.

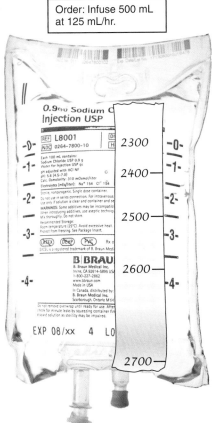

The flow meter is:
a. missing the start time.
b. missing the end time.
c. incorrect hourly marking.

16.

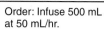

Order: Infuse 500 mL at 50 mL/hr.

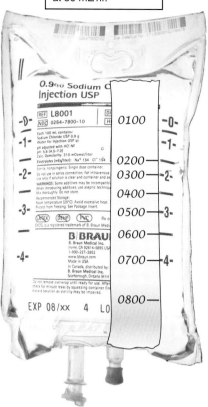

The flow meter is:
a. missing the start time.
b. missing the end time.
c. incorrect hourly marking.

17.

Order: Infuse 500 mL at 150 mL/hr.

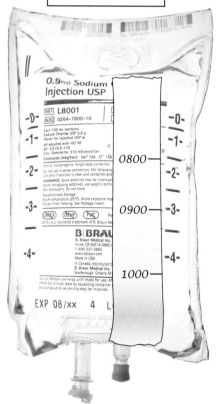

The flow meter is:
a. missing the start time.
b. missing the end time.
c. incorrect hourly marking.

18. The physician orders 500 mL IV to infuse at 63 mL/hr. The nurse starts the IV at 0130 and completes the flow meter with the start time, the hourly fluid level based on the mL/hr, and end time.

FloMeter™
PAT. NO. 3,517,450

For use on LIFECARE®
500ml Container

STARTING TIME 0130

Drops/min.	Rate/Hr.			
	3	4	6	8

Place arrow even with 0 ml. Approximate ml. only

Date: ___
Rm #: ___

0 →

0230

100—

0330

0430

200—

0530

300—

0630

0730

400—

0830

Solution: ___
Bottl. #:1

Ending Time:
0926

Patient: ___
Nurse: ___
Med. Added: ___

CAT. NO. FM-A4II-500

Select all the answers that apply to the flow meter.

a. The hourly fluid level is marked correctly.
b. The end time is correct.
c. The infusion time is 7 hours.
d. The end time should be 0826.
e. By 0730, approximately 375 mL have infused.

Complete the flow meter with the start time, the hourly time, and the completion time.

19. 1 liter D₅W is started at 150 mL/hr at 1830.

20. 1,000 mL 0.9% NaCl is started at 125 mL/hr at 1345.

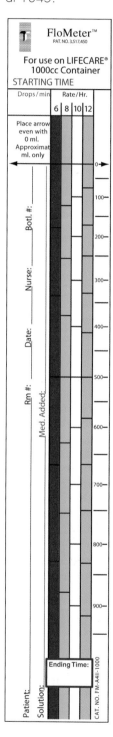

CHAPTER 16

Administering Direct IV Medications

LEARNING OUTCOMES

Interpret drug reference information about dilution and rate of administration of direct IV medications.

Calculate the amount of diluent to add to direct IV medications.

Calculate the rate of administration of direct IV medications.

When medications are administered by the direct IV route, the dose of medication is injected directly into a vein where it is absorbed and begins to act immediately. The sudden high concentration of the IV drug in the bloodstream is beneficial to the patient, but can also pose potential safety risks, as any adverse effects will appear immediately. To ensure patient safety, the nurse must be vigilant in the assessment of both the therapeutic and the adverse effects during and after the direct IV administration of the medication.

As with any medication, the physician orders the drug, dose, route, and time or frequency of administration of a direct IV medication. In addition to the usual practices for safe medication administration, to correctly implement the direct IV order the nurse needs to know:

- any recommended instructions for dilution of the medication
- the rate of administration for the direct IV medication

Drug Reference Information About Direct IV Medications

Most drug references include a special section on dilution and rate of administration for direct IV medications. The direct IV route can be worded in many ways and must not be confused with IV medications administered by continuous or intermittent infusion (Table 16-1).

Although drug references use a variety of terms to refer to the direct IV route, most physicians order direct IV medications using the terms "IV Push" or "IVP."

Table 16-1. Terms That Indicate the Direct IV Route Versus IV Infusion

DIRECT IV	IV INFUSION
Direct IV	Infusion
IV injection	IV infusion
Direct IV injection	Intermittent infusion
IV push	Continuous infusion
IVP	
IV bolus	
Bolus injection	

Dilution of Medications Given by Direct IV Route

Medications given by the direct IV route can be given diluted or undiluted. The primary purpose for dilution is to make the medication less irritating to the vein. The **dilution** of any direct IV medication is determined by the drug manufacturer. Before administering any direct IV medication, the nurse must check the package insert, drug reference, and/or institutional policies regarding dilution of the drug.

DIRECT IV MEDICATIONS ADMINISTERED UNDILUTED

Some medications given by the direct IV route can be administered without adding any **diluent.** Notice how the sample drug references in Figure 16-1 clearly state when a direct IV medication is to be given undiluted.

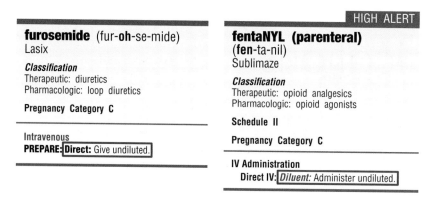

Figure 16-1. Direct IV medications that are administered undiluted.

When a direct IV medication is to be administered undiluted, the nurse calculates the dosage to be given (as with any medication), then draws up that amount in the syringe and administers it to the patient. There is no additional math calculation needed.

DIRECT IV MEDICATIONS DILUTED PRIOR TO ADMINISTRATION

If an IV medication is to be diluted prior to administration, a specified amount and type of diluent is added to the dose of medication in the syringe. The most common diluent solutions are normal saline and sterile water for injection, although other solutions are sometimes recommended. Instructions for dilution can be grouped into four main categories that specify:

1. A specific volume of diluent to be added to the medication
2. Dilution with an equal volume of drug and diluent
3. A concentration for the diluted medication
4. Dilution instructions based on diagnosis, age, or weight

Each of these four categories of dilution are discussed separately.

Regardless of the type of dilution instructions, the nurse first calculates the ordered drug dosage, and then calculates the amount of diluent needed. To draw up the medication, the nurse follows the following procedure:

1. Add air to the diluent vial.
2. Add air to the medication vial.
3. Draw up the correct amount of medication into the syringe.
4. Draw up the correct amount of diluent into the syringe (Fig. 16-2).

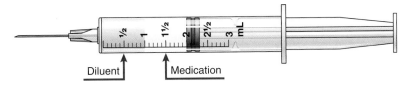

Diluent   Medication

Figure 16-2. Dilution of medication in a syringe.

Dilution Instructions: Adding a Specific Volume of Diluent

Drug references may specify that regardless of the dose of medication ordered, a specific volume of diluent is to be added to the medication (Fig. 16-3).

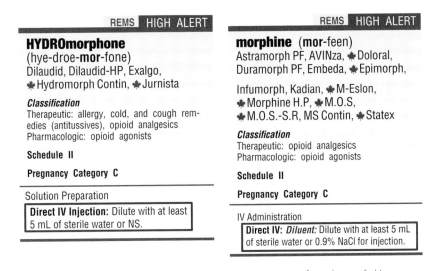

Figure 16-3. Direct IV medications that require a specific volume of diluent.

The direct IV information indicates that hydromorphone and morphine need to be diluted with 5 mL of sterile water or normal saline prior to administration by the direct IV route. The volume of diluent does not depend on the dose of medication ordered. For example, if the physician ordered either 0.75 mg, 1 mg, or 1.5 mg of hydromorphone, the nurse would calculate the ordered dosage, draw up the medication, and then add 5 mL of diluent to the syringe.

Dilution Instructions: Adding an Equal Volume of Diluent

Drug reference information may specify that the direct IV medication be diluted in a volume of diluent that is equal to the volume of medication in the syringe. Look at the example in Figure 16-4 that shows dilution instructions for lorazepam.

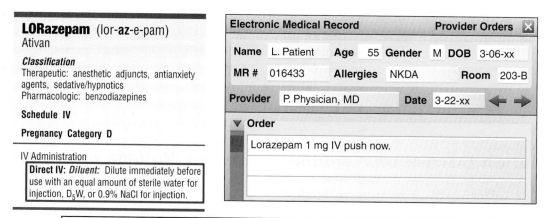

LORazepam (lor-az-e-pam)
Ativan

Classification
Therapeutic: anesthetic adjuncts, antianxiety agents, sedative/hypnotics
Pharmacologic: benzodiazepines

Schedule IV

Pregnancy Category D

IV Administration
Direct IV: *Diluent:* Dilute immediately before use with an equal amount of sterile water for injection, D₅W, or 0.9% NaCl for injection.

Electronic Medical Record	Provider Orders ☒
Name L. Patient Age 55 Gender M DOB 3-06-xx	
MR # 016433 Allergies NKDA Room 203-B	
Provider P. Physician, MD Date 3-22-xx ⬅ ➡	
▼ Order	
Lorazepam 1 mg IV push now.	

Lorazepam 2 mg/mL is available from the pharmacy.
How much diluent would the nurse add to the medication in the syringe?

Figure 16-4. Direct IV medication requiring an equal volume of drug and diluent.

In the example above, the nurse must first calculate the dosage to be administered. Using the dosage strength of lorazepam 2 mg/mL, the nurse calculates that 1 mg of lorazepam is contained in 0.5 mL. Once the dosage has been calculated, the nurse would draw up the 0.5 mL of medication into the syringe. Next, the nurse would draw up an equal amount of diluent (0.5 mL). The total volume in the syringe would be 1 mL.

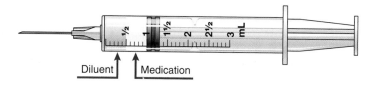

Diluent↑   Medication↑

Dilution Instructions: Direct IV Medication Written as a Concentration

A dilution can also be written as a ***concentration.*** Concentration specifies the amount of medication present in a solution. In drug references, concentration is expressed as a ratio: the first number is the amount of medication and the second number is the total volume of solution in the syringe (medication + diluent). See the example of dilution instructions in Figure 16-5.

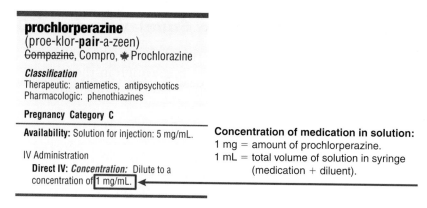

prochlorperazine
(proe-klor-**pair**-a-zeen)
~~Compazine~~, Compro, ✳ Prochlorazine

Classification
Therapeutic: antiemetics, antipsychotics
Pharmacologic: phenothiazines

Pregnancy Category C

Availability: Solution for injection: 5 mg/mL.

IV Administration
Direct IV: *Concentration:* Dilute to a concentration of 1 mg/mL.

Concentration of medication in solution:
1 mg = amount of prochlorperazine.
1 mL = total volume of solution in syringe (medication + diluent).

Figure 16-5. Direct IV medication in which dilution is expressed as a concentration.

The ordered dose of medication needs to be diluted so that the solution has a concentration of 1 mg/1 mL, that is, 1 mg of prochlorperazine for each mL of solution in the syringe (prochlorperazine + diluent). Notice that the drug reference does not indicate the volume of diluent to add to make the recommended concentration. This has to be calculated.

Calculations Needed When a Concentration Is Recommended

When dilution is written as a concentration, the nurse must calculate the volume of diluent to add to make the recommended concentration. Look at the following three examples of how to determine the volume of diluent to add for the ordered amount.

Example 1:

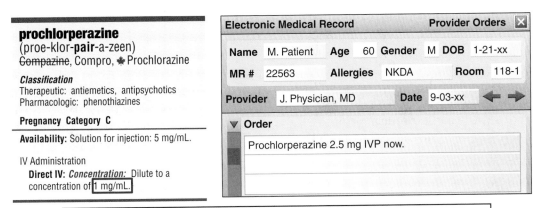

prochlorperazine
(proe-klor-**pair**-a-zeen)
~~Compazine~~, Compro, ✹ Prochlorazine

Classification
Therapeutic: antiemetics, antipsychotics
Pharmacologic: phenothiazines

Pregnancy Category C

Availability: Solution for injection: 5 mg/mL.

IV Administration
  Direct IV: *Concentration:* Dilute to a
  concentration of 1 mg/mL.

Electronic Medical Record		Provider Orders ☒
Name M. Patient	**Age** 60 **Gender** M	**DOB** 1-21-xx
MR # 22563	**Allergies** NKDA	**Room** 118-1
Provider J. Physician, MD	**Date** 9-03-xx	⬅ ➡

▼ **Order**

Prochlorperazine 2.5 mg IVP now.

Prochlorperazine 5 mg/mL is available from the pharmacy.
How much diluent would the nurse add to make a concentration of 1 mg/mL?

The physician's order is for 2.5 mg of prochlorperazine, and the available dosage strength of the medication is 5 mg/mL. The nurse calculates the dosage to be administered (2.5 mg is contained in 0.5 mL) and draws up 0.5 mL of prochlorperazine into the syringe. Next, the volume of diluent to add to make the concentration is calculated:

■ First, calculate the total volume of solution in the syringe (medication + diluent). To solve, set up the problem using the

  • concentration identified from the drug reference.
  • ordered dose from the physician's order.

■ Second, subtract the volume of the ordered medication from the total volume of solution in the syringe. The difference is the volume of diluent to add to the syringe.

The first calculation can be done using the ratio and proportion method or dimensional analysis. The formula $\dfrac{D}{H} \times Q = x$ cannot be used for dilution calculations. An alternate formula can be used:

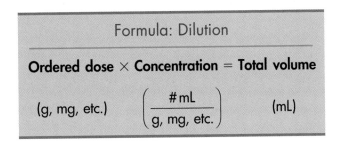

Formula: Dilution

$$\text{Ordered dose} \times \text{Concentration} = \text{Total volume}$$

(g, mg, etc.) $\left(\dfrac{\# \, mL}{g, \, mg, \, etc.} \right)$ (mL)

Here is how to solve the problem:

Linear Ratio & Proportion

First

$$\text{Known} :: \text{Unknown}$$

(concentration)   (ordered dose : total volume)

$$1 \text{ mg} : 1 \text{ mL} :: 2.5 \text{ mg} : x \text{ mL}$$

$$1x = 2.5$$

$$\frac{1x}{1} = \frac{2.5}{1}$$

$$x = 2.5 \text{ mL}$$

Second

$$\begin{array}{r} 2.5 \text{ mL (total volume in syringe)} \\ - 0.5 \text{ mL (volume of medication)} \\ \hline 2 \text{ mL (volume of diluent)} \end{array}$$

Dimensional Analysis

First

Ordered Amount	× Concentration =	Desired Amount (total volume)

$$\frac{2.5 \text{ mg}}{1} \times \frac{1 \text{ mL}}{1 \text{ mg}} = x \text{ mL}$$

$$\frac{2.5 \times 1 \text{ mL}}{1 \times 1} = \frac{2.5 \text{ mL}}{1} = 2.5 \text{ mL}$$

Second

$$\begin{array}{r} 2.5 \text{ mL (total volume in syringe)} \\ - 0.5 \text{ mL (volume of medication)} \\ \hline 2 \text{ mL (volume of diluent)} \end{array}$$

Fractional Ratio & Proportion

First

$$\text{Known} = \text{Unknown}$$

(concentration)   (ordered dose/total volume)

$$\frac{1 \text{ mg}}{1 \text{ mL}} \diagdown\diagup \frac{2.5 \text{ mg}}{x \text{ ml}} \begin{array}{l} \text{(ordered dose)} \\ \text{(total volume)} \end{array}$$

$$1x = 2.5$$

$$\frac{1x}{1} = \frac{2.5}{1}$$

$$x = 2.5 \text{ mL}$$

Second

$$\begin{array}{r} 2.5 \text{ mL (total volume in syringe)} \\ - 0.5 \text{ mL (volume of medication)} \\ \hline 2 \text{ mL (volume of diluent)} \end{array}$$

Formula: Dilution

First

Ordered dose × Concentration = Total volume

$$\text{(g, mg, etc.)} \quad \left(\frac{\# \text{mL}}{\text{g, mg, etc.}} \right) \quad \text{(mL)}$$

$$2.5 \text{ mg} \times \frac{1 \text{ mL}}{1 \text{ mg}} = x \text{ mL}$$

$$\frac{2.5 \text{ mg}}{1} \times \frac{1 \text{ mL}}{1 \text{ mg}} = x \text{ mL}$$

$$\frac{2.5}{1} = 2.5 \text{ mL}$$

Second

$$\begin{array}{r} 2.5 \text{ mL (total volume in syringe)} \\ - 0.5 \text{ mL (volume of medication)} \\ \hline 2 \text{ mL (volume of diluent)} \end{array}$$

The nurse adds 2 mL of diluent to the 0.5 mL of prochlorperazine in the syringe. The concentration is then the recommended 1 mg/mL (2.5 mg of prochlorperazine in 2.5 mL of solution).

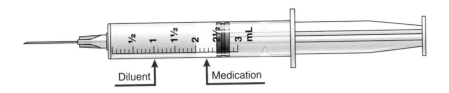

Diluent   Medication

⚠️ *The nurse must be careful to differentiate between the available dosage strength of the medication and the dilution concentration recommended in the drug reference.*

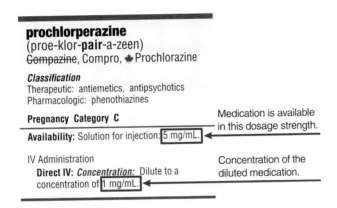

prochlorperazine
(proe-klor-**pair**-a-zeen)
~~Compazine~~, Compro, ✽Prochlorazine

Classification
Therapeutic: antiemetics, antipsychotics
Pharmacologic: phenothiazines

Pregnancy Category C

Availability: Solution for injection: 5 mg/mL.

Medication is available in this dosage strength.

IV Administration
   Direct IV: *Concentration:* Dilute to a concentration of 1 mg/mL.

Concentration of the diluted medication.

Example 2:

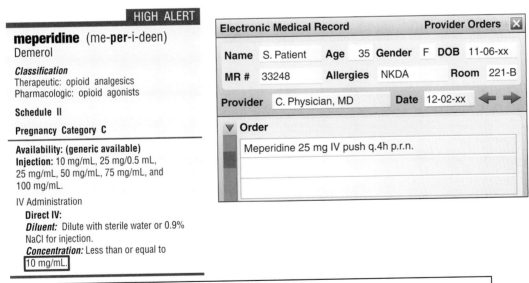

HIGH ALERT

meperidine (me-**per**-i-deen)
Demerol

Classification
Therapeutic: opioid analgesics
Pharmacologic: opioid agonists

Schedule II

Pregnancy Category C

Availability: (generic available)
Injection: 10 mg/mL, 25 mg/0.5 mL, 25 mg/mL, 50 mg/mL, 75 mg/mL, and 100 mg/mL.
IV Administration
   Direct IV:
   Diluent: Dilute with sterile water or 0.9% NaCl for injection.
   Concentration: Less than or equal to 10 mg/mL.

Electronic Medical Record   Provider Orders ☒

Name S. Patient   **Age** 35 **Gender** F **DOB** 11-06-xx

MR # 33248   **Allergies** NKDA   **Room** 221-B

Provider C. Physician, MD   **Date** 12-02-xx ⬅️ ➡️

▼ **Order**

Meperidine 25 mg IV push q.4h p.r.n.

Meperidine 25 mg/mL is available from the pharmacy.
How much diluent would the nurse add to make a concentration of 10 mg/mL?

The physician's order is for 25 mg of meperidine, and the dosage strength of meperidine 25 mg/mL is available. The nurse calculates the volume of medication to be administered (25 mg is contained in 1 mL). Notice how this volume of medication (1 mL) is subtracted from the total volume to arrive at the amount of diluent.

Linear Ratio & Proportion

First

Known :: Unknown

(concentration)   (ordered dose : total volume)

10 mg : 1 mL :: 25 mg : x mL

$$10x = 25$$

$$\frac{10x}{10} = \frac{25}{10}$$

$$x = 2.5 \text{ mL}$$

Second

2.5 mL (total volume in syringe)

$\underline{- 1 \text{ mL}}$ (volume of medication)

1.5 mL (volume of diluent)

Dimensional Analysis

First

$\begin{array}{c}\text{Ordered} \\ \text{Amount}\end{array} \times \text{Concentration} = \begin{array}{c}\text{Desired} \\ \text{Amount} \\ \text{(total volume)}\end{array}$

$$\frac{25 \text{ mg}}{1} \times \frac{1 \text{ mL}}{10 \text{ mg}} = x \text{ mL}$$

$$\frac{25 \times 1 \text{ mL}}{1 \times 10} = \frac{25 \text{ mL}}{10} = 2.5 \text{ mL}$$

Second

2.5 mL (total volume in syringe)

$\underline{- 1 \text{ mL}}$ (volume of medication)

1.5 mL (volume of diluent)

Fractional Ratio & Proportion

First

Known = Unknown

(concentration)   (ordered dose/total volume)

$$\frac{10 \text{ mg}}{1 \text{ mL}} \underset{\nwarrow}{\searrow} \frac{25 \text{ mg}}{x \text{ mL}} \begin{array}{l}\text{(ordered dose)} \\ \text{(total volume)}\end{array}$$

$$10x = 25$$

$$\frac{10x}{10} = \frac{25}{10}$$

$$x = 2.5 \text{ mL}$$

Second

2.5 mL (total volume in syringe)

$\underline{- 1 \text{ mL}}$ (volume of medication)

1.5 mL (volume of diluent)

Formula: Dilution

First

Ordered dose $\times$ Concentration = Total volume

(g, mg, etc.) $\left(\dfrac{\# \text{mL}}{\text{g, mg, etc.}}\right)$ (mL)

$$25 \text{ mg} \times \frac{1 \text{ mL}}{10 \text{ mg}} = x \text{ mL}$$

$$\frac{25 \text{ mg}}{1} \times \frac{1 \text{ mL}}{10 \text{ mg}} = x \text{ mL}$$

$$\frac{25}{10} = 2.5 \text{ mL}$$

Second

2.5 mL (total volume in syringe)

$\underline{- 1 \text{ mL}}$ (volume of medication)

1.5 mL (volume of diluent)

The nurse would add 1.5 mL of diluent to the 1 mL of meperidine in the syringe.

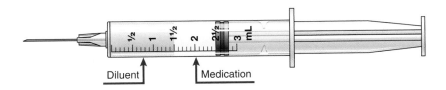

Example 3:

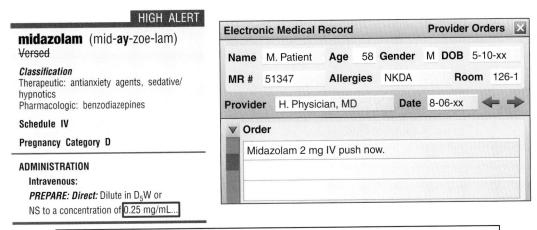

Using the dosage strength of midazolam 5 mg/mL, the nurse calculates the volume of medication to be administered (2 mg is contained in 0.4 mL). Notice how this volume of medication (0.4 mL) is subtracted from the total volume to arrive at the amount of diluent.

Linear Ratio & Proportion

First

$$\text{Known} :: \text{Unknown}$$

(concentration)   (ordered dose : total volume)

$$0.25 \text{ mg} : 1 \text{ mL} :: 2 \text{ mg} : x \text{ mL}$$

$$0.25x = 2$$

$$\frac{0.25x}{0.25} = \frac{2}{0.25}$$

$$x = 8 \text{ mL}$$

Second

$$8 \text{ mL (total volume in syringe)}$$
$$\underline{- 0.4 \text{ mL}} \text{ (volume of medication)}$$
$$7.6 \text{ mL (volume of diluent)}$$

Dimensional Analysis

First

$$\begin{array}{c}\text{Ordered} \\ \text{Amount}\end{array} \times \text{Concentration} = \begin{array}{c}\text{Desired} \\ \text{Amount} \\ \text{(total volume)}\end{array}$$

$$\frac{2 \text{ mg}}{1} \times \frac{1 \text{ mL}}{0.25 \text{ mg}} = x \text{ mL}$$

$$\frac{2 \times 1 \text{ mL}}{1 \times 0.25} = \frac{2 \text{ mL}}{0.25} = 8 \text{ mL}$$

Second

$$8 \text{ mL (total volume in syringe)}$$
$$\underline{- 0.4 \text{ mL}} \text{ (volume of medication)}$$
$$7.6 \text{ mL (volume of diluent)}$$

Fractional Ratio & Proportion

First

$$\text{Known} = \text{Unknown}$$

(concentration)   (ordered dose : total volume)

$$\frac{0.25 \text{ mg}}{1 \text{ mL}} \diagup\!\!\!\diagdown \frac{2 \text{ mg}}{x \text{ mL}} \begin{array}{l}\text{(ordered dose)} \\ \text{(total volume)}\end{array}$$

$$0.25x = 2$$

$$\frac{0.25x}{0.25} = \frac{2}{0.25}$$

$$x = 8 \text{ mL}$$

Second

$$8 \text{ mL (total volume in syringe)}$$
$$\underline{- 0.4 \text{ mL}} \text{ (volume of medication)}$$
$$7.6 \text{ mL (volume of diluent)}$$

Formula: Dilution

First

Ordered dose × Concentration = Total volume

(g, mg, etc.) $\left(\dfrac{\# \text{ mL}}{\text{g, mg, etc.}} \right)$ (mL)

$$2 \text{ mg} \times \frac{1 \text{ mL}}{0.25 \text{ mg}} = x \text{ mL}$$

$$\frac{2 \text{ mg}}{1} \times \frac{1 \text{ mL}}{0.25 \text{ mg}} = x \text{ mL}$$

$$\frac{2}{0.25} = 8 \text{ mL}$$

Second

$$8 \text{ mL (total volume in syringe)}$$
$$\underline{- 0.4 \text{ mL}} \text{ (volume of medication)}$$
$$7.6 \text{ mL (volume of diluent)}$$

The nurse would add 7.6 mL of diluent to the midazolam in the syringe.

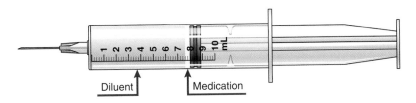

Dilution Instructions Based on Diagnosis, Age, or Weight

Instructions for dilution can vary based on factors specific to the individual patient. For example, the same medication may be given undiluted for one diagnostic indication and diluted if the drug is given for a different diagnosis. Sometimes the age or weight of the patient will determine if the direct IV medication is to be diluted or how much diluent to add. Look at the examples in Figure 16-6.

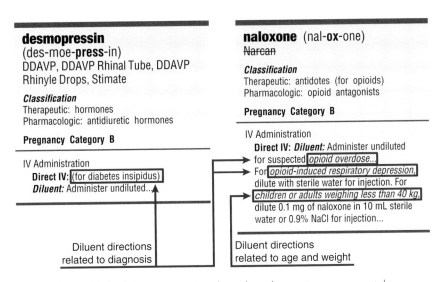

Figure 16-6. Dilution instructions based on diagnosis, age, or weight.

For example, if a patient has a suspected opioid overdose, a direct IV dose of naloxone would be administered undiluted. If the patient has opioid-induced respiratory depression, the direct IV dose of naloxone would be diluted with sterile water for injection or 0.9% NaCl for injection. The nurse has to carefully read the drug reference information for the specific dilution instructions related to the patient's diagnosis, age, weight, and clinical condition.

APPLY LEARNED KNOWLEDGE 16-1

Calculate the correct amount of diluent to add to the following medications.

1. *Order:* Lorazepam 2 mg direct IV q.12h prn.
   Available dosage strength: 2 mg/mL
   Drug reference information: **Direct IV: Diluent:** Dilute immediately before use with an equal amount of sterile water for injection, D_5W, or 0.9% NaCl for injection.

   _____

2. *Order:* Midazolam 2 mg direct IV now
   Available dosage strength: 1 mg/1 mL
   Drug reference information: **midazolam** (mid-**ay**-zoe-lam), **High Alert,** **Intravenous: PREPARE: Direct:** Dilute in D_5W or NS to a concentration of 0.25 mg/mL.

   _____

3. *Order:* Famotidine 20 mg direct IV q.12h
   Available dosage strength: 10 mg/mL
   Drug reference information: **Direct IV: Concentration:** Dilute to a concentration of 4 mg/mL.

   _____

4. *Order:* Prochlorperazine 2.5 mg direct IV now.
   Available dosage strength: 5 mg/mL
   Drug reference information: **Direct IV: Concentration:** Dilute to a concentration of 1 mg/mL.

   _____

5. *Order:* DiphenhydrAMINE 25 mg direct IV now.
   Available dosage strength: 50 mg/mL
   Drug reference information: **Direct IV: Diluent:** May be further diluted in 0.9% NaCl, 0.45% NaCl, D_5W, D10W, dextrose/saline combinations, Ringer's solution, LR, and dextrose/Ringer's combinations. **Concentration:** 25 mg/mL.

   _____

Rate of Administration for Direct IV Medications

In addition to knowing how to read and interpret instructions for dilution of direct IV medications, the nurse also needs to know the specific rate of administration for the ordered drug. Medications administered by the direct IV route are given over seconds or minutes. How quickly the direct IV medication is injected can affect the onset of therapeutic effects as well as any adverse effects of the medication. For this reason, each direct IV medication has its own optimal *rate of administration.* This is not something that the physician orders or the nurse estimates; rather, the rate of administration is researched for each direct IV drug administered. See Figure 16-7 for examples of rate of administration found in the drug reference. Notice that certain direct IV medications can have adverse effects if administered too slowly or too rapidly.

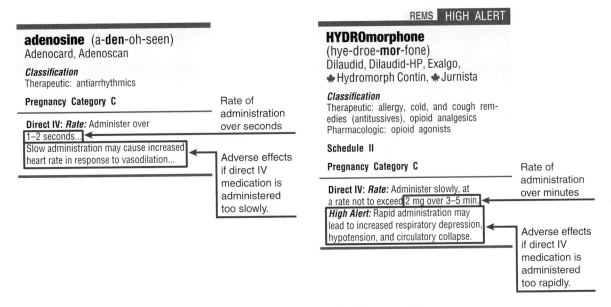

Figure 16-7. Rate of administration for direct IV medications.

 With some medications, a direct IV injection that is too rapid causes the appearance of sudden adverse effects, such as:

- *Hypotension*
- *Irregular pulse*
- *Syncope*
- *Tightness in the chest*
- *Facial flushing*
- *Severe headache*
- *Cardiac arrest*

These symptoms are characteristic of the adverse reaction called **speed shock.**

Look, for example, at the drug reference information about IV morphine in which speed shock is referenced: Speed shock is an emergency situation that requires immediate supportive care to stabilize the patient or immediate administration of an **antidote** (if available). Prevention of speed shock is a patient safety priority: the nurse must follow the recommended rate of administration for all direct IV medications.

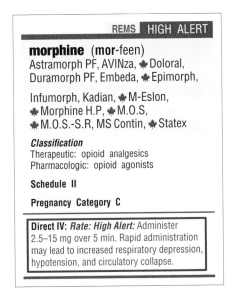

How the Rate of Administration Is Written in the Drug Reference

When a physician orders a direct IV medication, the nurse must look up the rate of administration.

Information in the drug reference can be written in one of several formats:

1. Non-dose dependent rate of administration
2. Dose dependent rate of administration
3. Age or diagnosis dependent rate of administration

NON-DOSE DEPENDENT RATE OF ADMINISTRATION

The rate of administration may be specified without regard for the dose of medication ordered. Look at the examples of this in Figure 16-8:

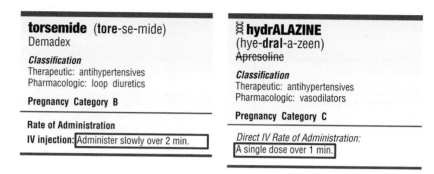

Figure 16-8. Non-dose dependent rate of administration.

For these two examples, regardless of the dose of medication ordered, the direct IV dose is given over 2 minutes or 1 minute, respectively. There is no math calculation needed for rate of administration that is written for all doses of a medication.

DOSE DEPENDENT RATE OF ADMINISTRATION

With many medications, the rate of administration depends on the dose of medication ordered. The ordered dose can exactly match the dose specified in the recommended rate of administration, or the ordered dose can be more than or less than the dose specified in the recommended rate of administration.

If the Ordered Dose Is the Same as the Dose Recommended for Rate of Administration

Look at the example in Figure 16-9. In this example, the ordered dose (1 mg) matches the dose recommended in the drug reference for rate of administration (1 mg/min).

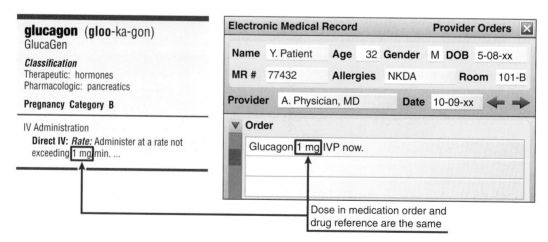

Figure 16-9. Dose dependent rate of administration: Doses match.

If the ordered dose matches the dose recommended for the rate of administration, no calculation is needed. In this example, the nurse refers to the drug reference and simply administers the ordered dose over 1 minute.

If the Ordered Dose Is More Than the Dose Specified for Rate of Administration

If the ordered dose is more than the dose specified in the drug reference, then a simple calculation can be done to determine the rate of administration. Look at the following two examples. In Example #1, the ordered dose (10 mg) is more than the dose identified for the rate of administration (5 mg/min) (Fig. 16-10).

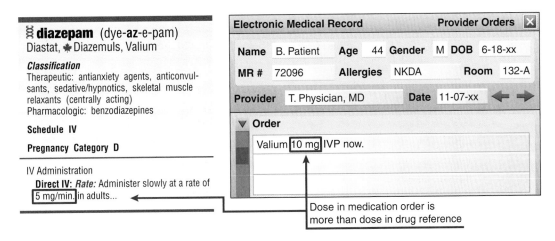

Figure 16-10. Dose dependent rate of administration: Dose more than in drug reference.

Calculating the rate of administration for 10 mg of direct IV Valium can be done by simple addition: The first 5 mg is given over 1 minute, and the second 5 mg is given over 1 minute. The 10 mg dose is administered over 2 minutes.

Calculation: 5 mg → 1 minute

+ 5 mg → 1 minute

10 mg → 2 minutes

Example 2:

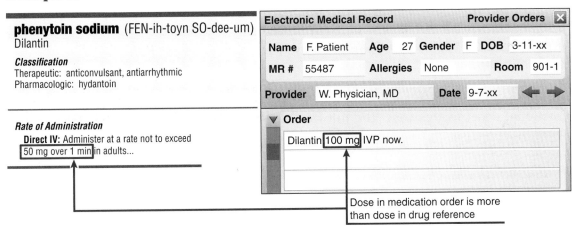

Calculating the rate of administration for 100 mg of direct IV Dilantin can be done by simple addition: The first 50 mg is given over 1 minute, and the second 50 mg is given over 1 minute. The 100 mg dose is administered over 2 minutes.

50 mg → 1 minute

+ 50 mg → 1 minute

100 mg → 2 minutes

Calculating the rate of administration is also possible using ratio and proportion and dimensional analysis. The formula $\dfrac{D}{H} \times Q = x$ cannot be used.

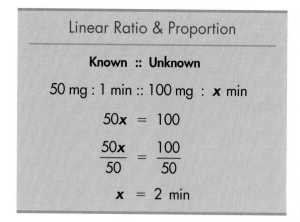

Linear Ratio & Proportion

Known :: Unknown

50 mg : 1 min :: 100 mg : **x** min

$$50x = 100$$

$$\frac{50x}{50} = \frac{100}{50}$$

$$x = 2 \text{ min}$$

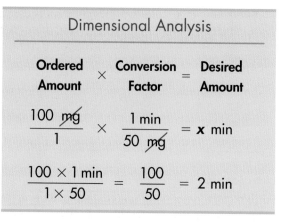

Dimensional Analysis

Ordered Amount	×	Conversion Factor	=	Desired Amount

$$\frac{100 \cancel{mg}}{1} \times \frac{1 \text{ min}}{50 \cancel{mg}} = x \text{ min}$$

$$\frac{100 \times 1 \text{ min}}{1 \times 50} = \frac{100}{50} = 2 \text{ min}$$

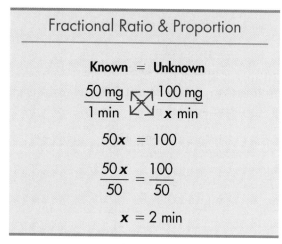

Fractional Ratio & Proportion

Known = Unknown

$$\frac{50 \text{ mg}}{1 \text{ min}} \quad \frac{100 \text{ mg}}{x \text{ min}}$$

$$50x = 100$$

$$\frac{50x}{50} = \frac{100}{50}$$

$$x = 2 \text{ min}$$

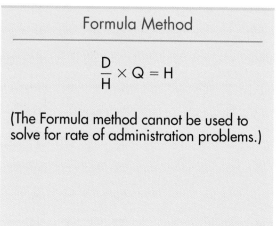

Formula Method

$$\frac{D}{H} \times Q = H$$

(The Formula method cannot be used to solve for rate of administration problems.)

If the Ordered Dose Is Less Than the Dose Recommended for Rate of Administration

The ordered dose may be less than, or a fraction of, the dose specified in the drug reference. There may be no specific information given about the rate of administration for a fractional dose. In this case, the full rate of administration time is used. Look at the example in Figure 16-11.

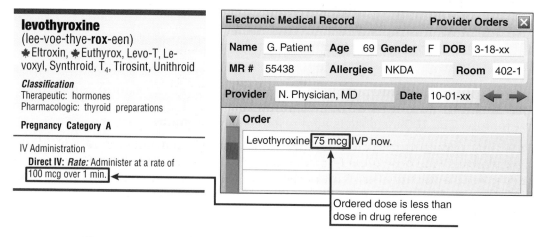

Figure 16-11. Dose dependent rate of administration: Dose less than in drug reference.

The ordered dose of 75 mcg is less than, or a fraction of, the dose recommended in the drug reference (100 mcg over 1 minute). Because there is no information in the drug reference about rate of administration for a fractional dose, the ordered dose of 75 mcg is given over the full minute.

$$\text{Calculation: } 75 \text{ mcg} \rightarrow 1 \text{ minute}$$

If the Ordered Dose Contains a Fraction of the Dose Recommended for Rate of Administration

Any time the ordered dose contains a fraction of the dose recommended for the rate of administration, the fractional part of the ordered dose is given over the full recommended time. Look at the example in Figure 16-12 in which the ordered dose contains a fraction of the specified dose in the drug reference:

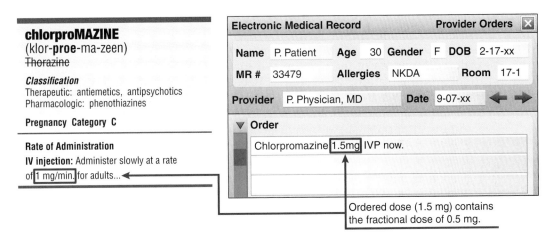

Figure 16-12. Dose dependent rate of administration: Fraction of recommended dose.

The total ordered dose of Chlorpromazine is 1.5 mg. Because the rate of administration in the drug reference is for 1 mg doses, the nurse will administer the fractional dose of 0.5 mg over the same amount of time as the full dose: the first 1 mg is given over 1 minute, and the remaining 0.5 mg is also given over the full 1 minute. The 1.5 mg dose is administered over 2 minutes.

$$
\begin{array}{rcl}
\text{Calculation:} \quad 1 \text{ mg} & \rightarrow & 1 \text{ minute} \\
\underline{+\ 0.5 \text{ mg}} & \rightarrow & \underline{1 \text{ minute}} \\
1.5 \text{ mg} & \rightarrow & 2 \text{ minutes}
\end{array}
$$

Some drug references use the term **"*fraction thereof*"** to denote the rate of administration for a fractional dose of an IV medication. The term "fraction thereof" means a part of the whole, or a fractional amount of the whole. This wording emphasizes the need to give fractional doses over the full rate of administration time. Look at the example from a drug reference book (Fig. 16-13).

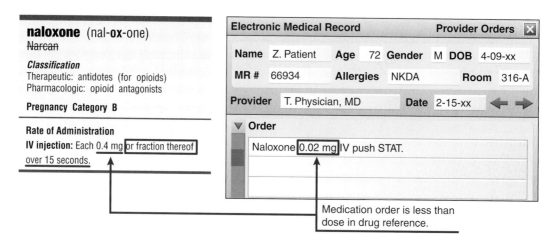

Figure 16-13. Use of term "fraction thereof" for rate of administration in drug reference.

In the example, the wording "fraction thereof" refers to any dose that is less than 0.4 mg. All ordered amounts of medication 0.4 mg or smaller are to be administered at the same rate of administration: 15 seconds. Because the ordered amount (0.02 mg) is less than (or a fraction of) 0.4 mg, the ordered amount is given over the full 15 seconds.

Calculation: 0.02 mg → 15 seconds

AGE OR DIAGNOSIS DEPENDENT RATE OF ADMINISTRATION

An IV drug can be used to treat several different symptoms or diseases, and the indications for use may affect the rate of administration. In addition, the rate of administration can be dependent on the age of the patient. Look at Figure 16-14:

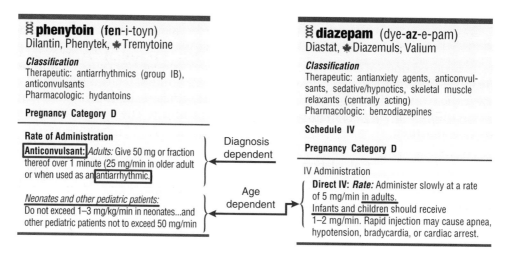

Figure 16-14. Age and diagnosis dependent rate of administration.

If the drug reference lists a range of time for direct IV administration (as in the rate for neonates and other pediatric patients in the example for phenytoin sodium), the nurse makes the choice based on the patient's age, diagnosis, and clinical condition.

APPLY LEARNED KNOWLEDGE 16-2

Calculate the rate of administration for the following direct IV medications.

1. *Order:* Dolasetron 12.5 mg direct IV now.
   Drug reference information: **Direct IV: *Rate:*** Administer 25 mg over at least 30 seconds.

   _____

2. *Order:* Thiamine 50 mg IVP TID.
   Drug reference information: **IV Administration: DIRECT:** Administer at a rate of 100 mg over 5 min.

   _____

3. *Order:* Diphenhydramine hydrochloride 35 mg IV injection q.6h prn.
   Drug reference information: **RATE OF ADMINISTRATION:** IV Injection: 25 mg or fraction thereof over 1 minute. Extend injection time in nonemergency situations and pediatric patients.

   _____

4. *Order:* Lorazepam 1.8 mg direct IV now.
   Drug reference information: **IV Injection:** Rate: Each 2 mg or fraction thereof over 1 to 5 minutes.

   _____

5. *Order:* Acetazolamide sodium 750 mg IVP q.12h.
   Drug reference information: **IV Administration:** 500 mg or fraction thereof over at least 1 minute or added to IV fluids to be given over 4 to 8 hours.

   _____

 CLINICAL REASONING 16-1
The physician writes the following order for the patient, and the nurse has the following drug available from the pharmacy:

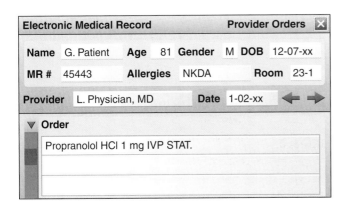

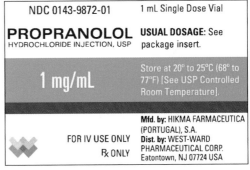

The drug reference for propanol states the following:
The nurse calculates the dose, draws up 1 mL of pro-pranolol, and adds 9 mL of D₅W to the syringe. The nurse administers the IV medication over 1 minute. The nurse's actions are (select all that apply):

A. Correct in calculating the dosage of the medication.
B. Correct in calculating the amount of diluent to add to the syringe.
C. Correct in calculating the rate of administration.
D. Incorrect; the rate of administration should be 10 minutes.
E. Incorrect; the rate of administration should be 2 minutes.

HIGH ALERT

✗ propranolol
(proe-**pran**-oh-lole)
Inderal, Inderal LA, InnoPran XL

Classification
Therapeutic: antianginals, antiarrhythmics (Class II), antihypertensives, vascular head-ache suppressants
Pharmacologic: beta blockers

Pregnancy Category C

IV Administration
 Direct IV:
 Diluent: Administer undiluted or dilute...
 Concentration: ...0.1 mg/mL.
 Rate: Administer at 0.5 mg/min for adults to avoid hypotension and cardiac arrest; do not exceeed 1 mg/min.
 Pedi: Administer over 10 min.

The nurse administering an IV medication has the responsibility to correctly interpret information from the drug reference about both the dilution and the rate of administration of the medication. As a patient advocate, the nurse carefully assesses the patient during the administration of the direct IV medication, monitoring for both therapeutic and adverse effects. These actions not only promote the Six Rights of Medication Administration, but are also essential to the safety of the patient receiving medication by the direct IV route.

Developing Competency

Use the information from the drug references to answer the following questions.

1. The order is for dipyridamole 40 mg IVP now. The dipyridamole is labeled 5 mg/mL. How many mL of diluent will the nurse add to the ordered dose? _____

dipyridamole
(dye-peer-**id**-a-mole)
✦Apo-Dipyridamole, Dipridacot,✦ Novodipiradol, Persantine, Persantine IV

Classification
Therapeutic: antiplatelet agents, diagnostic agents (coronary vasodilators)
Pharmacologic: platelet adhesion inhibitors

Pregnancy Category B

Dilution: Each 1 mL (5mg) must be diluted with a minimum of 2 mL D₅W, D₅½NS, or D₅NS...

Rate of Administration
Give a single dose over 4 min...

2. What is the rate of administration for the ordered dose of dipyridamole? _____

3. The order is for flumazenil 0.2 mg IVP now. The patient is 8 years old. What is the rate of administration for the ordered dose of flumazenil? _____

flumazenil (flu-**maz**-e-nil)
✽ Anexate, Romazicon

Classification
Therapeutic: antidotes

Pregnancy Category C

IV Administration
    Direct IV: *Rate:* Administer each dose over 15–30 sec into free-flowing IV in a large vein. Do not exceed 0.2 mg/min in children or 0.5 mg/min. in adults.

4. The patient is to receive Haldol 2 mg direct IV now. Haldol 5 mg/mL is available. What is the rate of administration for the ordered dose of Haldol? _____

haloperidol (ha-loe-**per**-i-dole)
Haldol, Haldol Decanoate

Classification
Therapeutic: antipsychotics
Pharmacologic: butyrophenones

Pregnancy Category C

IV Administration
    Direct IV:
    Diluent: May be administered undiluted for rapid control of acute psychosis or delirium.
    Concentration: 5 mg/mL.
    Rate: Administer at a rate of 5 mg/min.

5. The patient is to receive Methergine 0.2 mg direct IV now. Methergine 0.2 mg/mL is available. If the nurse dilutes the medication, how many mL of 0.9% NaCl will be added to the syringe? _____

methylergonovine
(meth-ill-er-goe-**noe**-veen)
Methergine

Classification
Therapeutic: oxytocic
Pharmacologic: ergot alkaloids

Pregnancy Category C

Dilution: Give undiluted or diluted in 5 mL of NS.

Rate of Administration
Give 0.2 mg or fraction thereof over 60 sec.

6. What is the rate of administration for the ordered dose of Methergine? _____

7. The order is for morphine 1 mg IVP q.15 minutes. How many mL of diluent will the nurse add to the medication?

_____

REMS **HIGH ALERT**

morphine (mor-feen)
Astramorph PF, AVINza, ✽Doloral,
Duramorph PF, Embeda, ✽Epimorph,

Infumorph, Kadian, ✽M-Eslon,
✽Morphine H.P, ✽M.O.S,
✽M.O.S.-S.R, MS Contin, ✽Statex

Classification
Therapeutic: opioid analgesics
Pharmacologic: opioid agonists

Schedule II

Pregnancy Category C

IV Administration
  Direct IV:
  Diluent: Dilute with at least 5 mL of sterile
  water or 0.9% NaCl for injection.
  Concentration: 0.5–5 mg/mL.
  Rate: High Alert: Administer 2.5–15 mg
  over 5 min. Rapid administration may
  lead to increased respiratory depression,
  hypotension, and circulatory collapse.

8. What is the rate of administration for the ordered dose of morphine?   _____

9. The order is for 2.5 mg of phentolamine direct IV now. What is the rate of administration for this ordered dose?

_____

phentolamine
(fen-**tole**-a-meen)
Oraverse, Regitine, ✽Rogitine

Classification
Therapeutic: agents for pheochromocytoma
Pharmacologic: alpha-adrenergic blockers

Pregnancy Category C

Rate of Administration
Each 5 mg or fraction thereof over 1 min.

10. What is the rate of administration for glycopyrrolate 0.3 mg direct IV?   _____

glycopyrrolate
(glye-koe-**pye**-roe-late)
Cuvposa, Robinul, Robinul-Forte

Classification
Therapeutic: antispasmodics
Pharmacologic: anticholinergics

**Pregnancy Category B (oral, parenteral),
C (oral solution)**

Rate of Administration
0.2 mg or fraction thereof over 1 to 2 min.

11. The patient is to receive doxorubicin 30 mg direct IV now. Doxorubicin 2 mg/mL is available. How many mL of 0.9% NaCl will be added to the syringe? _____

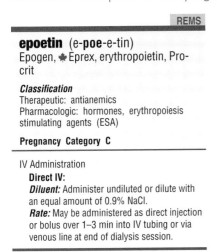

HIGH ALERT

DOXOrubicin
(dox-oh-**roo**-bi-sin)
~~Adriamycin~~, ✦Caelyx, ✦Myocet

Classification
Therapeutic: antineoplastics
Pharmacologic: anthracyclines

Pregnancy Category D

IV Administration
Direct IV:
Diluent: Dilute each 10 mg with 5 mL 0.9% NaCl (nonbacteriostatic) for injection. Shake to dissolve completely.
Concentration: 2 mg/mL
Rate: Administer each dose over 3–5 min... Facial flushing and erythema along involved vein frequently occur when administration is too rapid.

12. What is the rate of administration for the ordered dose of doxorubicin? _____

13. The dialysis nurse is to administer epoetin 2,500 units IVP at the end of dialysis. Epoetin is available in the dosage strength of 10,000 units/mL. If the nurse chooses to dilute the medication, how many mL of 0.9% NaCl will the nurse add to the epoetin in the syringe? _____

REMS

epoetin (e-**poe**-e-tin)
Epogen, ✦Eprex, erythropoietin, Procrit

Classification
Therapeutic: antianemics
Pharmacologic: hormones, erythropoiesis stimulating agents (ESA)

Pregnancy Category C

IV Administration
Direct IV:
Diluent: Administer undiluted or dilute with an equal amount of 0.9% NaCl.
Rate: May be administered as direct injection or bolus over 1–3 min into IV tubing or via venous line at end of dialysis session.

14. What is the most rapid rate of administration for the ordered dose of epoetin? _____

15. Should the ordered dose of Reglan be diluted? _____

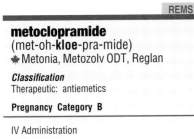

REMS

metoclopramide
(met-oh-**kloe**-pra-mide)
✦Metonia, Metozolv ODT, Reglan

Classification
Therapeutic: antiemetics

Pregnancy Category B

IV Administration
Direct IV:
Diluent: May be given undiluted if dose does not exceed 10 mg...
Rate: Too rapid IV injection will cause intense anxiety, restlessness, and then drowsiness.
IV injection: 10 mg or fraction thereof over 2 min. Reduce rate of injection in pediatric patients.

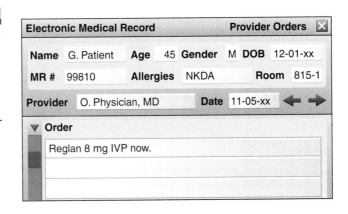

Electronic Medical Record		Provider Orders ☒
Name G. Patient	**Age** 45 **Gender** M	**DOB** 12-01-xx
MR # 99810	**Allergies** NKDA	**Room** 815-1
Provider O. Physician, MD	**Date** 11-05-xx	⬅ ➡

▼ **Order**

Reglan 8 mg IVP now.

16. What is the rate of administration for the ordered dose of Reglan? _____

17. Should the ordered dose of ascorbic acid be diluted prior to administration? _____

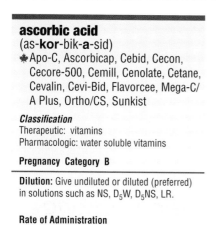

ascorbic acid
(as-**kor**-bik-**a**-sid)
✽Apo-C, Ascorbicap, Cebid, Cecon, Cecore-500, Cemill, Cenolate, Cetane, Cevalin, Cevi-Bid, Flavorcee, Mega-C/A Plus, Ortho/CS, Sunkist

Classification
Therapeutic: vitamins
Pharmacologic: water soluble vitamins

Pregnancy Category B

Dilution: Give undiluted or diluted (preferred) in solutions such as NS, D₅W, D₅NS, LR.

Rate of Administration
IV injection: 100 mg or fraction thereof over 1 min.

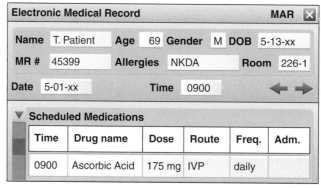

Electronic Medical Record					MAR

Name T. Patient **Age** 69 **Gender** M **DOB** 5-13-xx
MR # 45399 **Allergies** NKDA **Room** 226-1
Date 5-01-xx **Time** 0900

Scheduled Medications

Time	Drug name	Dose	Route	Freq.	Adm.
0900	Ascorbic Acid	175 mg	IVP	daily	

18. What is the rate of administration for the ordered dose of ascorbic acid? _____

19. The patient is to receive palonosetron 0.5 mg direct IV now. What is the rate of administration for the ordered dose of palonosetron? _____

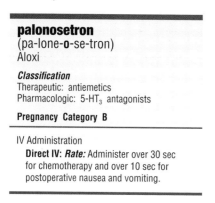

palonosetron
(pa-lone-**o**-se-tron)
Aloxi

Classification
Therapeutic: antiemetics
Pharmacologic: 5-HT₃ antagonists

Pregnancy Category B

IV Administration
Direct IV: *Rate:* Administer over 30 sec for chemotherapy and over 10 sec for postoperative nausea and vomiting.

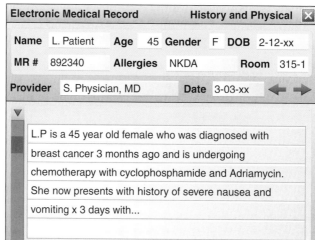

Electronic Medical Record		History and Physical

Name L. Patient **Age** 45 **Gender** F **DOB** 2-12-xx
MR # 892340 **Allergies** NKDA **Room** 315-1
Provider S. Physician, MD **Date** 3-03-xx

L.P is a 45 year old female who was diagnosed with
breast cancer 3 months ago and is undergoing
chemotherapy with cyclophosphamide and Adriamycin.
She now presents with history of severe nausea and
vomiting x 3 days with...

20. The ordered dose is magnesium sulfate 1 gram IVP stat. What is the rate of administration for this ordered dose?

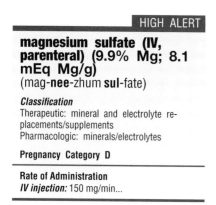

HIGH ALERT

magnesium sulfate (IV, parenteral) (9.9% Mg; 8.1 mEq Mg/g)
(mag-**nee**-zhum **sul**-fate)

Classification
Therapeutic: mineral and electrolyte replacements/supplements
Pharmacologic: minerals/electrolytes

Pregnancy Category D

Rate of Administration
IV injection: 150 mg/min...

IV Therapy and Administration of Intravenous Medications

Unit Review—Evaluate for Clinical Decision Making

*For each question, use your clinical judgment to determine whether the nurse's decision is **Correct** or **Incorrect**. For incorrect problems, write the correct answer.*

1. MD order: 1 L D$_5$/0.9% NS q.12h.
The nurse starts the IV and sets the rate on the pump at 83 mL/hr.
The rate set on the IV pump is:

Correct	Incorrect	Answer: _____

2. MD order: Famotidine 20 mg IVPB q.12h.
Pharmacy sends:

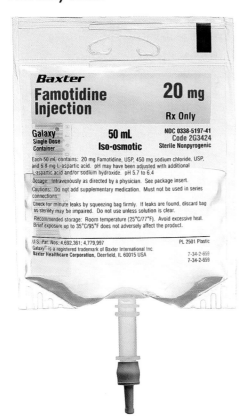

The nurse is to infuse the Famotidine over 15 minutes, and sets the IV pump to 100 mL/hr.
The rate set on the IV pump is:

Correct	Incorrect	Answer: _____

3. MD order: 500 mL 0.9% NaCl q.10h.
The nurse starts the IV by gravity and sets the rate at 50 gtt/min using a pedi IV tubing.
The IV rate is:

Correct	Incorrect	Answer: _____

4. MD order: 1 L LR @ 125 mL/hr.
IV Tubing:

Non-DEHP CONTINU-FLO Solution Set   2H6519

10 10 drops/mL Approx.

105" (2.7 m)
2 Injection Sites, Male Luer Lock Adapter

For use with COLLEAGUE and FLO-GARD 6201 and 6301 series pumps.

Fluid path is sterile, nonpyrogenic.
Cautions: Do not use if tip protectors (1) are not in place. Do not place on sterile field.
Directions: Use aseptic technique
Close regulating clamp (7). Insert spike (2) into solution container. Fill drip chamber (3) to fill line. Open regulating clamp (7). If flow does not start, squeeze plastic container. Invert and tap check valve (4) to purge air during priming. Prime set, purge air. Close regulating clamp (7) until roller meets bottom of frame. Attach male Luer adapter (8) to INTERLINK cannula or vascular access device using a firm push and twist motion and then engage the Luer lock collar to prevent accidental disconnection. Swab septum of injection site (5) with antiseptic prior to access. Access INTERLINK injection site (5) (identified by a colored ring) with INTERLINK cannula. See cannula directions.
To properly set flow, always close regulating clamp (7) until roller meets bottom of frame, then reopen to establish flow rate. Repeat procedure if adjusting clamp from fully open position.

Cautions:
Do not allow air to be trapped in set. Puncturing set components may cause air embolism. If needle must be used, insert small gauge needle into perimeter of septum. Do not disconnect administration set, syringe or other component from cannula while cannula is still connected to INTERLINK injection site. When used with FLO-GARD pumps, reduction in delivery accuracy may occur at programmed flow rates higher than 250 mL/hr or infusion times longer than 8 hours.
Rx Only. Single use only. Do not resterilize.
Notes:
This product does not contain natural rubber latex.
To stop flow without disturbing regulating device (7), close slide clamp (6). For secondary medication administration, use upper Y-Injection site (5) only. See directions for use with secondary medication set. When used in gravity mode or with COLLEAGUE pumps, replace per CDC guidelines. When used with FLO-GARD pumps, replace after 24 hours. Lengths are approximate.
For Product Information 1-800-933-0303

Baxter
Manufactured by an affiliate of Baxter Healthcare Corporation
Deerfield, IL 60015 USA
Made in Costa Rica
07-36-47-090

Baxter, INTERLINK, COLLEAGUE, CONTINU-FLO and FLO-GARD are trademarks of Baxter International Inc.
U.S. Pat. Nos. 4,662,599; 5,290,239; 5,300,044; 5,871,500; 6,569,125; 6,605,076

LDPE

**BAR CODE POSITION ONLY
085412000527

The nurse starts the IV by gravity and sets the rate at 21 gtt/min.
The IV rate is:

Correct	Incorrect	Answer: _____

5. MD order: 1 L D_5/0.45% NS q.12h.
During the handoff report, the evening shift nurse informs the night nurse that the IV was started at 1700, has been infusing well, and will be completed at 0400.
The reported completion time of the IV is:

Correct	Incorrect	Answer: _____

6. MD order: 1 L 0.9% NaCl at 125 mL/hr.
During the handoff report, the day shift nurse informs the evening shift nurse that an IV was started at 0900, has been infusing well, and the IV will be completed at 1700.
The reported completion time of the IV is:

Correct	Incorrect	Answer: _____

7. MD order: 1 L D$_5$W at 75 mL/hr.

During the handoff report, the night shift nurse informs the day shift nurse that an IV was started at 0100, infiltrated at 0500, and the remaining 700 mL was restarted at the same rate at 0600. The IV will be completed at 1520.

The reported completion time of the IV is:

Correct	Incorrect	Answer: _____

8. MD order: 1 L D$_5$/0.9% NaCl to infuse at 150 mL/hr for the first 3 hours then decrease rate to 100 mL/hr. Discontinue IV after liter has infused.

During the handoff report, the day shift nurse informs the evening shift nurse that an IV was started at 0800, and the rate was decreased to 100 mL/hr at 1100. The IV is infusing well and should be discontinued at 1730.

The reported completion time of the IV is:

Correct	Incorrect	Answer: _____

9. MD order: 500 mL D$_5$W to infuse over 4 hours.

The IV is started at 1900 and the flow meter is labeled and attached to the IV bag.

The flow meter is labeled correctly:

Correct	Incorrect	Answer: _____

10. **MD order:** Midazolam 0.5 mg direct IV now.
    Pharmacy sends: Midazolam 1 mg/mL
    Rate: Administer slowly over at least 2-5 min.
    Drug reference:

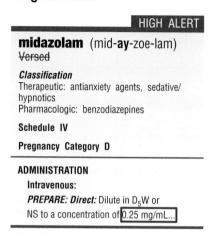

The nurse calculates the ordered dose, draws up 0.5 mL of
midazolam into a 3 mL syringe, and adds 1.5 mL of D$_5$W to
dilute the medication to a concentration of 0.25 mg/mL. The
nurse then administers the direct IV midazolam over 2 minutes.
The nurse's calculation of the ordered dose, amount of diluent
added, and rate of direct IV administration are:

Correct	Incorrect	Answer: _____

Verifying Safe Dose and Critical Care Calculations

V erifying safe dose and calculating dosages for drugs used in the critical care setting require the nurse to select relevant drug reference information and calculate
dosages that may require multiple steps. This unit teaches you to interpret information from the drug reference about recommended doses, verify that an ordered dose
of medication is safe to administer, and calculate and titrate high alert IV medications
based on the physiological response of the patient.

 APPLICATION TO NURSING PRACTICE
*Best practice requires the nurse to interpret information from the drug reference and
use clinical decision making to determine whether an ordered dose is a safe dose.*

diltiazem (dil-**tye**-a-zem)
Cardizem, Cardizem CD, Cardizem LA,
Cartia XT, Dilacor XR, Taztia XT, Tiazac

Classification
Therapeutic: antianginals, antiarrhythmics
(class IV), antihypertensives
Pharmacologic: calcium channel blockers

Pregnancy Category C

Route/Dosage

IV (Adults): 0.25 mg/kg; may repeat in 15 min
with a dose of 0.35 mg/kg. May follow with
continuous infusion at 10 mg/hr (range 5–15
mg/hr) for up to 24 hr.

   *The nurse must interpret the infor-
mation in the drug reference, apply it
to the individual patient, evaluate
whether the dose is safe to administer,
and monitor the patient's response to
the drug.*

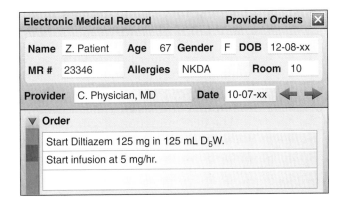

Electronic Medical Record					Provider Orders	❌
Name Z. Patient		**Age** 67	**Gender** F	**DOB** 12-08-xx		
MR # 23346		**Allergies** NKDA			**Room** 10	
Provider C. Physician, MD			**Date** 10-07-xx	⬅ ➡		

▼ **Order**

Start Diltiazem 125 mg in 125 mL D$_5$W.

Start infusion at 5 mg/hr.

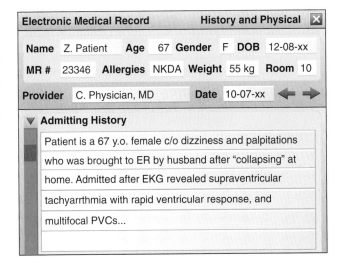

Electronic Medical Record				History and Physical	❌
Name Z. Patient	**Age** 67	**Gender** F	**DOB** 12-08-xx		
MR # 23346	**Allergies** NKDA	**Weight** 55 kg	**Room** 10		
Provider C. Physician, MD		**Date** 10-07-xx	⬅ ➡		

▼ **Admitting History**

Patient is a 67 y.o. female c/o dizziness and palpitations

who was brought to ER by husband after "collapsing" at

home. Admitted after EKG revealed supraventricular

tachyarrthmia with rapid ventricular response, and

multifocal PVCs...

CHAPTER 17

Verifying Safe Dose

LEARNING OUTCOMES

*Identify and interpret information regarding the recommended dose
in drug references.*

Calculate and verify safe dose based on body weight.

Calculate and verify safe dose based on body surface area.

One of the Six Rights of Medication Administration, the "right dose," requires the nurse to verify that the ordered dose of a medication is a safe dose for the individual patient. This is done by comparing the ordered dose of a drug with the ***recommended dose,*** the typical dose given to achieve a particular therapeutic effect. The recommended dose is determined by the drug manufacturer and is stated in the drug reference. After comparing the ordered dose with the recommended dose, the nurse uses critical thinking skills to determine whether the ordered dose of a medication is safe to administer. An ordered dose of medication is considered a safe dose if it is the same as or less than the recommended dose.

The determination of safe dose by the nurse is an essential part of safe medication administration practice. The nurse is the last member of the health care team to verify that the patient is receiving the right dose of medication. Verification of safe dose should be done by the nurse prior to administration of every drug.

Safe Dose Versus Effective Dose

A differentiation must be made between a ***safe dose*** and an ***effective dose.*** A dose is considered safe when the amount of drug is equal to or less than the dose recommended in the drug reference. A dose is considered effective when the amount of drug is enough to produce the desired therapeutic effect. Safe doses are not always effective doses. For example, one-half of an acetaminophen tablet may be safe, but not effective, in lowering a fever.

Doses more or less than the drug manufacturer's recommended dose may be ordered by the physician in special circumstances. For example, patients with liver disease may need to have a lower dose of a drug to prevent toxicity, and patients with a serious infection may need a higher dose of a drug to combat the infection. It is not within the nurse's scope of practice to determine the dose of a medication. However, safe practice and patient advocacy require that the nurse consult with the physician to clarify any order that is different from the drug manufacturer's recommended dose.

Although this chapter focuses on calculations related to safe dose, it is important that the nurse consider both safe dose and effective dose when evaluating a medication order.

The Recommended Dose in Drug References

The drug reference, package insert, or drug label state the recommended dose using headings such as "Dosage," "Dosage and Administration," or "Usual Dose." Several terms can be used in the drug reference to further differentiate a recommended dose (Table 17-1).

Table 17-1. Terms Related to Recommended Dose

TERM	DEFINITION
Single dose	A dose of medication administered at one time.
Total daily dose	The total amount of medication to be given in 24 hours.
Divided dose	Fractional portions of a total daily dose administered at specified intervals, such as every 6 hours.
Initial dose	The first dose of a drug given to a patient.
Loading dose	An initial large dose of medication administered to quickly achieve therapeutic levels in the body.
Maintenance dose	The dose required to sustain the desired effect of the drug; long-term therapy dose.
Dosage range	The minimum and maximum safe and effective dose.

TYPES OF RECOMMENDED DOSES

Recommended doses can be divided into several different types, including:

- a standard dose or dosage range.
- a weight-based dose or dosage range (usually measured in kg).
- a dose based on the patient's body surface area (BSA) (usually measured in m²).

Examples of each type of recommended dose are provided in Table 17-2.

Table 17-2. Types of Recommended Doses

RECOMMENDED DOSE	EXAMPLES OF RECOMMENDED DOSE AND DOSAGE RANGE	
Standard dose	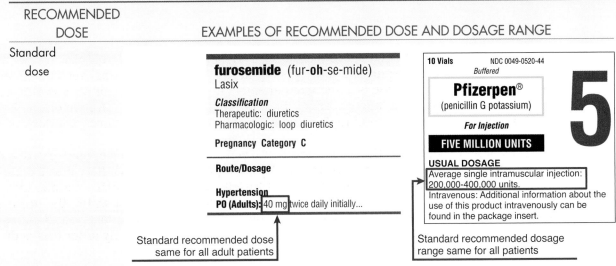	

Continued

Table 17-2. Types of Recommended Doses—*cont'd*

RECOMMENDED DOSE	EXAMPLES OF RECOMMENDED DOSE AND DOSAGE RANGE
Weight-based dose	
Dose based on body surface area (BSA)	

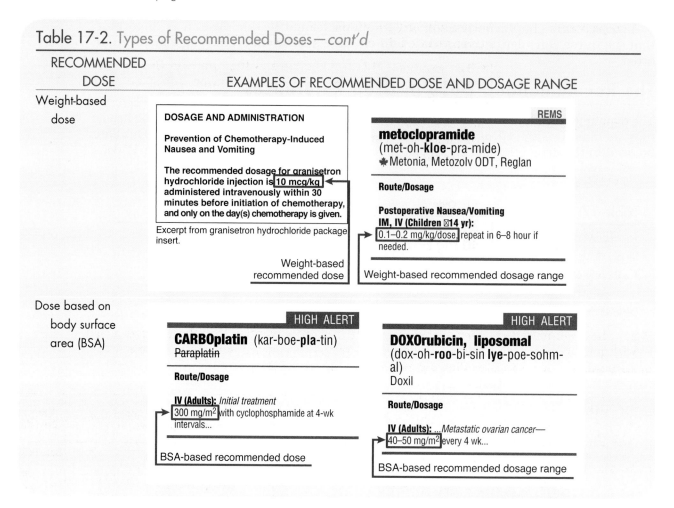

Standard Recommended Dose

When the drug reference lists a standard recommended dose without regard to the patient's size or weight, the nurse simply compares the ordered dose with the drug manufacturer's recommended dose. The nurse then makes a clinical decision about whether the ordered dose is a safe dose. Look at this decision-making process in the following example in Figure 17-1.

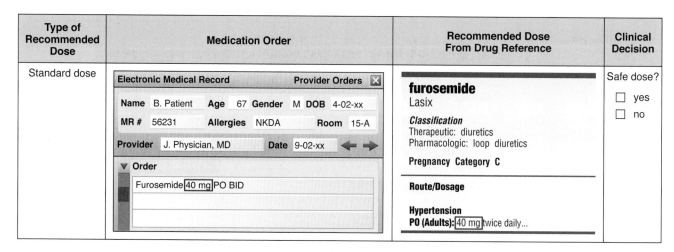

Figure 17-1. Verifying safe dose for a standard recommended dose.

Comparison:	Medication order = 40 mg BID Recommended dose = 40 mg twice daily

In this example, the ordered dose is the same as the recommended dose. Notice that the administration schedule also matches (twice a day).

Clinical decision: The nurse makes the clinical decision that the ordered dose of furosemide is a safe dose to administer as it matches the recommended dose from the drug reference.

Summary:

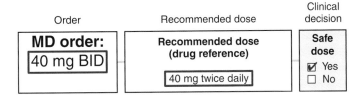

Standard Recommended Dosage Range

When the recommended dose is a dosage range, the nurse verifies that the ordered dose is within this dosage range. If so, the ordered dose is considered safe. Look at this decision-making process in the following example in Figure 17-2.

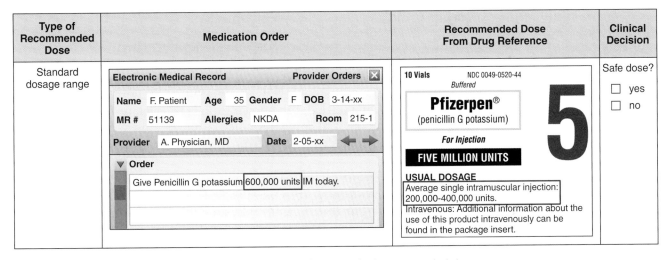

Figure 17-2. Verifying safe dose for a standard recommended dosage range.

Comparison: Medication order = 600,000 units today (single dose)
Recommended dose = 200,000 to 400,000 units (single dose)

In this example, the ordered dose is outside of the recommended dosage range.

Clinical decision: The nurse makes the clinical decision that the ordered dose of Penicillin G Potassium is not a safe dose as it is more than is recommended by the drug reference. Safe practice requires the nurse to consult the physician to clarify the order prior to administering the medication.

Summary:

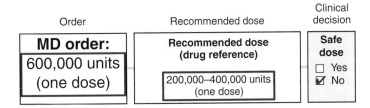

If the amount of drug ordered is not within the recommended dosage range in the drug reference, the nurse must contact the physician to clarify the dose. Communication between the physician and the nurse will ensure that the patient receives the right dose of medication.

Weight-Based Dosing

Weight-based dosing is standard practice with pediatric and oncology medications, and is frequently used for medications given to specialized patient populations, such as the older adult or the critically ill adult. With **weight-based dosing,** the drug manufacturer determines that the recommended dose of a medication should not be the same for all patients, but should vary according to the weight of the patient. The recommended dose is stated as an amount of drug per kilogram (or pound) of body weight (for example, 1 mg/kg).

The nurse must calculate a recommended dose that is weight-based for each patient, based on that patient's weight. If a conversion between lb and kg is needed, the nurse recalls the following equivalent measurement: 2.2 lb = 1 kg.

CALCULATING AND VERIFYING SAFE DOSE BASED ON WEIGHT

To verify safe dose when a recommended dose is based on weight, the nurse needs to gather the following information:

- Weight of the patient (usually in kg)
- Medication order
- Weight-based dosing information from the drug reference

After this information is gathered, the nurse uses the following steps:

1. Convert the patient's weight from lb to kg if necessary.
2. Calculate the weight-based recommended dose for the individual patient.

   If using the ratio and proportion method, the known ratio is the weight-based dose from the drug reference. The dimensional analysis calculation begins with the patient's weight (rather than the ordered amount), and the weight-based dose from the drug

   reference is used as the conversion factor. The formula method $\dfrac{D}{H} \times Q = x$ cannot

   be used for weight-based problems. Instead, a simple multiplication formula can be used to calculate the recommended dose:

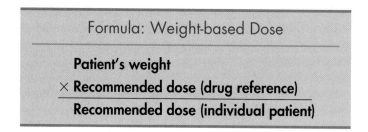

Formula: Weight-based Dose

$$\frac{\text{Patient's weight}}{\times \text{Recommended dose (drug reference)}}$$
$$\text{Recommended dose (individual patient)}$$

3. Compare the recommended dose for the individual patient with the ordered dose.
4. Make a clinical decision regarding safe dose.

Now apply these steps to the example of a weight-based recommended dose in Figure 17-3.

Type of Recommended Dose	Medication Order	Recommended Dose From Drug Reference	Clinical Decision
Weight-based dose	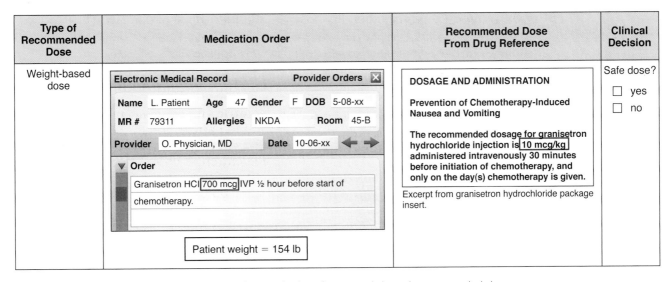 **Electronic Medical Record** — **Provider Orders** ⊠ **Name** L. Patient **Age** 47 **Gender** F **DOB** 5-08-xx **MR #** 79311 **Allergies** NKDA **Room** 45-B **Provider** O. Physician, MD **Date** 10-06-xx ⬅ ➡ ▼ **Order** Granisetron HCl 700 mcg IVP ½ hour before start of chemotherapy. Patient weight = 154 lb	**DOSAGE AND ADMINISTRATION** **Prevention of Chemotherapy-Induced Nausea and Vomiting** The recommended dosage for granisetron hydrochloride injection is 10 mcg/kg administered intravenously 30 minutes before initiation of chemotherapy, and only on the day(s) chemotherapy is given. Excerpt from granisetron hydrochloride package insert.	Safe dose? ☐ yes ☐ no

Figure 17-3. Verifying safe dose for a weight-based recommended dose.

Step 1: Convert the patient's weight from lb to kg if necessary.

The patient's weight is given in pounds (154 lb). The nurse converts 154 lb to 70 kg.

Step 2: Calculate the weight-based recommended dose for the individual patient.

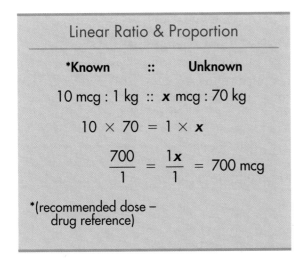

Linear Ratio & Proportion

*Known :: Unknown

$$10 \text{ mcg} : 1 \text{ kg} :: x \text{ mcg} : 70 \text{ kg}$$

$$10 \times 70 = 1 \times x$$

$$\frac{700}{1} = \frac{1x}{1} = 700 \text{ mcg}$$

*(recommended dose – drug reference)

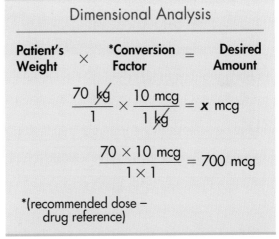

Dimensional Analysis

Patient's Weight × *Conversion Factor = Desired Amount

$$\frac{70 \text{ kg}}{1} \times \frac{10 \text{ mcg}}{1 \text{ kg}} = x \text{ mcg}$$

$$\frac{70 \times 10 \text{ mcg}}{1 \times 1} = 700 \text{ mcg}$$

*(recommended dose – drug reference)

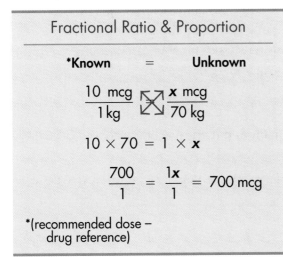

Fractional Ratio & Proportion

*Known = Unknown

$$\frac{10 \text{ mcg}}{1 \text{ kg}} \qquad \frac{x \text{ mcg}}{70 \text{ kg}}$$

$$10 \times 70 = 1 \times x$$

$$\frac{700}{1} = \frac{1x}{1} = 700 \text{ mcg}$$

*(recommended dose – drug reference)

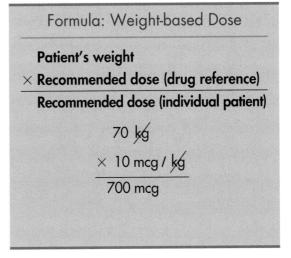

Formula: Weight-based Dose

Patient's weight
× Recommended dose (drug reference)
―――――――――――――――――
Recommended dose (individual patient)

$$\frac{70 \text{ kg} \times 10 \text{ mcg} / \text{kg}}{700 \text{ mcg}}$$

Step 3: Compare the recommended dose for the individual patient with the ordered dose.

Medication order = 700 mcg (single dose)

Recommended dose for this patient from the drug reference = 700 mcg (single dose)

Step 4: Make a clinical decision regarding safe dose.

Decision: Because the ordered dose is the same as the recommended dose, it is a safe dose for this patient.

The process is summarized in the following diagram:

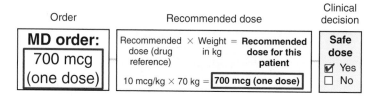

Figure 17-4 provides another example of how to calculate and verify safe dose for a weight-based recommended dose.

Medication Order   **Drug Reference Information**

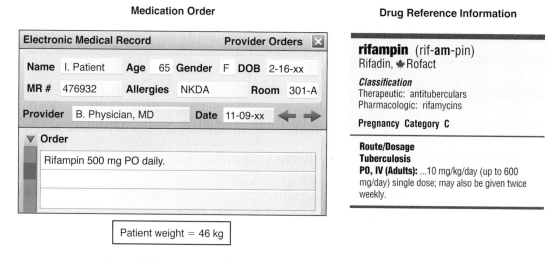

Figure 17-4. Verifying safe dose for a weight-based recommended dose.

Step 1: Convert the patient's weight from lb to kg if necessary.

The patient's weight is given in kilograms (46 kg). No conversion step is needed.

Step 2: Calculate the weight-based recommended dose for the individual patient.

Only the formula for weight-based dose will be shown for this calculation.

Formula: Weight-based Dose	
46 kg	(pt's weight)
× 10 mg/kg	(recommended dose – drug reference)
460 mg	(recommended dose – individual patient)

Step 3: Compare the recommended dose for the individual patient with the ordered dose.

Medication order = 500 mg daily

Recommended dose for this patient from the drug reference = 460 mg daily

Step 4: Make a clinical decision regarding safe dose.

Decision: Because the ordered dose is more than the weight-based recommended dose, it is not a safe dose for this patient. (The ordered dose of 500 mg is less than the maximum dose from the drug reference. The recommended weight-based dose for this patient, however, is 460 mg per day.) The nurse would need to contact the physician to clarify why the ordered dose exceeds the weight-based recommended dose.

Summary:

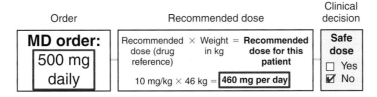

See Figure 17-5 for another example of how the steps are applied to verifying safe dose for a weight-based recommended dose. In this example, note the patient's age, as the recommended dose differs depending on the patient's age.

Medication Order

Drug Reference Information

Electronic Medical Record — **Provider Orders** ☒

| Name | L. Patient | Age | 11 | Gender | M | DOB | 4-10-xx |

| MR # | 134342 | Allergies | NKDA | Room | 114-A |

| Provider | M. Physician, MD | Date | 9-11-xx | ← → |

▼ **Order**

Ceftibuten 300 mg PO daily.

Patient weight = 35 kg

CEPHALOSPORINS — THIRD GENERATION

ceftibuten (sef-tye-**byoo**-ten)
Cedax

Classification
Therapeutic: anti-infectives
Pharmacologic: third-generation cephalosporins

Pregnancy Category B

Route/Dosage

PO (Adults and Children greater than or equal to 12 yr): 400 mg q.24h for 10 days.

PO (Children 6 mo–12 yr): 9 mg/kg q.24h for 10 days (maximum dose = 400 mg/day).

Figure 17-5. Verifying safe dose for a weight-based recommended dose based on age.

Step 1: Convert the patient's weight from lb to kg if necessary.

The patient's weight is given in kilograms (35 kg). No conversion step is needed.

Step 2: Calculate the weight-based recommended dose for the individual patient.

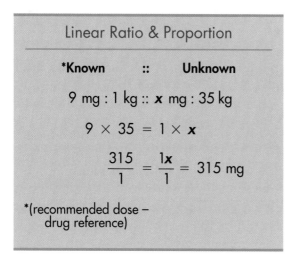

Linear Ratio & Proportion

*Known :: Unknown

9 mg : 1 kg :: **x** mg : 35 kg

9 × 35 = 1 × **x**

$$\frac{315}{1} = \frac{1x}{1} = 315 \text{ mg}$$

*(recommended dose – drug reference)

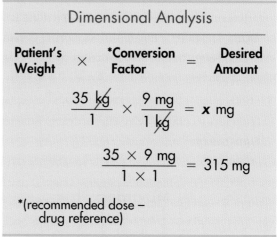

Dimensional Analysis

Patient's Weight × *Conversion Factor = Desired Amount

$$\frac{35 \text{ kg}}{1} \times \frac{9 \text{ mg}}{1 \text{ kg}} = x \text{ mg}$$

$$\frac{35 \times 9 \text{ mg}}{1 \times 1} = 315 \text{ mg}$$

*(recommended dose – drug reference)

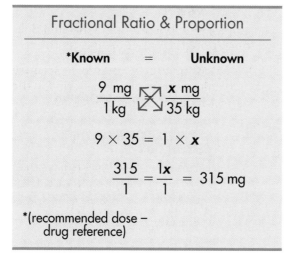

Fractional Ratio & Proportion

*Known = Unknown

$$\frac{9 \text{ mg}}{1 \text{ kg}} \diagup\kern-1.2em\diagdown \frac{x \text{ mg}}{35 \text{ kg}}$$

9 × 35 = 1 × **x**

$$\frac{315}{1} = \frac{1x}{1} = 315 \text{ mg}$$

*(recommended dose – drug reference)

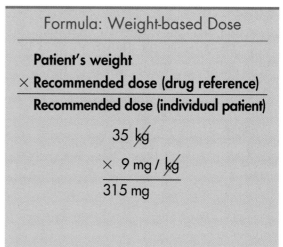

Formula: Weight-based Dose

Patient's weight

$$\frac{\times \textbf{ Recommended dose (drug reference)}}{\textbf{Recommended dose (individual patient)}}$$

$$\frac{35 \text{ kg} \times 9 \text{ mg} / \text{kg}}{315 \text{ mg}}$$

Step 3: Compare the recommended dose for the individual patient with the ordered dose.

Medication order = 300 mg daily

Recommended dose for this patient from the drug reference = 315 mg daily

Step 4: Make a clinical decision regarding safe dose.

Decision: Because the ordered dose is less than the weight-based recommended dose (and does not exceed 400 mg/day), it is a safe dose for this patient.

Summary:

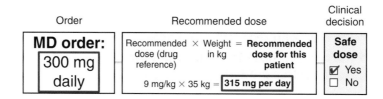

Order	Recommended dose	Clinical decision
MD order: 300 mg daily	Recommended × Weight = Recommended dose (drug reference) in kg dose for this patient 9 mg/kg × 35 kg = 315 mg per day	**Safe dose** ☑ Yes ☐ No

Finally, Figure 17-6 presents another example of how to calculate and verify if an ordered dose based on weight is a safe dose. This example involves a recommended dose stated as a dosage range.

Medication Order   **Drug Reference Information**

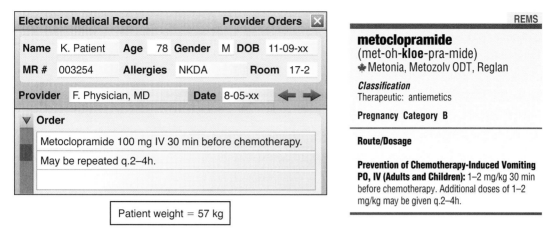

Figure 17-6. Verifying safe dose for a weight-based recommended dosage range.

Step 1: Convert the patient's weight from lb to kg if necessary.

The patient's weight is given in kilograms (57 kg). No conversion step is needed.

Step 2: Calculate the weight-based recommended dose for the individual patient.

Only the formula for weight-based dose will be shown for this calculation. Because the recommended dose is stated as a range, two calculations are done: one for the lowest recommended dose, and one for the highest recommended dose.

Formula: Weight-based Dose

Calculation: (lowest dose)	$\begin{array}{r} 57 \text{ kg} \\ \times\ 1 \text{ mg/kg} \\ \hline 57 \text{ mg} \end{array}$	(pt's weight) (lowest recommended dose – drug reference) (lowest recommended dose – individual patient)
Calculation: (highest dose)	$\begin{array}{r} 57 \text{ kg} \\ \times\ 2 \text{ mg/kg} \\ \hline 114 \text{ mg} \end{array}$	(pt's weight) (highest recommended dose – drug reference) (highest recommended dose – individual patient)

Step 3: Compare the recommended dose for the individual patient with the ordered dose.

Medication order = 100 mg (single dose)

Recommended dosage range for this patient from the drug reference = 57 mg to 114 mg (single dose)

Step 4: Make a clinical decision regarding safe dose.

Decision: Because the ordered dose is within the weight-based recommended dosage range, it is a safe dose for this patient.

Summary:

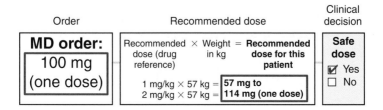

The nurse needs to be very careful to draw the correct conclusion once the math is done.

If the ordered dose is equal to or less than the recommended dose, then the dose is considered safe, and the nurse can give the medication. If the ordered dose is more than the recommended dose, then the nurse needs to clarify the order with the physician prior to administering the medication.

APPLY LEARNED KNOWLEDGE 17-1

Use the medication order and the information about weight-based recommended dose from the drug reference to answer the following questions.

1. **Order:** Administer 150 mcg IVP daily.
   Patient weight: 50 kg
   Drug reference: Dosage and Administration: Adult: 2.5 mcg/kg IV every 24 hours.

   Calculate the weight-based recommended dose for this patient. _____

   Is the ordered dose a safe dose? _____

2. **Order:** Give 650 mg PO daily.
   Patient weight: 187 lb
   Drug reference: Usual Adult Dosage: 8 mg/kg PO daily.

   Calculate the weight-based recommended dose for this patient. _____

   Is the ordered dose a safe dose? _____

3. **Order:** Administer 50 mg IVP now.
   Patient weight: 65 kg
   Drug reference: Dosage: Administer 0.2 to 0.4 mg/kg IV q.4h. prn nausea.

   Calculate the weight-based recommended dosage range for this patient. _____

   Is the ordered dose a safe dose? _____

4. **Order:** Administer 4.5 mcg IVP BID.
   Patient weight: 110 lb
   Drug reference: Usual Dose: 0.1 mcg/kg IV twice daily.

   Calculate the weight-based recommended dose for this patient. _____

   Is the ordered dose a safe dose? _____

5. **Order:** Administer 1.5 g PO daily.
   Patient weight: 80 kg
   Drug reference: Dosage and Administration: Adult: 0.02 g/kg PO every 24 hours.

   Calculate the weight-based recommended dose for this patient. _____

   Is the ordered dose a safe dose? _____

Variation in Weight-Based Recommended Dose: Total Daily Dose That Must Be Divided

With some medications, the weight-based recommended dose is stated as a total daily dose that is divided into several individual doses throughout the day. Look at the example from a drug label in Figure 17-7.

The weight-based recommended dose on the Vibramycin label is a total daily dose. Notice how the total daily dose must be divided into 2 equal individual doses on the first day of administering the medication, given q.12h.

Figure 17-8 shows another example:

The weight-based recommended dosage range on the ampicillin label is a total daily dose. Notice how the total daily dose must be divided into 3 or 4 equal individual doses, given either q.8h (if the total dose is divided into 3 individual doses) or q.6h (if the total dose is divided into 4 individual doses).

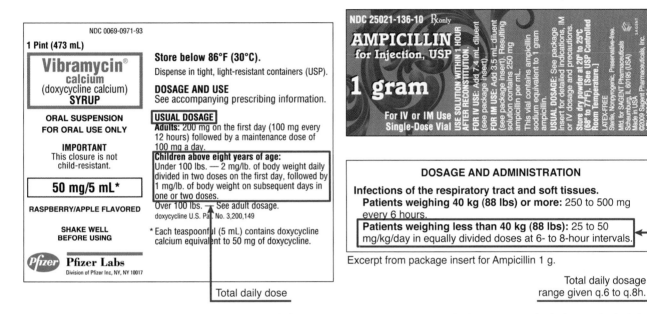

Figure 17-7. Total daily dose divided into individual doses.

Figure 17-8. Total daily dosage range divided into individual doses.

Calculating and Verifying Safe Dose With a Recommended Total Daily Dose

Calculating safe dose when the weight-based recommended dose is written as a total daily dose requires one extra step: dividing the total daily dose into individual doses. This is done by dividing the total daily dose by the number of individual doses to be administered in 24 hours. The recommended individual dose is then compared with the medication order to determine whether the dose is safe. See the example in Figure 17-9.

Medication Order

Drug Reference Information

Electronic Medical Record				Provider Orders	☒
Name T. Patient	**Age** 12	**Gender** M	**DOB** 12-04-xx		
MR # 90556	**Allergies** NKDA		**Room** 415-2		
Provider A. Physician, MD		**Date** 3-19-xx	← →		

▼ **Order**

Ampicillin 250 mg IVP q.6h.

Ampicillin sodium

Usual dosage: Children less than 40 kg: 25–50 mg/kg/day in equally divided doses at 6-hour intervals.

Patient weight = 40 kg

Figure 17-9. Verifying safe dose for recommended total daily dosage range.

Step 1: Convert the patient's weight from lb to kg if necessary.

The patient's weight is given in kilograms (40 kg). No conversion step is needed.

Step 2a: Calculate the weight-based recommended total daily dose for the individual patient.

Only the formula for weight-based dose will be shown for this calculation. Because the recommended dose is stated as a range, two calculations are done: one for the lowest recommended daily dose, and one for the highest recommended daily dose.

Formula: Total Daily Dosage Range

Calculation: (lowest dose)

$$\frac{40 \text{ kg} \times 25 \text{ mg/kg/day}}{1000 \text{ mg/day}}$$

(pt's weight)
(lowest recommended daily dose – drug reference)
(lowest total daily recommended dose – individual pt)

Calculation: (highest dose)

$$\frac{40 \text{ kg} \times 50 \text{ mg/kg/day}}{2000 \text{ mg/day}}$$

(pt's weight)
(highest recommended daily dose – drug reference)
(highest total daily recommended dose – individual pt)

The recommended total daily dosage range for this patient (based on the patient's weight) is between 1,000 to 2,000 mg per day.

Step 2b: Divide the recommended total daily dose (lowest and highest) into individual doses.

It is important to remember that the recommended dosage range is for the total daily dose. Both the lowest and the highest total daily dose must be divided by the number of times the drug will be administered to the patient in 24 hours. In the example in Figure 17-9, the dose is to be given q.6h, so the patient will receive four equal individual doses in a day.

Formula: Individual Dose From Total Daily Dose

Calculation: (lowest dose)

$$4\overline{)1000 \text{ mg}} = 250 \text{ mg}$$

(lowest total daily dose ÷ by # doses in 24 hr = lowest individual dose)

Calculation: (highest dose)

$$4\overline{)2000 \text{ mg}} = 500 \text{ mg}$$

(highest total daily dose ÷ by # doses in 24 hr = highest individual dose)

The recommended individual dose for this patient (based on the patient's weight) is between 250 to 500 mg per dose.

Step 3: Compare the recommended dose for the individual patient with the ordered dose.

Medication order = 250 mg q.6h

Recommended dosage range for this patient from the drug reference = 250 mg to 500 mg q.6h

Step 4: Make a clinical decision regarding safe dose.

Decision: Because the ordered dose is within the recommended dosage range, it is a safe dose for this patient.

Summary:

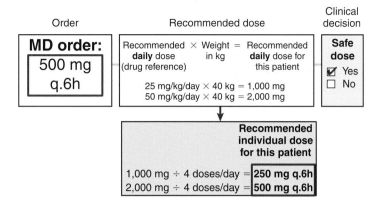

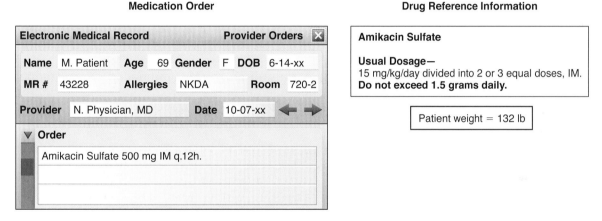

Here is another example in Figure 17-10 showing how to calculate and verify safe dose when the drug reference states the recommended dose as a total daily dose to be divided into individual doses:

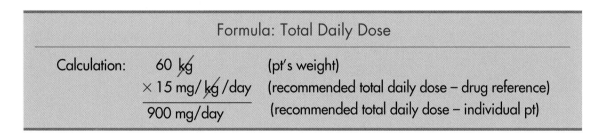

Figure 17-10. Verifying safe dose for recommended dose as a total daily dose.

Step 1: Convert the patient's weight from lb to kg if necessary.

The patient's weight is 132 lb (conversion step needed →132 lb = 60 kg)

Step 2a: Calculate the weight-based recommended total daily dose for the individual patient.

Only the formula for total daily dose will be shown for this calculation.

Formula: Total Daily Dose	
Calculation: 60 k̶g̶	(pt's weight)
× 15 mg/ k̶g̶ /day	(recommended total daily dose – drug reference)
───────── 900 mg/day	(recommended total daily dose – individual pt)

The recommended total daily dose for this patient (based on the patient's weight) is 900 mg per day.

Step 2b: Divide the recommended total daily dose into individual doses.

Next, the total daily dose needs to be divided by the number of individual doses to be administered in 24 hours. The drug reference states that the total daily dose can be given in 2 or 3 divided doses. Because the physician ordered the medication to be given twice a day (q.12h), it is logical to divide the recommended total daily dose by 2 to get the individual dose.

Formula: Individual Dose From Total Daily Dose

Calculation: $\dfrac{450 \text{ mg}}{2\overline{)900 \text{ mg}}}$ (total daily dose ÷ by 2 doses in 24 hr = individual dose)

The recommended individual dose for this patient (based on the patient's weight) is 450 mg per dose.

Step 3: Compare the recommended dose for the individual patient with the ordered dose.

Medication order = 500 mg q.12h

Recommended dose for this patient from the drug reference = 450 mg q.12h

Step 4: Make a clinical decision regarding safe dose.

Decision: Because the ordered dose is more than the recommended dose, it is not considered a safe dose. The nurse will need to contact the physician to clarify the order.

Summary:

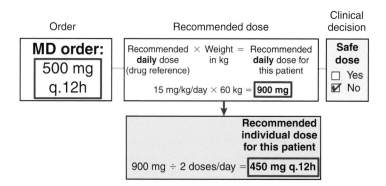

APPLY LEARNED KNOWLEDGE 17-2

Use the medication order and the information from the drug label or package insert to answer the following questions.

1. **Order:** Administer amoxicillin oral suspension 150 mg PO q.8h.

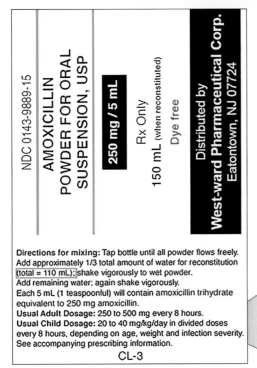

Usual Adult Dosage:
250 to 500 mg every 8 hours.
Usual Child Dosage:
20 to 40 mg/kg/day in divided doses every 8 hours, depending on age, weight, and infection severity. See accompanying prescribing information.

Patient is 5 y.o. and weighs 21 kg.

Calculate the weight-based recommended dosage range for q.8h administration to this patient. _____

Is the ordered dose a safe dose? _____

2. **Order:** Granisetron hydrochloride 0.8 mg IVP 30 min before chemotherapy.

DOSAGE AND ADMINISTRATION

Prevention of Chemotherapy-Induced Nausea and Vomiting

The recommended dosage for granisetron hydrochloride injection is 10 mcg/kg administered intravenously 30 minutes before initiation of chemotherapy, and only on the day(s) chemotherapy is given.

Pediatric Patients

The recommended dose in pediatric patients 2 to 16 years of age is 10 mcg/kg (see **CLINICAL TRIALS**). Pediatric patients under 2 years of age have not been studied.

Geriatric Patients, Renal Failure Patients or Hepatically Impaired Patients

No dosage adjustment is recommended (see **CLINICAL PHARMACOLOGY: Pharmacokinetics**).

Excerpt from granisetron hydrochloride package insert.

Patient is 49 y.o. and weighs 78 kg.

Calculate the weight-based recommended dose for this patient. _____

Is the ordered dose a safe dose? _____

Continued

APPLY LEARNED KNOWLEDGE 17-2—cont'd

3. Order: 300 mcg IV push granisetron hydrochloride 30 min before chemotherapy.
Patient is 9 y.o. and weighs 68 lb.

Calculate the weight-based recommended dose for this patient. _____

Is the ordered dose a safe dose? _____

4. Order: Start fluconazole 300 mg PO today only; followed by fluconazole 125 mg PO daily for 2 weeks.

> **Oropharyngeal candidiasis**
> The recommended dosage of fluconazole for oropharyngeal
> candidiasis in children is 6 mg/kg on the first day, followed by
> 3 mg/kg once daily. Treatment should be administered for at least
> 2 weeks to decrease the likelihood of relapse.

Excerpt from fluconazole package insert.

Patient is 13 y.o. and weighs 45 kg.

Calculate the weight-based recommended dose for this patient. _____

Is the ordered dose a safe dose? _____

5. Order: Initial dose of diltiazem hydrochloride 20 mg IV push now.

> **DOSAGE AND ADMINISTRATION**
> **Direct Intravenous Single Injections (Bolus)**
> The initial dose of diltiazem hydrochloride injection should be
> 0.25 mg/kg actual body weight as a bolus administered over 2
> minutes (20 mg is a reasonable dose for the average patient).

Excerpt from diltiazem hydrochloride package insert.

Patient is 69 y.o. and weighs 58 kg.

Calculate the weight-based recommended initial dose for this patient. _____

Is the ordered dose a safe dose? _____

Recommended Dose Based on Body Surface Area

The drug manufacturer may list the recommended dose of a medication as an amount of drug per **body surface area.** Body surface area **(BSA),** a measurement of the total surface of the patient's body, is measured in meters squared (m^2). Body surface area takes into account both the height and weight of the patient. Many oncology drugs, drugs used for children, and some drugs used for critically ill adults have recommended doses based on body surface area. As with weight-based dosing, a recommended dose that is based on body surface area must be calculated for each patient, based on that patient's BSA.

 The current practice of using body-surface area to establish recommended doses for anticancer drugs was implemented half a century ago. Recently, questions about the efficacy of BSA-dosing have been raised in the professional literature. Further research is needed to validate whether dosing based on BSA is more accurate than weight-based dosing or using a standard dose.

DETERMINING THE PATIENT'S BSA

In most clinical settings, the patient's BSA is calculated by the physician ordering the medication and is written on the patient's medical record. When verifying safe dose, the nurse uses the patient's BSA in the calculation, so it is important that the written BSA is accurate.

Safe practice requires the nurse to validate that the BSA written in the patient's medical record is correct. BSA must always be based on current height and weight measurements.

There are two common methods that can be used to calculate a patient's BSA: use of a standard BSA formula or use of a nomogram. The nurse can use either of these two methods when validating the accuracy of BSA written in the patient's medical record.

USE OF A FORMULA TO DETERMINE BSA

To calculate BSA using a formula, all that is needed is the patient's weight and height and a calculator with a square root function. Here are the standard formulas for calculating BSA, one using metric measurements and the other using household measurements for height and weight:

Formula: BSA Using Metric Measurements	Formula: BSA Using Household Measurements
$BSA (m^2) = \sqrt{\dfrac{wt\ (kg) \times ht\ (cm)}{3600}}$	$BSA (m^2) = \sqrt{\dfrac{wt\ (lb) \times ht\ (in)}{3131}}$

 Notice that the main difference in the two BSA formulas is the denominator within the square root sign.

Here is an example of how to calculate BSA using height and weight measurements from the metric system. To solve, first multiply the numerators of the fraction within the square root sign, then divide the product of the multiplication by the denominator of the fraction. Finally, press the square root symbol (√) on the calculator. The answer to this square root calculation is the BSA. The BSA should be rounded to the hundredths place, if necessary.

Formula: BSA Using Metric Measurements

Weight: 46 kg   Height: 105 cm

Square root problem set up:

$$BSA (m^2) = \sqrt{\frac{46\ kg \times 105\ cm}{3600}}$$

Calculate within the square root sign:
- first multiple the numbers in the numerator,
- then divide the product by the denominator.

$$= \sqrt{\frac{4830}{3600}} = \sqrt{1.341}$$

Press the square root symbol (√) on the calculator.

$$= \sqrt{1.341} = 1.158$$

Round square root calculation to the hundredths place for the BSA.

$$1.158 = 1.16\ m^2$$

$$BSA = 1.16\ m^2$$

The following shows an example of how to calculate BSA using height and weight measurements from the household system:

Formula: BSA Using Household Measurements

Weight: 100 lb   Height: 62 in

Square root problem set up:

$$\text{BSA (m}^2) = \sqrt{\dfrac{100 \text{ lb} \times 62 \text{ in}}{3131}}$$

Calculate within the square root sign:
- first multiple the numbers in the numerator,
- then divide the product by the denominator.

$$= \sqrt{\dfrac{6200}{3131}} = \sqrt{1.98}$$

Press the square root symbol ($\sqrt{\ }$) on the calculator.

$$= \sqrt{1.98} = 1.407$$

Round square root calculation to the hundredths place for the BSA.

$$1.407 = 1.41 \text{ m}^2$$

$$\text{BSA} = 1.41 \text{ m}^2$$

USE OF A NOMOGRAM TO DETERMINE BSA

The second common method of determining a patient's BSA is the use of a nomogram. A **nomogram** is a graph or chart that shows the relationship between different numerical variables, such as height and weight. A nomogram can be used to estimate BSA for the patient. An example of a weight and height-based nomogram is the **West Nomogram,** which is used for children (Fig. 17-11).

To read the West Nomogram, a straight line is drawn from the child's height, in the left-hand column, to the child's weight, in the right-hand column. The intersecting line on the surface area (SA) column provides an estimate of the child's BSA. The **Nomogram for Children of Normal Height for Weight,** which is in a box in the West Nomogram, can be used if a child is of normal height for his or her weight, as determined by standardized growth and development charts. In this nomogram, only the weight of the child is used to determine the body surface area. A ruler or other exact straight-edged item is used, as any slight imperfection in the edge will cause an error in estimating the BSA.

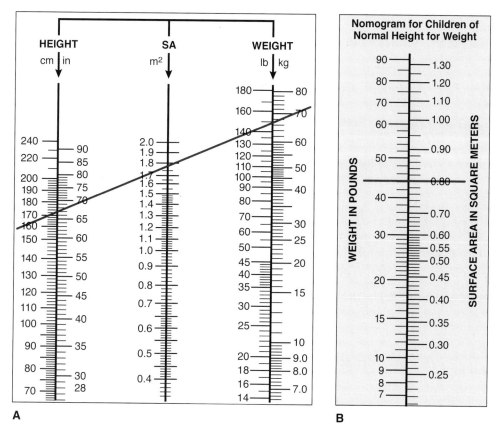

Figure 17-11. The West Nomogram. (A) BSA estimated to be 1.78 m². (B) BSA estimated to be 0.80 m².

CALCULATING AND VERIFYING SAFE DOSE BASED ON BSA

To verify safe dose when the recommended dose is based on BSA, the nurse needs to gather the following information:

- BSA of the patient (usually in m²) from the medical record
- Medication order
- Recommended dose from the drug reference

The method used to check for safe dose using a patient's BSA is similar to the method used for weight-based dosing. These are the steps the nurse can use to calculate a BSA-based recommended dose and verify whether the ordered dose is safe:

1. Validate (or calculate) the patient's BSA.
2. Calculate the BSA-based recommended dose for the individual patient.

   If using the ratio and proportion method, the known ratio is the BSA-based dose from the drug reference. The dimensional analysis calculation begins with the patient's BSA (rather than the ordered amount). The recommended dose from the drug reference is the conversion factor. The formula method $\dfrac{D}{H} \times Q = x$ cannot be used for BSA-based problems. Instead, a simple formula to calculate a BSA-based dose can be used:

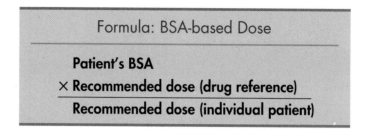

Formula: BSA-based Dose

$$\text{Patient's BSA} \times \frac{\text{Recommended dose (drug reference)}}{\text{Recommended dose (individual patient)}}$$

Work the calculation to the thousandths place (if needed), and round the answer to the hundredths place.

3. Compare the recommended dose for the individual patient with the ordered dose.

4. Make a clinical decision regarding safe dose.

Now apply these steps to the example of BSA-based recommended dose in Figure 17-12:

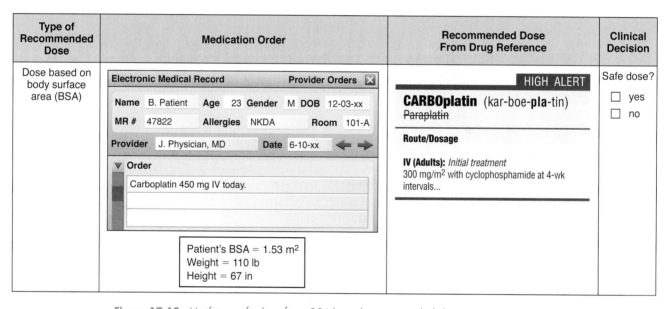

Type of Recommended Dose	Medication Order		Recommended Dose From Drug Reference	Clinical Decision
Dose based on body surface area (BSA)	**Electronic Medical Record**	**Provider Orders** ✖	HIGH ALERT	Safe dose?
	Name B. Patient Age 23 Gender M DOB 12-03-xx		**CARBOplatin** (kar-boe-**pla**-tin)	☐ yes
	MR # 47822 Allergies NKDA Room 101-A		~~Paraplatin~~	☐ no
	Provider J. Physician, MD Date 6-10-xx ⬅ ➡		**Route/Dosage**	
	▼ Order		**IV (Adults):** *Initial treatment* 300 mg/m² with cyclophosphamide at 4-wk intervals...	
	Carboplatin 450 mg IV today.			
	Patient's BSA = 1.53 m² Weight = 110 lb Height = 67 in			

Figure 17-12. Verifying safe dose for a BSA-based recommended dose.

Step 1: Validate (or calculate) the patient's BSA.

The patient's stated BSA is 1.53 m². Use the BSA formula with household measurements to validate the BSA:

$$\text{BSA (m}^2) = \sqrt{\frac{110 \times 67}{3131}} = \sqrt{\frac{7370}{3131}} = \sqrt{2.354} = 1.534$$

$$\text{BSA} = 1.53 \text{ m}^2$$

The stated BSA is correct. Now the nurse can verify safe dose.

Step 2: Calculate the BSA-based recommended dose for the individual patient.

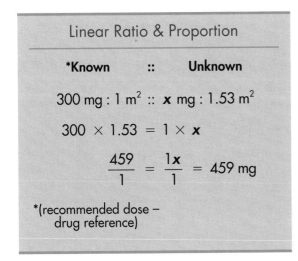

Linear Ratio & Proportion

*Known :: Unknown

$300 \text{ mg} : 1 \text{ m}^2 :: x \text{ mg} : 1.53 \text{ m}^2$

$300 \times 1.53 = 1 \times x$

$\dfrac{459}{1} = \dfrac{1x}{1} = 459 \text{ mg}$

*(recommended dose –
drug reference)

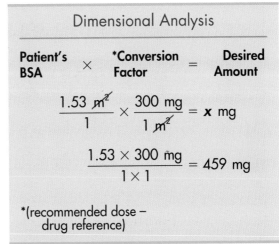

Dimensional Analysis

| Patient's BSA | × | *Conversion Factor | = | Desired Amount |

$\dfrac{1.53 \text{ m}^2}{1} \times \dfrac{300 \text{ mg}}{1 \text{ m}^2} = x \text{ mg}$

$\dfrac{1.53 \times 300 \text{ mg}}{1 \times 1} = 459 \text{ mg}$

*(recommended dose –
drug reference)

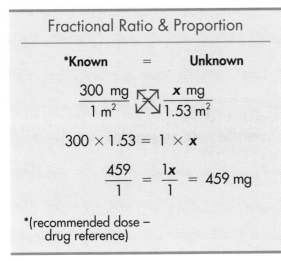

Fractional Ratio & Proportion

*Known = Unknown

$\dfrac{300 \text{ mg}}{1 \text{ m}^2} \quad \dfrac{x \text{ mg}}{1.53 \text{ m}^2}$

$300 \times 1.53 = 1 \times x$

$\dfrac{459}{1} = \dfrac{1x}{1} = 459 \text{ mg}$

*(recommended dose –
drug reference)

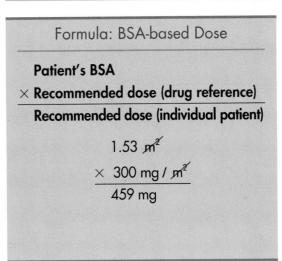

Formula: BSA-based Dose

**Patient's BSA
× Recommended dose (drug reference)**
Recommended dose (individual patient)

$\dfrac{1.53 \text{ m}^2 \times 300 \text{ mg} / \text{m}^2}{459 \text{ mg}}$

Step 3: Compare the recommended dose for the individual patient with the ordered dose.

Medication order = 450 mg (single dose)

Recommended dose for this patient from the drug reference = 459 mg (single dose)

Step 4: Make a clinical decision regarding safe dose.

Decision: Because the ordered dose is less than the recommended dose, it is a safe dose for this patient.

Summary:

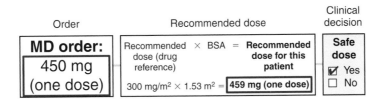

Order	Recommended dose	Clinical decision
MD order: 450 mg (one dose)	Recommended × BSA = Recommended dose (drug reference) dose for this patient 300 mg/m² × 1.53 m² = **459 mg (one dose)**	**Safe dose** ☑ Yes ☐ No

See Figure 17-13 for another example of how to apply the steps to verify safe dose based on BSA.

Medication Order

Drug Reference Information

Electronic Medical Record   **Provider Orders** ☒

Name Y. Patient   **Age** 39 **Gender** F **DOB** 9-05-xx

MR # 77643   **Allergies** NKDA   **Room** 220-A

Provider N. Physician, MD   **Date** 10-07-xx ⬅ ➡

▼ **Order**

Daunorubicin HCl 100 mg IV daily.

Patient's BSA = 1.62 m²
Weight = 55 kg
Height = 171 cm

HIGH ALERT

DAUNOrubicin hydrochloride
(daw-noe-**roo**-bi-sin **hye**-dro-**klor**-ide)
Cerubidine

Route/Dosage

Other dose regimens are used. In adults, cumulative dose should not exceed 550 mg/m² (450 mg/m² if previous chest radiation).

IV (Adults less than 60 yr): 45 mg/m²/day in first course, then for 2 days of second course (as part of combination regimen)...

Figure 17-13. Verifying safe dose for a BSA-based recommended dose.

Step 1: Validate (or calculate) the patient's BSA.

The patient's stated BSA is 1.62 m². Use the BSA formula with metric measurements to validate the BSA:

$$\text{BSA (m}^2) = \sqrt{\frac{55 \times 171}{3600}} = \sqrt{\frac{9405}{3600}} = \sqrt{2.613} = 1.616$$

$$\text{BSA} = 1.62 \text{ m}^2$$

The stated BSA is correct. Now the nurse can verify safe dose.

Step 2: Calculate the BSA-based recommended dose for the individual patient.

Only the multiplication method will be shown for this calculation.

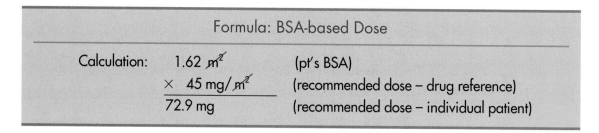

Formula: BSA-based Dose

Calculation:	1.62 m²	(pt's BSA)
	× 45 mg/m²	(recommended dose – drug reference)
	72.9 mg	(recommended dose – individual patient)

Step 3: Compare the recommended dose for the individual patient with the ordered dose.

Medication order = 100 mg daily

Recommended dose for this patient from the drug reference = 72.9 mg/day

Step 4: Make a clinical decision regarding safe dose.

Decision: Because the ordered dose is more than the recommended dose, it is not considered a safe dose for this patient. The nurse will need to contact the physician to clarify the order.

Summary:

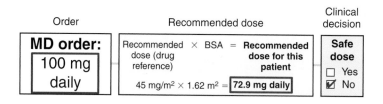

Order	Recommended dose	Clinical decision
MD order: 100 mg daily	Recommended × BSA = Recommended dose (drug reference) dose for this patient 45 mg/m² × 1.62 m² = 72.9 mg daily	**Safe dose** ☐ Yes ☑ No

APPLY LEARNED KNOWLEDGE 17-3

Use the medication order and the information about recommended dose from the drug label or package insert to answer the following questions.

1. **Order:** Daunorubicin hydrochloride 80 mg IV.

> **Representative Dose Schedules and Combination for the Approved Indication of Remission Induction in Adult Acute Nonlymphocytic Leukemia**
>
> For patients 60 years of age and above, daunorubicin hydrochloride 30 mg/m^2/day IV on days 1, 2, and 3 of the first course and on days...

Excerpt from daunorubcin hydrochloride package insert.

Patient is 67 y.o. and has a BSA of 1.9 m^2.

Calculate the BSA-based recommended dose for this patient. _____

Is the ordered dose a safe dose? _____

2. **Order:** Daunorubicin hydrochloride 50 mg IV.
   Patient is 83 y.o. and has a BSA of 1.7 m^2.

Calculate the BSA-based recommended dose for this patient. _____

Is the ordered dose a safe dose? _____

3. **Order:** Bleomycin 2 units IV for first two doses of chemotherapy. If no adverse reaction, give bleomycin 40 units weekly.

> **DOSAGE AND ADMINISTRATION**
>
> **BECAUSE OF THE POSSIBILITY OF AN ANAPHYLACTOID REACTION, LYMPHOMA PATIENTS SHOULD BE TREATED WITH 2 UNITS OR LESS FOR THE FIRST TWO DOSES. IF NO ACUTE REACTION OCCURS, THEN THE REGULAR DOSAGE SCHEDULE MAY BE FOLLOWED.**
>
> The following dose schedule is recommended: **Squamous cell carcinoma, non-Hodgkin's lymphoma, testicular carcinoma**— 0.25 to 0.50 units/kg (10 to 20 units/m^2) given intravenously, intramuscularly, or subcutaneously weekly or twice weekly.
>
> Hodgkin's Disease—0.25 to 0.50 units/kg (10 to 20 units/m^2) given intravenously, intramuscularly, or subcutaneously weekly or twice weekly. After a 50% response, a maintenance dose of 1 unit daily or 5 units weekly intravenously or intramuscularly should be given.
>
> Pulmonary toxicity of bleomycin appears to be dose related with a striking increase when the total dose is over 400 units. Total doses over 400 units should be given with great caution.
>
> **Note: When bleomycin for injection is used in combination with other antineoplastic agents, pulmonary toxicities may occur at lower doses.**

Excerpt from bleomycin package insert.

Patient is 39 y.o. with non-Hodgkin's lymphoma with a BSA of 2.1 m^2.

Calculate the BSA-based recommended dose for this patient. _____

Is the ordered dose a safe dose? _____

Continued

APPLY LEARNED KNOWLEDGE 17-3—cont'd

4. **Order:** Bleomycin 2 units IV today and next Tuesday. If no adverse reactions develop, give bleomycin 50 units weekly on Tuesdays.

Patient is 22 y.o. with a BSA of 1.75 m² who has testicular carcinoma.

Calculate the BSA-based recommended dose for this patient. _____

Is the ordered dose a safe dose? _____

5.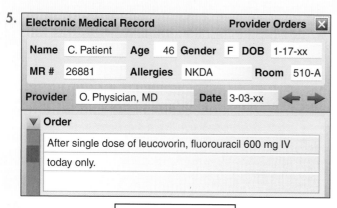

Patient's BSA = 1.8 m²

Calculate the BSA-based recommended dose for this patient. _____

Is the ordered dose a safe dose? _____

CLINICAL REASONING 17-1

The physician ordered an initial dose of valproic acid for a 12-year-old patient with complex partial seizures who weighs 40 kg. The nurse uses the drug reference to verify that the ordered dose is safe for the patient, and administers the 500 mg of valproic acid.

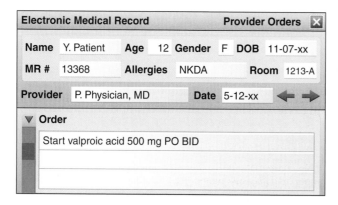

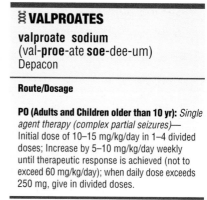

The administration of the valproic acid is:

A. *Correct; 500 mg is a safe dose to administer.*

B. *Not correct; the ordered dose should be given more frequently than BID.*

C. *Not correct; the nurse should call the physician because 500 mg is more than the recommended dose and is not a safe dose.*

D. *Not correct; the nurse should call the physician because 500 mg is less than the recommended dose and is not a safe dose.*

The verification of safe dose is a priority intervention of the nurse as patient advocate. To be considered safe, an ordered dose must not exceed the manufacturer's recommended dose of the medication. Because recommended doses can be stated as standard doses, total daily doses, doses based on weight, or doses based on BSA, the nurse must read and interpret the drug reference carefully. The nurse must use critical thinking to decide whether an ordered dose is safe. Safe practice requires verification of safe dose prior to the administration of each medication.

Developing Competency

Use the information from the drug references to answer the following questions.

1. The drug reference states the following:

DAPTOmycin (dap-to-**mye**-sin)
Cubicin

Classification
Therapeutic: anti-infectives
Pharmacologic: cyclic lipopeptide antibacterial agents

Pregnancy Category B

Route/Dosage

IV (Adults): 4 mg/kg every 24 hr.

Which of the following applies to this drug?
a. The recommended adult IV dose of daptomycin has to be calculated.
b. A conversion is needed if the patient's weight is in lb.
c. If the physician ordered this drug for a 15-year-old who weighs 50 kg, the recommended dose would be 200 mg every 24 hours.
d. If the physician ordered this drug for a 79-year-old who weighs 82 kg, the recommended dose would be 328 mg every 24 hours.

2. The drug reference states the following:

Diltiazem hydrochloride

DOSAGE AND ADMINISTRATION

Direct Intravenous Single Injection (Bolus)

The initial dose of diltiazem hydrochloride injection should be 0.25 mg/kg actual body weight as a bolus administered over 2 minutes (20 mg is a reasonable dose for the average patient).

Excerpt from diltiazem hydrochloride package insert.

Which of the following applies to this drug?
a. The recommended initial dose of diltiazem is a weight-based dose.
b. The recommended initial dose of diltiazem hydrochloride is the same for all patients.
c. If the physician ordered this drug for a patient who weighs 110 lb, the recommended initial IV dose would be 12.5 mg.
d. If the physician ordered this drug for a patient who weighs 75 kg, the recommended dose would be 18.75 mg.

3. **Usual dose:** IM (Children 8–12 yr): 0.3 mg

IM (Children 3–8 yr): 0.2 mg

IM (Children 7 mo–3 yr): 0.15 mg

If the nurse is to administer this drug to a 7-year-old child, it would be correct to give:
a. 0.15 mg
b. 0.2 mg
c. 0.3 mg

4.

CEPHALOSPORINS—SECOND GENERATION

cefOXitin (se-**fox**-i-tin)
Mefoxin

Classification
Therapeutic: anti-infectives
Pharmacologic: second-generation cephalo-
sporins

Pregnancy Category B

Route/Dosage

IM, IV (Adults): *Most infections—1 g q 6–8 hr...*

IM, IV (Children and Infants older than 3 mo):
Most infections—13.3–26.7 mg/kg q 4hr...

What is the recommended dosage range for cefoxitin for a 3-year old patient who weighs 33 lb?   _____

For the following questions, review the medication order, patient information, and medication label to determine whether the ordered dose is safe for the patient.

5. The doctor orders a maintenance dose of doxycycline calcium syrup 2 tsp PO daily. The pharmacy sends the following medication. Using the recommended dose printed on the drug label, is the ordered dose a safe dose to administer to an 85-year-old patient?

Vibramycin®
calcium
(doxycycline calcium)
SYRUP

Store below 86°F (30°C).

Dispense in tight, light-resistant containers (USP).

DOSAGE AND USE
See accompanying prescribing information.

USUAL DOSAGE
Adults: 200 mg on the first day (100 mg every 12 hours) followed by a maintenance dose of 100 mg a day.
Children above eight years of age:
Under 100 lbs. — 2 mg/lb. of body weight daily divided in two doses on the first day, followed by 1 mg/lb. of body weight on subsequent days in one or two doses.
Over 100 lbs. — See adult dosage.
doxycycline U.S. Pat. No. 3,200,149

* Each teaspoonful (5 mL) contains doxycycline calcium equivalent to 50 mg of doxycycline.

6. The doctor orders paclitaxel 330 mg IV infusion administered over 3 hours for a patient with newly diagnosed ovarian cancer who has a BSA of 1.9 m². The package insert for paclitaxel states the following under Dosage and Administration: Is the ordered dose a safe dose for this patient?   _____

For previously untreated patients with carcinoma of the ovary, one of the following recommended regimens maybe given every 3 weeks...

1. Paclitaxel injection administered intravenously over 3 hours at at a dose of 175 mg/m² followed by cisplatin...
2. Paclitaxel injection administered intravenously over 24 hours at a dose of 135 mg/m² followed by cisplatin...

Excerpt from Paclitaxel package insert.

7. The order is for cefoxitin 1.5 g IV q.4h for a 12-year-old patient who weighs 88 lb. *(Refer to the Cefoxitin drug information in question 4.)*

Is this a safe dose for this patient? _____

8. The following medication is available from the pharmacy. The order is for 1 g qid. IV. Is the ordered dose a safe dose? _____

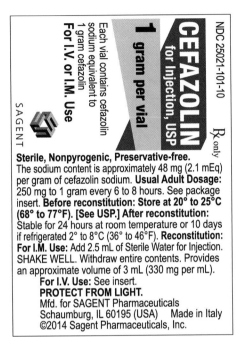

9. The nurse is preparing 0900 medications for the patient. Is the ordered dose a safe dose? _____

Electronic Medical Record   **MAR** ☒

| Name | D. Patient | Age | 74 | Gender | M | DOB | 8-21-xx |

| MR # | 96442 | Allergies | NKDA | Room | 401-1 |

| Date | 11-07-xx | Time | 0900 | ← → |

▼ **Scheduled Medications**

Time	Drug name	Dose	Route	Freq.	Adm.
0900	Bupropion	100 mg	PO	TID	

REMS

buPROPion (byoo-**proe**-pee-on)

Route/Dosage

Depression
PO (Adults): *Immediate-release*—100 mg twice daily initially; after 3 days may increase to 100 mg 3 times day...

10. The order is for 0.15 g of DOXOrubicin HCl Injection IV every 21 days for a patient who has a BSA of 1.7 m². Is the ordered dose a safe dose?   _____

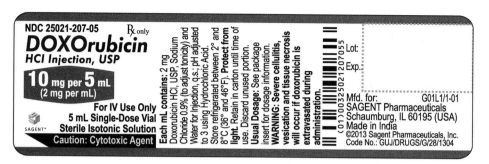

DOSAGE AND ADMINISTRATION

- Single agent: 60 to 75 mg/m² given intravenously every 21 days (2.1).
- In combination therapy: 40 to 75 mg/m² given intravenously every 21 to 28 days (2.1).
- Discontinue doxorubicin HCl in patients who develop signs or symptoms of cardiomyopathy (2.2).
- Reduce dose in patients with hepatic impairment (2.2).

Excerpt from package insert for DOXOrubicin.

11. The order is for 20 million International Units of interferon alfa-2b subcut three times a week for a patient with malignant melanoma who has a BSA of 1.75 m². The patient is in the fifth week of chemotherapy treatment with interferon alfa-2b. The following information is available in the drug reference:

Malignant melanoma: Usual dose, induction: 20 million International Units/m² daily for 5 days of each week for 4 weeks, followed by subcut maintenance dosing. . . .

Malignant melanoma: Usual dose, maintenance: 10 million units/m² subcut 3 times weekly for up to 6 months.

Is the ordered dose a safe dose?   _____

12. The order is for decitabine 27 mg IV over 3 hours q.8h for 3 days for a patient who weighs 130 lb and is 5 feet 9 inches tall. The patient's body surface area is documented as 1.8 m². The drug reference states the following: "Usual dose: 15 mg/m² as an infusion over 3 hours."

Is the ordered dose a safe dose?   _____

13. What is a safe dose of Dilantin for a 7-year-old patient who weighs 66 lb? Is the following order safe for this patient: "Start Dilantin 50 mg PO q.8h."   _____

Store at room temperature between 68°F to 77°F (20°C to 25°C). Protect from moisture.

DOSAGE AND USE
Pediatric patients, 5 mg/kg daily in two or three equally divided doses initially, with subsequent dosage individualized to a maximum of 300 mg daily. See package insert for full prescribing information.

NOT FOR ONCE-A-DAY DOSING
Chewable, flavored for pediatric patients. Dilantin Infatabs can be either chewed thoroughly before being swallowed or swallowed whole.
Store so that pediatric patients cannot eat these flavored tablets as candy.

Dispense in tight (USP), child-resistant container.

Each tablet contains 50 mg phenytoin, USP.

Manufactured by:
Pfizer Pharmaceuticals Ltd.
Vega Baja, PR 00694

ALWAYS DISPENSE WITH ACCOMPANYING MEDICATION GUIDE

Pfizer   NDC 0071-0007-24

INFATABS®

Dilantin®

Phenytoin Chewable Tablets, USP

50 mg

100 Tablets   **Rx only**

14. The patient has community-acquired pneumonia. The physician ordered azithromycin 500 mg PO daily for 10 days after the patient had received IV azithromycin for 2 days. Is the ordered dose a safe dose? _____

> **DOSAGE AND ADMINISTRATION**
> **(see INDICATIONS AND USAGE and CLINICAL PHARMACOLOGY.)**
>
> The recommended dose of azithromycin for injection for the treatment of adult patients with community-acquired pneumonia due to the indicated organisms is: 500 mg as a single daily dose by the intravenous route for at least two days. Intravenous therapy should be followed by azithromycin by the oral route at a single, daily dose of 500 mg, administered as two 250-mg tablets to complete a 7- to 10-day course of therapy. The timing of the switch to oral therapy should be done at the discretion of the physician and in accordance with clinical response.

Excerpt from azithromycin package insert.

15. The nurse is preparing to administer the following initial oral dose of amiodarone to the patient who has been receiving IV amiodarone for 8 days. Is the ordered dose a safe dose? _____

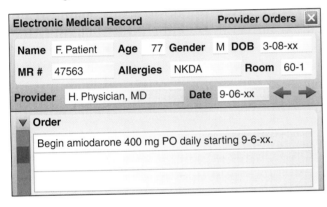

The following table provides suggested doses of oral amiodarone to be initiated after varying durations of amiodarone hydrochloride injection administration. These recommendations are made on the basis of a comparable total body amount of amiodarone delivered by the intravenous and oral routes, based on 50% bioavailability of oral amiodarone.

RECOMMENDATIONS FOR ORAL DOSAGE AFTER IV INFUSION

Duration of Amiodarone Hydrochloride Injection Infusion#	Initial Daily Dose of Oral Amiodarone
<1 week	800-1600 mg
1-3 weeks	600-800 mg
>3 weeks*	400 mg

Assuming a 720 mg/day infusion (0.5 mg/min).
* Amiodarone hydrochloride injection is not intended for maintenance treatment

Excerpt from amiodarone package insert.

16. The physician's order is for doxorubicin liposomal 90 mg IV every 4 weeks for a patient with ovarian cancer who has a BSA of 1.55 m². Is the ordered dose a safe dose? _____

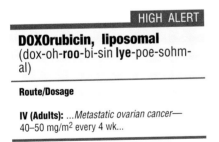

HIGH ALERT

DOXOrubicin, liposomal
(dox-oh-**roo**-bi-sin **lye**-poe-sohm-al)

Route/Dosage

IV (Adults): ...*Metastatic ovarian cancer—* 40–50 mg/m² every 4 wk...

17. The patient is 12 days old, has a gestational age of 29 weeks, and weighs 3 kg. The pediatrician orders fluconazole 30 mg q.72h IV for this neonate. Does the ordered dose fall within the recommendations of the drug manufacturer? _____

Dosage and Administration in Children
The following dose equivalency scheme should generally provide equivalent exposure in pediatric and adult patients:

Pediatric Patients	Adults
3 mg/kg	100 mg
6 mg/kg	200 mg
12* mg/kg	400 mg

*Some older children may have clearances similar to that of adults. Absolute doses exceeding 600 mg/day are not recommended.

Experience with fluconazole in neonates is limited to pharmacokinetic studies in premature newborns.

(See **CLINICAL PHARMACOLOGY**.) Based on the prolonged half-life seen in premature newborns (gestational age 26 to 29 weeks), these children, in the first two weeks of life, should receive the same dosage (mg/kg) as in older children, but administered every 72 hours. After the first two weeks, these children should be dosed once daily. No information regarding fluconazole pharmacokinetics in full-term newborns is available.

Excerpt from fluconazole package insert.

18. The physician writes an order for eribulin 2 mg IV today (the first day of the chemotherapy cycle for this drug) for a 54-year-old patient with breast cancer. The patient's BSA is 1.46 m^2. Today's lab results include a platelet count of 19,000/mm^3. Should the nurse administer the dose of eribulin to the patient? _____

---

eribulin (e-rib-yoo-lin)
Halaven

Classification
Therapeutic: antineoplastics
Pharmacologic: antimicrotubulars

Pregnancy Category D

Route/Dosage

IV (Adults): 1.4 mg/m^2 on days 1 and 8 of a 21-day cycle; dose modifications required for hepatic impairment, moderate renal impairment, neutropenia, thrombocytopenia, or peripheral neuropathy...
• *Permanently reduce 1.4 mg/m^2 eribulin dose to 1.1 mg/m^2 if:* ...platelets <25,000/mm^3, platelets <50,000/mm^3 requiring transfusion...

19. The home care nurse is visiting a family with a child who was just discharged from the hospital after having a seizure. The child is 9 years old and weighs 28 kg. The discharge medications include clonazepam 0.375 mg PO BID. Is the ordered dose a safe dose? _____

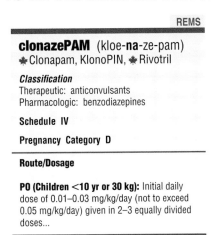

REMS

clonazePAM (kloe-na-ze-pam)
✿ Clonapam, KlonoPIN, ✿ Rivotril

Classification
Therapeutic: anticonvulsants
Pharmacologic: benzodiazepines

Schedule IV

Pregnancy Category D

Route/Dosage

PO (Children <10 yr or 30 kg): Initial daily dose of 0.01–0.03 mg/kg/day (not to exceed 0.05 mg/kg/day) given in 2–3 equally divided doses...

20. On 11-9-xx, the nurse administered 6 mg methotrexate PO to the patient with leukemia who has a BSA of 1.9 m². On 11-12-xx, the nurse administered methotrexate 40 mg PO to the patient. Were the nurse's actions correct? _____

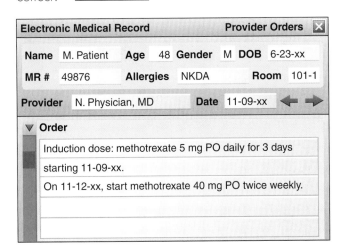

Electronic Medical Record — Provider Orders ☒

Name M. Patient   Age 48   Gender M   DOB 6-23-xx

MR # 49876   Allergies NKDA   Room 101-1

Provider N. Physician, MD   Date 11-09-xx ⬅ ➡

▼ Order

Induction dose: methotrexate 5 mg PO daily for 3 days starting 11-09-xx.

On 11-12-xx, start methotrexate 40 mg PO twice weekly.

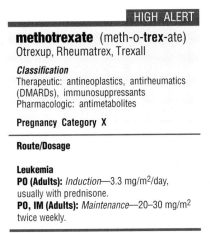

HIGH ALERT

methotrexate (meth-o-**trex**-ate)
Otrexup, Rheumatrex, Trexall

Classification
Therapeutic: antineoplastics, antirheumatics (DMARDs), immunosuppressants
Pharmacologic: antimetabolites

Pregnancy Category X

Route/Dosage

Leukemia
PO (Adults): *Induction*—3.3 mg/m²/day, usually with prednisone.
PO, IM (Adults): *Maintenance*—20–30 mg/m² twice weekly.

CHAPTER 18

Titration of Intravenous Medications

LEARNING OUTCOMES

Discuss the concept of titration.

Identify the components of a titration order.

Solve problems related to setting up an initial titration infusion.

Solve problems related to adjusting a titration infusion rate.

Critically ill patients are often given potent **high alert** medications by IV infusion through a process called **titration.** This process involves "titrating" the dose of medication by adjusting (increasing or decreasing) the IV rate of the infusion to achieve a desired physiological response in the patient. Many of the drugs administered by titration have a narrow **therapeutic index** or margin of safety. This means that the margin between a safe dose and a toxic or lethal dose is very small. Titration provides a process for determining the minimum amount of a drug that is required to attain a desired physiological response in the patient while remaining within the margin of safety.

Safe Nursing Practice and Titration of IV Medications

Because titrated IV medications may be adjusted frequently, (i.e., q.5 min, q.15 min), the nurse must be knowledgeable about the drug's onset of action, duration, elimination, and therapeutic effects. Knowledge of expected and adverse drug effects is critical in providing safe care to the patient. Titrated medications administered by the IV route will have a rapid onset of action, usually a few seconds or minutes, necessitating continuous monitoring for the drug's immediate physiological effect on the patient. The duration of action is influenced by the drug's **half-life.** The half-life refers to the amount of time it takes for one-half of the strength of a drug to be eliminated from the body. Drugs with a short half-life (see Fig. 18-1) are

**NITROGLYCERIN IN DEXTROSE (nitroglycerin) injection
CLINICAL PHARMACOLOGY**

The principal pharmacological action of nitroglycerin is relaxation of vascular smooth muscle and consequent dilatation of peripheral arteries and veins, especially the latter...

Pharmacokinetics:
The volume of distribution of nitroglycerin is about 3 L/kg, and nitroglycerin is cleared from this volume at extremely rapid rates, with a resulting serum half-life of about 3 minutes..

Excerpted from **NITROGLYCERIN IN DEXTROSE (nitroglycerin) injection package insert (© Baxter Healthcare Corporation).**

Figure 18-1. Nitroglycerin in Dextrose injection and half-life of the drug.

eliminated from the body more quickly than drugs with a longer half-life, requiring more frequent administration of the drug to maintain a therapeutic serum concentration. Like-wise, the longer a drug's half-life, the longer it takes for the body to eliminate the drug, and there is more active drug available for a longer period of time.

The administration of any titrated drug warrants the implementation of practices that promote safe care, including double-checking with another licensed professional for verifi-cation of titrated doses, use of smart pumps, and communicating assessment findings.

Differentiating IV Infusion Orders

Recognizing the different types of IV orders assists the nurse to calculate the correct infusion rate and to implement appropriate nursing interventions for assessing and monitoring the patient (see Table 18-1). Recall that the order for a primary IV includes the IV solution and the frequency of administration or hourly infusion rate. The IV piggyback (IVPB) order iden-tifies the drug, the drug dose, and the frequency of administration. Because titration involves the administration of small doses of medication that stimulate a physiological response, the nurse can readily identify the titration order by the following two components:

■ The strength of the ordered drug in a specific volume of IV fluid

■ The amount of drug administered over time (minutes or hours)

Table 18-1. Differentiating IV Infusion Orders

TYPE OF IV ORDER	PURPOSE	HOW THE ORDER IS WRITTEN
Titration	Administration of small amounts of IV medica-tion, titrated based on the patient's physio-logical response.	Strength of medication (mg, mcg, g, units, and so on) over time (minutes or hours).
Primary IV	Continuous IV fluid administration for hydration and fluid and electrolyte replacement.	Volume of fluid ordered as a continuous infusion.

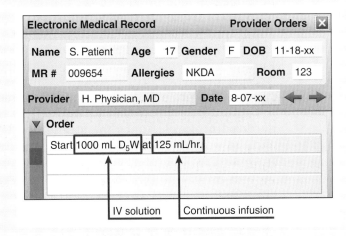

Continued

Table 18-1. Differentiating IV Infusion Orders—cont'd

TYPE OF IV ORDER	PURPOSE	HOW THE ORDER IS WRITTEN
IVPB	Intermittent administration of IV medications.	Medication is mixed in a small volume of fluid and administer as ordered.

Electronic Medical Record — **Provider Orders** ☒

Name　E. Patient　Age　40　Gender　M　DOB　2-26-xx

MR #　56709　Allergies　NKDA　Room　314

Provider　E. Physician, MD　Date　2-17-xx　⬅　➡

▼ **Order**

500 mg ampicillin | IVPB q.4h

Drug and dose　|　Intravenous piggyback medication

When a medication is to be administered by titration, the strength of the drug and the type and volume of IV fluid are ordered by the physician based on the patient's clinical condition. Ready-to-use IV bags are available for some drugs in standard concentrations. Certain drugs are stable for just a few hours; therefore, the pharmacist will prepare the ordered IV bag prior to administration.

Order for the Titration of Medications

There are two methods by which medications by IV infusion may be titrated in clinical practice:

1. Titration per protocol
2. Titration with parameters

The orders for both methods of titration contain the strength of the drug in a specific volume of IV solution and the titration dose administered over time (minutes or hours). The physician determines the titration method most appropriate for the patient.

TITRATION PER PROTOCOL

Protocols used in the titration of medications are collaboratively developed by physicians, pharmacists, and nurses for the purpose of standardizing procedures for the safe administration of the drug. Titration drug protocols identify the criteria (i.e., laboratory test results) for increasing or decreasing the dose of the drug. Protocols may also include information regarding the roles and responsibilities of the physician, pharmacist, and nurse; nursing interventions; monitoring requirements; and appropriate interventions for treating an adverse drug reaction. Examples of drugs titrated based on a standard protocol include heparin, insulin, oxytocin, and amiodarone.

Figure 18-2 demonstrates a physician's order for titration of heparin based on a standardized protocol. Notice the strength of the drug, the type and volume of IV solution, and the titration dose. In this order, the titration of heparin per protocol starts with the results of the laboratory test (aPTT). The nurse will refer to the heparin titration protocol to increase or decrease the dose of the drug based on the results of the required laboratory test.

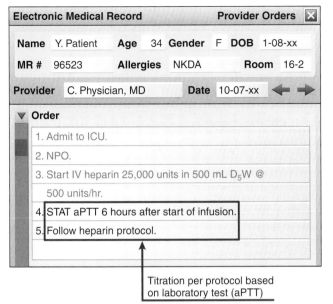

Electronic Medical Record	Provider Orders ☒

Name Y. Patient **Age** 34 **Gender** F **DOB** 1-08-xx

MR # 96523 **Allergies** NKDA **Room** 16-2

Provider C. Physician, MD **Date** 10-07-xx ⬅ ➡

▼ **Order**

1. Admit to ICU.

2. NPO.

3. Start IV heparin 25,000 units in 500 mL D₅W @ 500 units/hr.

4. STAT aPTT 6 hours after start of infusion.

5. Follow heparin protocol.

Titration per protocol based on laboratory test (aPTT)

HEParin Dose Titration Protocol	
aPTT (seconds)	**Infusion**
<34	↑ 100 units/hr
34–44	↑ 100 units/hr
45–54	↑ 50 units/hr
55–70	Keep at current rate
71–85	↓ 100 units/hr
86–100	↓ 150 units/hr
101–125	↓ 200 units/hr
>125	Notify MD STAT

Figure 18-2. A protocol for the titration of heparin.

Here is an example of a clinical situation in which the heparin titration protocol is used:

The nurse starts the heparin infusion at 1300 and the result of the aPTT laboratory test at 1900 is 40 seconds. Following the heparin titration protocol, the nurse will increase the heparin dose 100 units per hour so that the patient receives 600 units of heparin per hour. The nurse will refer to the protocol to determine when a follow-up aPTT test is to be done, and for patient monitoring and reporting requirements.

TITRATION WITH PARAMETERS

Unlike the titration per protocol, the physician's order for titration with parameters order includes guidelines for observing specific individualized physiological changes in the patient (such as blood pressure, heart rate, ECG pattern) that guide the nurse in the titration of the drug. Figure 18-3 gives two clinical examples of titration by parameters.

Management of blood pressure

A patient has a BP of 84/48. A medication to raise BP is started at 100 mcg/min (15 mL/hr). Fifteen minutes later, the BP is 92/58. The infusion rate of the medication is increased to 200 mcg/min (30 mL/hr). The patient's blood pressure is maintained at 106/73 on the 200 mcg/min dose.

Management of chest pain

A patient has severe chest pain. A vasodilator medication is started at 5 mcg/min (6 mL/hr). The patient states that the chest pain is gone within 5 minutes. The infusion rate of the medication is maintained at 6 mL/hr for 12 hours then decreased to 3 mL/hr. The patient remains free of chest pain.

Figure 18-3. Titrating IV medications with titration parameters.

To effectively and safely guide the nurse in titrating the drug and monitoring for the desired physiological response, the physician's order must communicate specific titration parameters. In reading a titration order, the nurse needs to identify the following five components:

1. Initial dose or infusion rate

2. Titration parameters (specific dose adjustment increments)

3. Time interval(s) for adjustment of dose and evaluation

4. Patient response or goal

5. Maximum and minimum dose limits

Titration of IV medications begins with the administration of an initial dose. The nurse monitors the patient and uses the titration parameters to adjust the dose at the ordered intervals. The dose will continue to be adjusted until the patient's goal (as defined in the order) is achieved, or the maximum dose limit has been reached (see Fig. 18-4). If the physiological response is not achieved within the titration parameters, the nurse needs to consult with the physician to reevaluate the order and/or the patient goals.

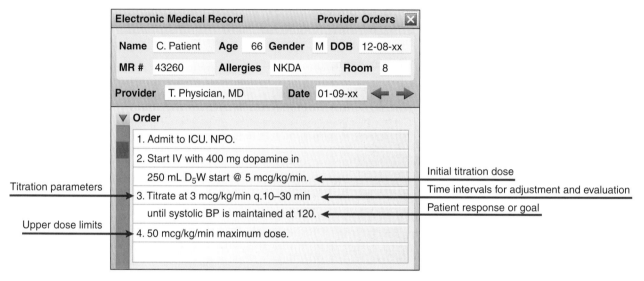

Figure 18-4. The physician's order with titration parameters.

APPLY LEARNED KNOWLEDGE 18-1

Use the physician's orders to answer each of the following questions.

1.

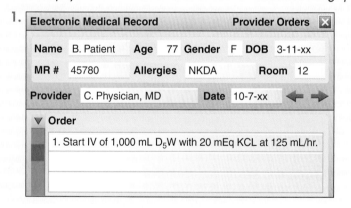

Select the statement(s) that apply to this order.

a. This is an order for a primary IV.

b. This is an order for titration of a drug.

c. This is an order for an IVPB.

APPLY LEARNED KNOWLEDGE 18-1—cont'd

2.

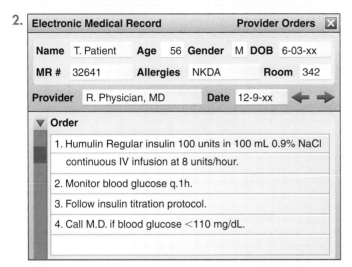

Electronic Medical Record		Provider Orders	☒

Name T. Patient **Age** 56 **Gender** M **DOB** 6-03-xx

MR # 32641 **Allergies** NKDA **Room** 342

Provider R. Physician, MD **Date** 12-9-xx ← →

▼ **Order**

1. Humulin Regular insulin 100 units in 100 mL 0.9% NaCl continuous IV infusion at 8 units/hour.
2. Monitor blood glucose q.1h.
3. Follow insulin titration protocol.
4. Call M.D. if blood glucose <110 mg/dL.

Select the statement(s) that apply to this order.
a. This is an order for an IVPB.
b. This is an order for titration of a drug.
c. The drug will be titrated per protocol.

3.

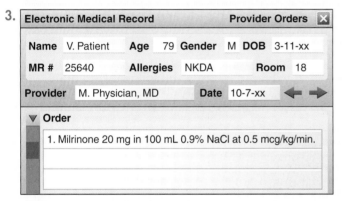

Electronic Medical Record		Provider Orders	☒

Name V. Patient **Age** 79 **Gender** M **DOB** 3-11-xx

MR # 25640 **Allergies** NKDA **Room** 18

Provider M. Physician, MD **Date** 10-7-xx ← →

▼ **Order**

1. Milrinone 20 mg in 100 mL 0.9% NaCl at 0.5 mcg/kg/min.

Select the components written in the titration order.
a. Initial dose or infusion rate
b. Titration parameter for adjustment of dose
c. Time interval for adjustment of dose
d. Patient response or goal
e. Maximum dose limits

4.

Electronic Medical Record		Provider Orders	☒

Name N. Patient **Age** 69 **Gender** F **DOB** 5-19-xx

MR # 45780 **Allergies** NKDA **Room** 11

Provider I. Physician, MD **Date** 2-14-xx ← →

▼ **Order**

1. Labetalol 400 mg in 200 mL 0.9% NaCl at 0.25 mg/min.
2. Titrate at 0.25 mg/min every 4 hours to keep systolic BP at ≥100.
3. Maximum dose 4 mg/min.

Select the components written in the titration order.
a. Initial dose or infusion rate
b. Titration parameter for adjustment of dose
c. Time interval for adjustment of dose
d. Patient response or goalk
e. Maximum dose limits

Continued

APPLY LEARNED KNOWLEDGE 18-1—cont'd

5.

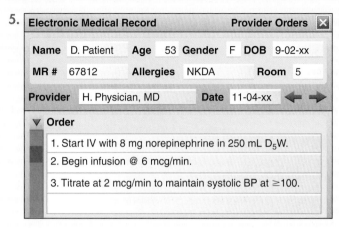

Electronic Medical Record	Provider Orders ☒

Name D. Patient   **Age** 53 **Gender** F **DOB** 9-02-xx

MR # 67812   **Allergies** NKDA   **Room** 5

Provider H. Physician, MD   **Date** 11-04-xx ← →

▼ **Order**

1. Start IV with 8 mg norepinephrine in 250 mL D$_5$W.
2. Begin infusion @ 6 mcg/min.
3. Titrate at 2 mcg/min to maintain systolic BP at ≥100.

Select the components written in the titration order.
a. Initial dose or infusion rate
b. Titration parameters for adjustment of dose
c. Time interval(s) for adjustment of dose
d. Patient response or goal
e. Maximum and minimum dose limits

Identifying the Information From the Titration Order

To accurately administer and periodically adjust the hourly volume (mL/hr) of a titrated drug, it is critical for the nurse to understand the information in the titration order. In working with a titration order, the nurse needs to identify the following components:

■ The strength of the drug
■ The specific IV fluid volume
■ The amount of the drug to be administered over time (hours and minutes)

Titration orders vary and may require several preliminary calculations including conversion of metric units of measurement, conversion of lb to kg (when working with weight-based orders), and conversion of minutes to hours (as IV infusion pumps are set in mL per hour). The nurse must systematically identify the components of the titration order and any preliminary calculations needed prior to solving for the hourly volume (mL/hr). Look at the various titration orders presented in Table 18-2.

Table 18-2. Identifying the Components Used in Calculating Titration Problems

SAMPLE TITRATION ORDER	COMPONENTS OF THE TITRATION PROBLEM	USING THE COMPONENTS, THE NURSE IDENTIFIES:
Lorazepam 100 mg in 100 mL D$_5$W at 0.2 mg/hr.	1. Strength of the drug: **100 mg** 2. Specific volume: **100 mL** 3. Amount of drug to be administered over time: **0.2 mg/hr**	• That the units of measurement are the same • That the problem can be set up and solved without any preliminary calculations
Epinephrine 2 mg in 250 mL D$_5$W @ 2 mcg/min.	1. Strength of the drug: **2 mg** 2. Specific volume: **250 mL** 3. Amount of drug to be administered over time: **2 mcg/min** ↑	• That the units of measurement are not the same; a metric conversion is needed • The need to calculate for the mL/hr (not minutes) to set on the IV pump

Table 18-2. Identifying the Components Used in Calculating Titration Problems—cont'd

SAMPLE TITRATION ORDER	COMPONENTS OF THE TITRATION PROBLEM	USING THE COMPONENTS, THE NURSE IDENTIFIES:
Dexmedetomidine 200 mcg in 50 mL 0.9% NaCl at 0.2 mcg/kg/hr	1. Strength of the drug: **200 mcg** 2. Specific volume: **50 mL** 3. Amount of drug to be administered over time: **0.2 mcg/kg/hr** ↑	• That the units of measurement are the same • That this is a weight-based titration order; the patient's weight in kg is needed for the calculation of the hourly rate
Nitroglycerine 50 mg in 250 mL D₅W at 5 mcg/min. Titrate at 5 mcg/min q.5 min until chest pain is relieved. Maximum dose: 200 mcg/min.	1. Strength of the drug: **50 mg** 2. Specific volume: **250 mL** 3. Amount of drug to be administered over time: **5 mcg/min** ↑	• That the units of measurement are not the same; a metric conversion is needed • The need to calculate for the mL/hr (not minutes) to set on the IV pump • The need to calculate (mL/hr) for the adjusted titration rate if the patient experiences chest pain (titrate infusion by 5 mcg/min q.5min) • The need to calculate (mL/hr) for the maximum dose that may be administered (200 mcg/min)

 Solving for the hourly volume (mL/hr) may require multiple conversions; therefore, the recommended standard of practice is that calculations for titrated drugs be verified for accuracy by another licensed health-care professional.

Solving for the Hourly Volume (mL/hr) for Titrated IV Medications

When solving titration problems, the nurse needs to calculate the infusion rate to set on the IV pump. To set up and solve for this hourly volume (mL/hr) for a titrated medication, the nurse needs to identify the following:

■ The total drug in the IV (total drug or **TD**)

■ The total volume of fluid in the IV bag (total volume or **TV**)

■ The amount of drug to be administered over time (hourly drug or **HD**)

Once this information is gathered, the problem can be set up using one of the methods of calculation. The number of mL/hr to set on the IV pump (hourly volume or **HV**) is the unknown in a titration problem.

With Ratio and Proportion, the TD and TV make up the known ratio, and the HD and HV make up the unknown ratio.

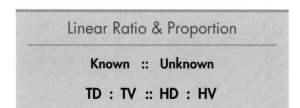

Linear Ratio & Proportion

Known :: Unknown

TD : TV :: HD : HV

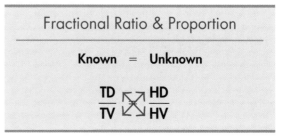

Fractional Ratio & Proportion

Known = Unknown

$$\frac{TD}{TV} \diagup\!\!\!\!\diagdown \frac{HD}{HV}$$

With Dimensional Analysis, the HD, TD, and TV are part of the Ordered Amount. Conversion factors are used as needed.

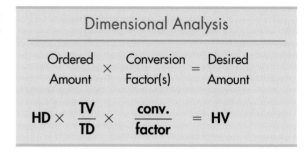

The Formula Method $\dfrac{D}{H} \times Q = x$ cannot be used; instead, a formula for titration can be substituted:

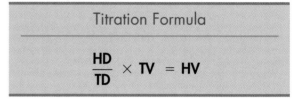

The titration order consists of specific information that guides the nurse in the administration of potent drugs. It is important for the nurse to thoroughly understand the titration order and carefully solve titration problems that contain:

■ The same units of measurement

■ Unlike units of measurement

■ Weight-based doses

■ Drugs ordered per minute

■ Adjustment of the titration dose

Each of these types of titration problems will be discussed separately.

SOLVING FOR HOURLY VOLUME (HV) WHEN UNITS OF MEASUREMENT ARE THE SAME

In Figure 18-5, the titration order for heparin identifies the TD, the TV, and the HD. The unit of measurement in the TD (units) is the same as the unit of measurement in the HD (units/hr) IV. The nurse will need to determine the hourly volume in mL/hr (HV) to set on the IV pump. Because the units of measurement are the same, no preliminary calculations are needed.

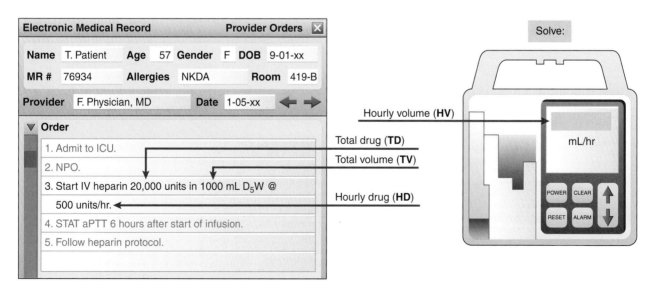

Figure 18-5. Solving for the hourly volume (mL/hr).

Here is how the problem is set up and solved:

Linear Ratio & Proportion

Known :: Unknown

TD : TV :: HD : HV

20,000 units : 1000 mL :: 500 units/hr : x mL/hr

$$20,000x = 500,000$$

$$\frac{20,000x}{20,000} = \frac{500,000}{20,000}$$

$$x = 25 \text{ mL/hr}$$

Dimensional Analysis

Ordered Amount	$\times$	Conversion Factor	$=$	Desired Amount

$$HD \times \frac{TV}{TD} \times \frac{\text{conv.}}{\text{factor}} = HV$$

$$\frac{500 \text{ units}}{1 \text{ hr}} \times \frac{1000 \text{ mL}}{20,000 \text{ units}} = x \text{ mL/hr}$$

$$\frac{500 \times 1000 \text{ mL}}{1 \text{ hr} \times 20,000} = x \text{ mL/hr}$$

$$x = 25 \text{ mL/hr}$$

Fractional Ratio & Proportion

Known = Unknown

$$\frac{TD}{TV} = \frac{HD}{HV}$$

$$\frac{20,000 \text{ units}}{1000 \text{ mL}} \diagup\!\!\!\diagdown \frac{500 \text{ units/hr}}{x \text{ mL/hr}}$$

$$20,000x = 500,000$$

$$\frac{20,000x}{20,000} = \frac{500,000}{20,000}$$

$$x = 25 \text{ mL/hr}$$

Titration Formula

$$\frac{HD}{TD} \times TV = HV$$

$$\frac{500 \text{ units/hr}}{20,000 \text{ units}} \times 1000 \text{ mL} = x \text{ mL/hr}$$

$$\frac{500}{20,000} \times 1000 = x \text{ mL/hr}$$

$$x = 25 \text{ mL/hr}$$

SOLVING FOR HOURLY VOLUME (HV) WHEN UNITS OF MEASUREMENT ARE NOT THE SAME

Sometimes the unit of measurement in the TD (the total drug in the IV) is not the same as the unit of measurement in the HD (the amount of drug to be administered per hour). With the ratio and proportion or the titration formula methods, a preliminary calculation must be done so that the units of measurement are the same before the nurse can solve for the HV (the hourly volume in mL/hr). With the dimensional analysis method, a conversion factor is used. Conversion between units of measurement is covered in Unit 3.

In the example shown in Figure 18-6, the unit of measurement in TD (g) is not the same as the unit of measurement in the HD (mg).

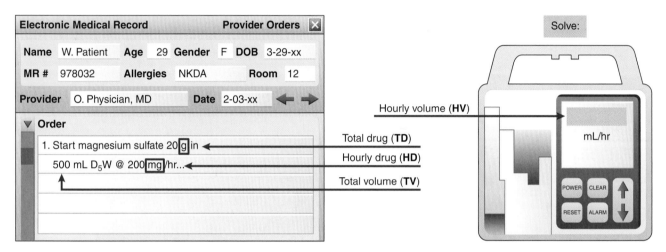

Figure 18-6. Converting the units of measurement.

Linear Ratio & Proportion

Known   ::   Unknown

Convert mg to g

$$200 \text{ mg/hr} = 0.2 \text{ g/hr}$$

Solve

TD : TV   ::   HD : HV

$$20 \text{ g} : 500 \text{ mL} :: 0.2 \text{ g/hr} : x \text{ mL/hr}$$

$$20x = 100$$

$$\frac{20x}{20} = \frac{100}{20}$$

$$x = 5 \text{ mL/hr}$$

Dimensional Analysis

$$\frac{\text{Ordered}}{\text{Amount}} \times \frac{\text{Conversion}}{\text{Factor(s)}} = \frac{\text{Desired}}{\text{Amount}}$$

$$\text{HD} \times \frac{\text{TV}}{\text{TD}} \times \frac{\text{conv.}}{\text{factor}} = \text{HV}$$

$$\frac{200 \text{ m\cancel{g}}}{1 \text{ hr}} \times \frac{500 \text{mL}}{20 \text{ \cancel{g}}} \times \frac{1 \text{ \cancel{g}}}{1000 \text{ m\cancel{g}}} = x \text{ mL/hr}$$

$$\frac{200 \times 500 \text{ mL} \times 1}{1 \text{ hr} \times 20 \times 1000} = x \text{ mL/hr}$$

$$x = 5 \text{ mL/hr}$$

Fractional Ratio & Proportion

Known   =   Unknown

Convert mg to g

$$200 \text{ mg/hr} = 0.2 \text{ g/hr}$$

Solve

$$\frac{\text{TD}}{\text{TV}} = \frac{\text{HD}}{\text{HV}}$$

$$\frac{20 \text{ g}}{500 \text{ mL}} \bowtie \frac{0.2 \text{ g/hr}}{x \text{ mL/hr}}$$

$$20x = 100$$

$$\frac{20x}{20} = \frac{100}{20}$$

$$x = 5 \text{ mL/hr}$$

Titration Formula

Convert mg to g

$$200 \text{ mg/hr} = 0.2 \text{ g/hr}$$

Solve

$$\frac{\text{HD}}{\text{TD}} \times \text{TV} = \text{HV}$$

$$\frac{0.2 \text{ \cancel{g}/hr}}{20 \text{ \cancel{g}}} \times 500 \text{ mL} = x \text{ mL/hr}$$

$$\frac{0.2}{20} \times 500 = x \text{ mL/hr}$$

$$x = 5 \text{ mL/hr}$$

APPLIED LEARNED KNOWLEDGE 18-2

Use the titration order to solve the following problems.

1. Order: Diltiazem HCl IV to infuse at 12 mg/hr
   IV: 0.125 g diltiazem HCl in 500 mL D$_5$W
   How many mL/hr will the nurse set on the IV pump? _____

2. Order: IV heparin to infuse at 800 units/hr
   IV: Heparin 20,000 units in 500 mL 0.9% NaCL
   How many mL/hr will the nurse set on the IV pump? _____

3. Order: Morphine sulfate IV to infuse at 3 mg/hr
   IV: 250 mg morphine sulfate in 500 mL D$_5$W
   How many mL/hr will the nurse set on the IV pump? _____

4. Order: Regular Humulin insulin IV infusion to infuse at 5 units/hr
   IV: Regular Humulin insulin 100 units in 1 L 0.9% NaCL
   How many mL/hr will the nurse set on the IV pump? _____

5. Order: IV aminophylline to infuse at 5 mg/hr
   IV: 0.5 g aminophylline in 500 mL D$_5$W
   How many mL/hr will the nurse set on the IV pump? _____

SOLVING FOR HOURLY VOLUME (ML/HR) WITH WEIGHT-BASED TITRATION ORDERS

Some titration drugs are ordered based on the patient's weight. To solve weight-based titration problems, the nurse needs to first calculate the weight-based dose for the individual patient. Weight-based medication orders are discussed in Chapter 17, Verifying Safe Dose. With the ratio and proportion or the titration formula methods, a preliminary calculation for the individual weight-based dose is required. Once this has been calculated, this individual weight-based dose is used as the hourly dose (HD) in the calculation. With the dimensional analysis method, the patient's weight is used in the setup. Review the titration order that follows in Figure 18-7.

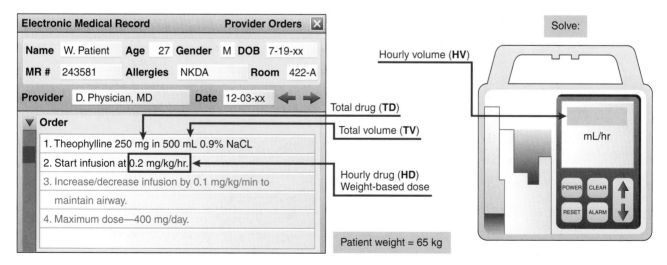

Figure 18-7. Weight-based titration order.

Here is how the problem is solved:

Linear Ratio & Proportion

Known :: Unknown

Solving for the weight-based dose

$$0.2 \text{ mg} : 1 \text{ kg} :: x \text{ mg} : 65 \text{ kg}$$

$$13 = 1x$$

$$x = 13 \text{ mg}$$

Weight-based dose is 13 mg/hr

Solve

$$\text{TD} : \text{TV} :: \text{HD} : \text{HV}$$

$$250 \text{ mg} : 500 \text{ mL} :: 13 \text{ mg/hr} : x \text{ mL/hr}$$

$$250x = 6500$$

$$\frac{250x}{250} = \frac{6500}{250}$$

$$x = 26 \text{ mL/hr}$$

Dimensional Analysis

$$\frac{\text{Ordered}}{\text{Amount}} \times \frac{\text{Conversion}}{\text{Factor(s)}} = \frac{\text{Desired}}{\text{Amount}}$$

$$\text{HD} \times \frac{\text{TV}}{\text{TD}} \times \frac{\text{conv.}}{\text{factor}} = \text{HV}$$

$$\frac{0.2 \text{ mg} / \cancel{\text{kg}}}{1 \text{ hr}} \times \frac{500 \text{ mL}}{250 \cancel{\text{mg}}} \times \frac{65 \cancel{\text{kg}}}{1} = x \text{ mL/hr}$$

$$\frac{0.2 \times 500 \times 65}{1 \text{ hr} \times 250 \times 1} = x \text{ mL/hr}$$

$$x = 26 \text{ mL/hr}$$

Fractional Ratio & Proportion

Known = Unknown

Solving for weight-based dose

$$\frac{0.2 \text{ mg}}{1 \text{ kg}} \diagdown\!\!\!\diagup \frac{x \text{ mg}}{65 \text{ kg}}$$

$$13 = 1x$$

$$x = 13 \text{ mg}$$

Weight-based dose is 13 mg/hr

Solve

$$\frac{\text{TD}}{\text{TV}} = \frac{\text{HD}}{\text{HV}}$$

$$\frac{250 \text{ mg}}{500 \text{ mL}} \diagdown\!\!\!\diagup \frac{13 \text{ mg/hr}}{x \text{ mL/hr}}$$

$$250x = 6500$$

$$\frac{250x}{250} = \frac{6500}{250}$$

$$x = 26 \text{ mL/hr}$$

Titration Formula

Solving for weight-based dose

$$\frac{0.2 \text{ mg}}{1 \cancel{\text{kg}}} \times 65 \cancel{\text{kg}} = 13 \text{ mg}$$

Weight-based dose is 13 mg/hr

Solve

$$\frac{\text{HD}}{\text{TD}} \times \text{TV} = \text{HV}$$

$$\frac{13 \text{ mg/hr}}{250 \cancel{\text{mg}}} \times 500 \text{ mL} = x \text{ mL/hr}$$

$$\frac{13}{250} \times 500 = x \text{ mL/hr}$$

$$x = 26 \text{ mL/hr}$$

SOLVING FOR HOURLY VOLUME (HV) WITH TITRATED MEDICATIONS ORDERED PER MINUTE

Some titrated medications are ordered as an amount of drug per minute. Because IV pumps are set by the number of mL/hour, drugs ordered per minute need to be converted to the amount of drug per hour (60 min = 1 hour). See the example in Figure 18-8.

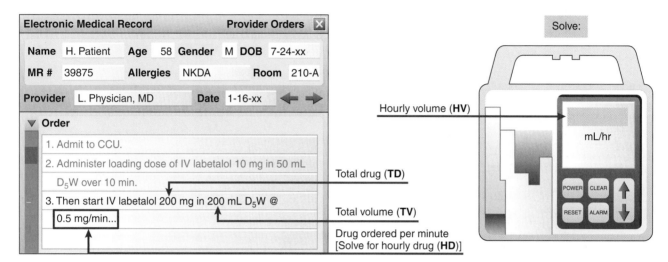

Figure 18-8. Drugs ordered per minute.

Here is how to solve the problem using the four methods:

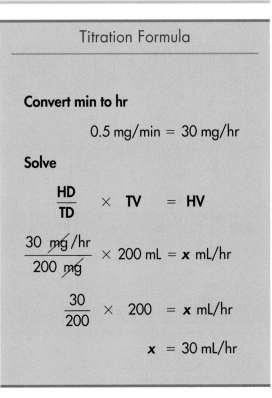

Linear Ratio & Proportion

Known :: Unknown

Convert min to hr

0.5 mg/min = 30 mg/hr

Solve

TD : TV :: HD : HV

200 mg : 200 mL :: 30 mg/hr : x mL/hr

200x = 6000

$$\frac{200x}{200} = \frac{6000}{200}$$

x = 30 mL/hr

Dimensional Analysis

$$\frac{\text{Ordered}}{\text{Amount}} \times \frac{\text{Conversion}}{\text{Factors}} = \frac{\text{Desired}}{\text{Amount}}$$

$$HD \times \frac{TV}{TD} \times \frac{\text{conv.}}{\text{factor}} = HV$$

$$\frac{0.5 \, \cancel{mg}}{1 \, \cancel{min}} \times \frac{200 mL}{200 \, \cancel{mg}} \times \frac{60 \, \cancel{min}}{1 \, hr} = x \, mL/hr$$

$$\frac{0.5 \times 200 \, mL \times 60}{1 \times 200 \times 1 \, hr} = x \, mL/hr$$

x = 30 mL/hr

Fractional Ratio & Proportion

Known = Unknown

Convert min to hr

0.5 mg/min = 30 mg/hr

Solve

$$\frac{TD}{TV} = \frac{HD}{HV}$$

$$\frac{200 \, mg}{200 \, mL} \diagdown\!\!\!\!\diagup \frac{30 \, mg/hr}{x \, mL/hr}$$

200x = 6000

$$\frac{200x}{200} = \frac{6000}{200}$$

x = 30 mL/hr

Titration Formula

Convert min to hr

0.5 mg/min = 30 mg/hr

Solve

$$\frac{HD}{TD} \times TV = HV$$

$$\frac{30 \, \cancel{mg}/hr}{200 \, \cancel{mg}} \times 200 \, mL = x \, mL/hr$$

$$\frac{30}{200} \times 200 = x \, mL/hr$$

x = 30 mL/hr

Solving for the Infusion Rate When Multiple Preliminary Calculations Are Required

Some titration problems require several calculations and conversions, such as calculating a weight-based titration dose, converting minutes to hours, and converting units of measurement so they are the same. With the dimensional analysis method, conversion factors are used. The other methods require a step-by-step approach in solving each preliminary calculation one at a time.

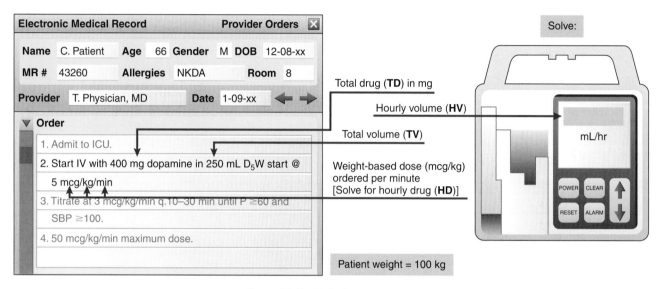

Figure 18-9. Multiple conversions.

In the example in Figure 18-9, several calculations are required. First, the individual weight-based dose needs to be calculated. The unit of measurement in the TD (mg) needs to be converted to the unit of measurement in the HD (mcg), or vice versa. Finally, the minutes need to be converted to hours. Once these calculations are done, the HV can be calculated. Notice how the answer is rounded to a whole number. Here is how to solve the problem using the four methods:

Linear Ratio & Proportion

Known :: Unknown

Calculate the weight-based dose
(wt = 100 kg)

5 mcg/kg/min = 500 mcg/min

Convert the units (mcg to mg)

500 mcg/min = 0.5 mg/min

Convert min to hr

0.5 mg/min = 30 mg/hr

Solve

TD : TV :: HD : HV

400 mg : 250 mL :: 30 mg/hr : x mL/hr

$$400x = 7500$$

$$\frac{400x}{400} = \frac{7500}{400}$$

$$x = 18.75 = 19 \text{ mL/hr}$$

Dimensional Analysis

$$\frac{\text{Ordered}}{\text{Amount}} \times \frac{\text{Conversion}}{\text{Factor(s)}} = \frac{\text{Desired}}{\text{Amount}}$$

$$\text{HD} \times \frac{\text{TV}}{\text{TD}} \times \frac{\text{conv.}}{\text{factor}} = \text{HV}$$

$$\frac{5 \text{ mcg} / \text{kg}}{1 \text{ min}} \times \frac{250 \text{mL}}{400 \text{ mg}} \times \frac{100 \text{ kg}}{1} \times$$

$$\frac{1 \text{ mg}}{1000 \text{ mcg}} \times \frac{60 \text{ min}}{1 \text{ hr}} = x \text{ mL/hr}$$

$$\frac{5 \times 250 \text{ mL} \times 100 \times 1 \times 60}{1 \times 400 \times 1 \times 1000 \times 1 \text{ hr}} = x \text{ mL/hr}$$

$$x = 18.75 = 19 \text{ mL/hr}$$

Fractional Ratio & Proportion

Known = Unknown

Calculate the weight-based dose
(wt = 100 kg)

5 mcg/kg/min = 500 mcg/min

Convert the units (mcg to mg)

500 mcg/min = 0.5 mg/min

Convert min to hr

0.5 mg/min = 30 mg/hr

Solve

$$\frac{\text{TD}}{\text{TV}} = \frac{\text{HD}}{\text{HV}}$$

$$\frac{400 \text{ mg}}{250 \text{ mL}} \diagup\!\!\!\!\diagdown \frac{30 \text{ mg/hr}}{x \text{ mL/hr}}$$

$$400x = 7500$$

$$\frac{400x}{400} = \frac{7500}{400}$$

$$x = 18.75 = 19 \text{ mL/hr}$$

Titration Formula

Calculate the weight-based dose
(wt = 100 kg)

5 mcg/kg/min = 500 mcg/min

Convert the units (mcg to mg)

500 mcg/min = 0.5 mg/min

Convert min to hr

0.5 mg/min = 30 mg/hr

Solve

$$\frac{\text{HD}}{\text{TD}} \times \text{TV} = \text{HV}$$

$$\frac{30 \text{ mg} /\text{hr}}{400 \text{ mg}} \times 250 \text{ mL} = x \text{ mL/hr}$$

$$\frac{30}{400} \times 250 = x \text{ mL/hr}$$

$$x = 18.75 = 19 \text{ mL/hr}$$

Adjusting the Titration Dose

Once the initial IV infusion is started, the nurse monitors the patient and adjusts the dose as specified in the titration order. The dose will continue to be adjusted (increased or decreased) to achieve the ordered patient goal or until the maximum dose limit has been reached. Consider the example in Figure 18-10.

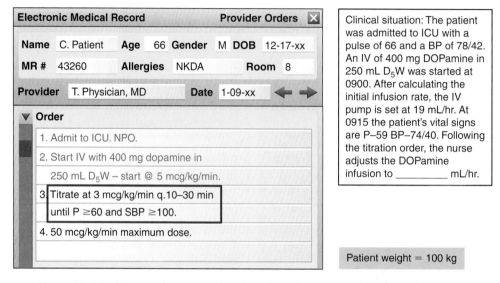

Figure 18-10. Adjusting the titration dose based on the patient's physiological response.

The 0915 vital signs do not meet the ordered patient goals. Implementing the titration order, the nurse increases the rate of the DOPamine IV infusion by 3 mcg/kg/min. To do this, the nurse must calculate the additional mL/hr to set on the IV pump. Here is the calculation:

Linear Ratio & Proportion

Known :: Unknown

Calculate the weight-based dose
(wt = 100 kg)

3 mcg/kg/min = 300 mcg/min

Convert the units (mcg to mg)

300 mcg/min = 0.3 mg/min

Convert min to hr

0.3 mg/min = 18 mg/hr

Solve

TD : TV :: HD : HV

400 mg : 250 mL :: 18 mg/hr : x mL/hr

400x = 4500

$$\frac{400x}{400} = \frac{4500}{400}$$

x = 11.25 = 11 mL/hr

Dimensional Analysis

$$\frac{\text{Ordered}}{\text{Amount}} \times \frac{\text{Conversion}}{\text{Factor(s)}} = \frac{\text{Desired}}{\text{Amount}}$$

$$HD \times \frac{TV}{TD} \times \frac{\text{conv.}}{\text{factor}} = HV$$

$$\frac{3\,\text{mcg}/\text{kg}}{1\,\text{min}} \times \frac{250\,\text{mL}}{400\,\text{mg}} \times \frac{100\,\text{kg}}{1} \times$$

$$\frac{1\,\text{mg}}{1000\,\text{mcg}} \times \frac{60\,\text{min}}{1\,\text{hr}} = x\,\text{mL/hr}$$

$$\frac{3 \times 250\,\text{mL} \times 100 \times 1 \times 60}{1 \times 400 \times 1 \times 1000 \times 1\,\text{hr}} = x\,\text{mL/hr}$$

x = 11.25 = 11 mL/hr

Fractional Ratio & Proportion

Known = Unknown

Calculate the weight-based dose
(wt = 100 kg)

3 mcg/kg/min = 300 mcg/min

Convert the units (mcg to mg)

300 mcg/min = 0.3 mg/min

Convert min to hr

0.3 mg/min = 18 mg/hr

Solve

$$\frac{TD}{TV} = \frac{HD}{HV}$$

$$\frac{400\,\text{mg}}{250\,\text{mL}} \diagdown\!\!\!\diagup \frac{18\,\text{mg/hr}}{x\,\text{mL/hr}}$$

400x = 4500

$$\frac{400x}{400} = \frac{4500}{400}$$

x = 11.25 = 11 mL/hr

Titration Formula

Calculate the weight-based dose
(wt = 100 kg)

3 mcg/kg/min = 300 mcg/min

Convert the units (mcg to mg)

300 mcg/min = 0.3 mg/min

Convert min to hr

0.3 mg/min = 18 mg/hr

Solve

$$\frac{HD}{TD} \times TV = HV$$

$$\frac{18\,\text{mg}/\text{hr}}{400\,\text{mg}} \times 250\,\text{mL} = x\,\text{mL/hr}$$

$$\frac{18}{400} \times 250 = x\,\text{mL/hr}$$

x = 11.25 = 11 mL/hr

Notice that the answer, 11.25 mL/hr, is rounded to a whole number, 11. The rate of the DOPamine infusion needs to be increased by 11 mL/hr. This 11 mL/hr is added to the initial infusion rate of 19 mL/hr. The adjusted IV rate is 30 mL/hr. The nurse will continue to assess the patient's vital signs every 10 to 30 minutes, and titrate the IV rate according to the physiological patient response.

CLINICAL REASONING 18.1

At 0500, the patient's BP is 84/46, and the physician writes an order for an IV DOPamine infusion. The nurse calculates the IV DOPamine infusion rate to set on the IV pump.

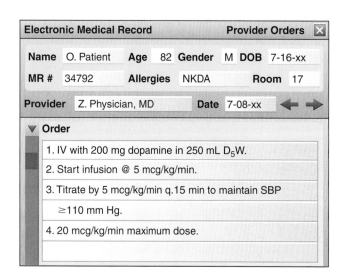

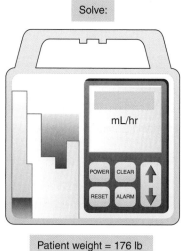

Solve:

mL/hr

Patient weight = 176 lb

Which of the following actions by the nurse is correct? (Select all that apply.)

A. Set the infusion rate on the IV pump at 20 mL/hr.
B. Set the infusion rate on the IV pump at 30 mL/hr.
C. Have a second nurse validate the calculation before starting the infusion.
D. Plan to increase the infusion rate by 5 mcg/kg/min in 15 minutes.
E. Recheck the patient's BP 15 minutes after the start of the infusion.

Patient safety is increased with the use of smart pumps. However, with the use of any IV infusion device, safe practice requires the nurse to thoroughly investigate any warning alerts or alarm sounds that may indicate unsafe dose settings, programming errors, or device malfunction.

Safe practice is an integral component of all patient care, especially in the administration of potent drugs. In the implementation of titration orders, the nurse needs to employ safe strategies at every point of care: understanding the titration order, working collaboratively with professional staff to verify drug calculations, and setting and adjusting IV pump rates accurately. The nurse must use critical decision-making skills in every step of the titration of medications.

Electronic Medical Record — Provider Orders

Name O. Patient Age 82 Gender M DOB 7-16-xx
MR # 34792 Allergies NKDA Room 17
Provider Z. Physician, MD Date 7-08-xx

Order
1. IV with 200 mg dopamine in 250 mL D_5W.
2. Start infusion @ 5 mcg/kg/min.
3. Titrate by 5 mcg/kg/min q.15 min to maintain SBP ≥110 mm Hg.
4. 20 mcg/kg/min maximum dose.

Developing Competency

Use the following titration order to answer questions 1 through 3.

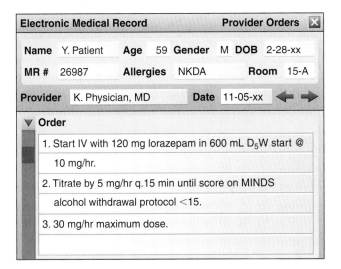

Electronic Medical Record   **Provider Orders** ☒

Name Y. Patient   **Age** 59 **Gender** M **DOB** 2-28-xx

MR # 26987   **Allergies** NKDA   **Room** 15-A

Provider K. Physician, MD   **Date** 11-05-xx ⬅ ➡

▼ **Order**

1. Start IV with 120 mg lorazepam in 600 mL D$_5$W start @ 10 mg/hr.

2. Titrate by 5 mg/hr q.15 min until score on MINDS alcohol withdrawal protocol <15.

3. 30 mg/hr maximum dose.

1. Identify the total drug (TD) in the titration order. _____

2. Identify the hourly drug (HD) in the initial titration order. _____

3. What is the initial rate in mL/hr that the nurse will set on the IV pump to start the infusion? _____

Use the following titration order to answer questions 4 through 6.

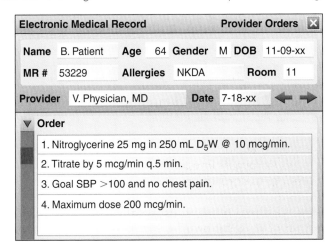

Electronic Medical Record   **Provider Orders** ☒

Name B. Patient   **Age** 64 **Gender** M **DOB** 11-09-xx

MR # 53229   **Allergies** NKDA   **Room** 11

Provider V. Physician, MD   **Date** 7-18-xx ⬅ ➡

▼ **Order**

1. Nitroglycerine 25 mg in 250 mL D$_5$W @ 10 mcg/min.

2. Titrate by 5 mcg/min q.5 min.

3. Goal SBP >100 and no chest pain.

4. Maximum dose 200 mcg/min.

4. Identify the units of measurement in the titration order.

TD: _____   HD: _____

5. The nurse will set up the initial infusion rate at _____ mL/hr.

6. The infusion was started at 1400. At 1405, the patient's SBP is 98 with complaints of chest pain. The nurse will increase the infusion rate by _____ mL/hr.

Use the following titration order to answer questions 7–8.

Electronic Medical Record	Provider Orders ☒
Name H. Patient **Age** 38 **Gender** M **DOB** 5-17-xx	
MR # 43260 **Allergies** NKDA **Room** 108-1	
Provider N. Physician, MD **Date** 7-10-xx ⬅ ➡	

▼ **Order**

1. IV orders: 2000 mcg fentanyl in 100 mL 0.9% NaCl @
   120 mcg/hr.
2. Titrate by 20 mcg/hr q.5 min to keep pain level ≤3.
4. Maximum dose 400 mcg/hr.

7. What is the initial infusion rate in mL/hr that the nurse will set on the IV pump? _____

8. If the patient's pain level is greater than 3, the nurse will increase the infusion rate by _____ mL/hr.

Use the following HEParin Dose Titration Protocol to answer questions 9 through 11.

HEParin Dose Titration Protocol	
aPTT (seconds)	**Infusion**
<34	↑ 100 units/hr
34–44	↑ 100 units/hr
45–54	↑ 50 units/hr
55–70	Keep at current rate
71–85	↓ 100 units/hr
86–100	↓ 150 units/hr
101–125	↓ 200 units/hr
>125	Notify MD STAT

9. At 0800, the nurse starts an IV of heparin 25,000 units in 1,000 mL D$_5$W to infuse at 400 units per hour. A heparin protocol is used to titrate the heparin infusion q.6h according to the aPTT lab results. The aPTT result at 1400 is 40 seconds. Calculate the adjusted infusion rate (mL/hr) that the nurse set on the IV pump at 1400. _____

10. The patient has an order for an IV of heparin 25,000 units in 1,000 mL D$_5$W to infuse at 600 units per hour. The heparin protocol is used to titrate the heparin infusion q.6h according to the aPTT lab results. The infusion is started at 1700, and the aPTT result at 2300 is 65 seconds. The nurse's clinical decision at 2300 is to: _____

11. Heparin 20,000 units in 1,000 mL D$_5$W is started to infuse at 500 units per hour. The heparin protocol is used to titrate the heparin infusion q.6h according to the aPTT lab results. The infusion is started at 1300, and the aPTT result at 1900 is 90 seconds. Calculate the adjusted infusion rate (mL/hr) that the nurse will set on the IV pump at 1900? _____

Use the following titration order to answer questions 12 through 14.

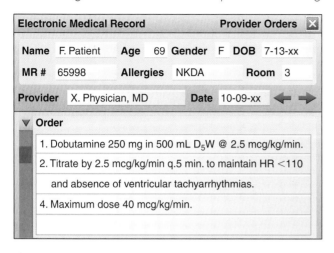

12. The DOBUTamine order is for a patient who weighs 60 kg. Identify the preliminary calculations.

(1) _____

(2) _____

(3) _____

13. The nurse begins the infusion at 1030. What is the initial infusion rate in mL/hr that the nurse will set on the IV pump? _____

14. At 1035 the patient's ECG shows ventricular tachyarrhythmias and the heart rate is 130 beats per minute. What is the adjusted rate in mL/hr that the nurse sets on the IV pump? _____

Use the following titration order to answer questions 15 through 17.

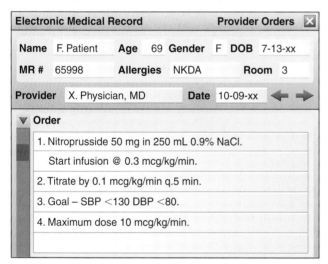

15. The patient weighs 176 lb. Identify the preliminary calculations.

(1) _____

(2) _____

(3) _____

(4) _____

16. What rate in mL/hr will the nurse set on the IV pump to start the infusion of nitroprusside? _____

17. Ten minutes after beginning the IV infusion of nitroprusside, the patient's BP is 180/94. The nurse adjusts the rate of the infusion. The nurse will increase the infusion rate by _____mL/hr.

Use the following titration order to answer questions 18 through 20.

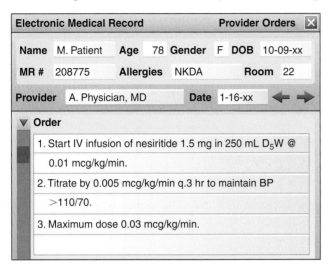

18. The patient weighs 70 kg. Identify the preliminary calculations.

(1) _____

(2) _____

(3) _____

19. What is the initial infusions rate in mL/hr that the nurse will set on the IV pump? _____

20. Three hours after beginning the IV infusion of nesiritide, the patient has a BP of 100/58. The nurse adjusts the rate of the infusion. The nurse will increase the infusion rate by _____ mL/hr.

Verifying Safe Dose and Critical Care Calculations

Unit Review—Evaluate for Clinical Decision Making

*For each question, use your clinical judgment to determine whether the nurse's decision is **Correct** or **Incorrect**. For incorrect problems, write the correct answer.*

1. The physician orders propranolol 160 mg PO twice daily for an adult with angina.
   Drug reference:

   HIGH ALERT

   ☒ propranolol
   (proe-**pran**-oh-lole)

   Route/Dosage

   PO (Adults): *Antianginal*—80–320 mg/day in 2-4 divided doses or once daily as extended/sustained-release capsules...

   The nurse determines that the ordered dose is a safe dose to administer. The nurse's decision is:

Correct	Incorrect	Answer: _____

2. The physician orders traMADol 100 mg PO q.6h for a 78-year-old patient.
   Drug reference:

   ---
   traMADol (tra-ma-dol)

   Route/Dosage

   Immediate-release
   PO (Adults >18 yr): *Rapid titration*—50–100 mg q 4–6 hr (not to exceed 400 mg/day [300 mg in patients >75 yr])...

   The nurse determines that the ordered dose is a safe dose to administer. The nurse's decision is:

Correct	Incorrect	Answer: _____

3. The physician orders cyclophosphamide 500 mg IV twice a week for a 35-year-old patient who weighs 176 lb.
Drug reference:

HIGH ALERT

cyclophosphamide
(sye-kloe-**fos**-fa-mide)

Route/Dosage

IV (Adults): 40–50 mg/kg in divided doses over 2–5 days *or* 10–15 mg/kg q. 7–10 days *or* 3–5 mg/kg twice weekly *or* 1.5–3 mg/kg/day...

The nurse determines that the ordered dose is a safe dose to administer. The nurse's decision is:

Correct	Incorrect	Answer: _____

4. The physician orders DOXOrubicin liposomal 50 mg IV monthly for a 48-year-old patient with ovarian cancer who has a BSA of 1.2 m^2.
Drug reference:

HIGH ALERT

DOXOrubicin, liposomal
(dox-oh-**roo**-bi-sin **lye**-poe-sohm-al)

Route/Dosage
Other regimens are used.

IV (Adults): *AIDS-related KS*—20 mg/m^2 every 3 wk; *Metastatic ovarian cancer*—40–50 mg/m^2 every 4 wk; *Multiple myeloma*—30 mg/m^2 on day 4 after following borezomib for up to 8 cycles.

The nurse determines that the ordered dose is a safe dose to administer. The nurse's decision is:

Correct	Incorrect	Answer: _____

5. The physician orders ganciclovir 13 mg IV q.12h for a newborn infant with congenital CMV infection. The infant weighs 6.6 lb.
Drug reference:

ganciclovir (gan-**sye**-kloe-vir)

Route/Dosage

IV (Neonates): *Congenital CMV infection*—12 mg/kg/day divided q.12 hr x 6 weeks.

The nurse determines that the ordered dose is a safe dose to administer. The nurse's decision is:

Correct	Incorrect	Answer: _____

6.

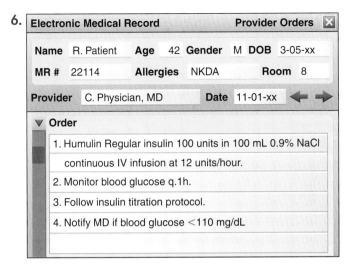

Electronic Medical Record | Provider Orders ☒

| Name | R. Patient | Age | 42 | Gender | M | DOB | 3-05-xx |

MR # 22114   Allergies NKDA   Room 8

Provider C. Physician, MD   Date 11-01-xx ⬅ ➡

▼ Order

1. Humulin Regular insulin 100 units in 100 mL 0.9% NaCl
   continuous IV infusion at 12 units/hour.
2. Monitor blood glucose q.1h.
3. Follow insulin titration protocol.
4. Notify MD if blood glucose <110 mg/dL

To begin the infusion, the nurse calculates the flow rate at
12 mL/hr.
The flow rate is verified by another nurse and the flow rate is:

Correct	Incorrect	Answer: _____

7.

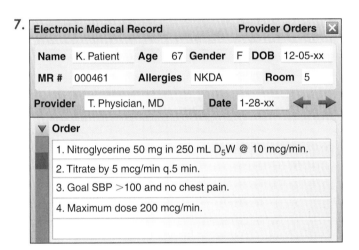

Electronic Medical Record | Provider Orders ☒

| Name | K. Patient | Age | 67 | Gender | F | DOB | 12-05-xx |

MR # 000461   Allergies NKDA   Room 5

Provider T. Physician, MD   Date 1-28-xx ⬅ ➡

▼ Order

1. Nitroglycerine 50 mg in 250 mL D$_5$W @ 10 mcg/min.
2. Titrate by 5 mcg/min q.5 min.
3. Goal SBP >100 and no chest pain.
4. Maximum dose 200 mcg/min.

The nurse calculates the flow rate at 30 mL/hr.
The flow rate is verified by another nurse and the flow rate is:

Correct	Incorrect	Answer: _____

Use the MD order and the HEParin Dose Titration Protocol for questions 8 through 10.

Electronic Medical Record — **Provider Orders** ☒

Name	O. Patient	Age	44	Gender	F	DOB	2-28-xx

MR #	45320	Allergies	NKDA	Room	112

Provider	C. Physician, MD	Date	4-09-xx	← →

▼ **Order**

1. Admit to ICU. NPO.

2. Start IV heparin 25,000 units in 500 mL D5W @ 400 units/hr.

3. Stat aPTT 6 hours after start of infusion.

4. aPTT 6 hours after any dose change.

5. Follow heparin protocol.

HEParin Dose Titration Protocol	
aPTT (seconds)	**Infusion**
<34	↑ 100 units/hr
34–44	↑ 100 units/hr
45–54	↑ 50 units/hr
55–70	Keep at current rate
71–85	↓ 100 units/hr
86–100	↓ 150 units/hr
101–125	↓ 200 units/hr
>125	Notify MD STAT

8. To begin the infusion at 0700, the nurse calculates a flow rate of 8 mL/hr.
The flow rate is verified by another nurse and the flow rate is:

Correct	Incorrect	Answer: _____

9. The 1300 aPTT result is 54 seconds. Following the heparin protocol, the nurse sets the infusion pump to 9 mL/hr.
The flow rate is verified by another nurse and the flow rate is:

Correct	Incorrect	Answer: _____

10. The 1900 aPTT result is 88 seconds. Following the heparin protocol, the nurse sets the infusion pump to 7 mL/hr.
The flow rate is verified by another nurse and the flow rate is:

Correct	Incorrect	Answer: _____

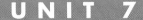

Intake and Output

Accurate documentation of a patient's intake and output provides important information regarding a patient's fluid status. This unit assists you to identify, calculate, and document the intake (oral and parenteral) and output based on the source (for example, urine, drainage, or emesis).

 APPLICATION TO NURSING PRACTICE

The nurse uses the electronic intake and output record to document the total intake for the shift and to review the patient's 24 hour totals. Careful calculation and documentation help to provide an accurate clinical picture of a patient's fluid needs.

Intake and Output Record ☒

Name S. Patient **Age** 64 **Gender** F **DOB** 2-17-xx

MR # 7128 **Allergies** PCN **Room** 115

Shift 2300–0700 **Date** 8-17-xx ← →

Intake				Output	
Oral	IV	IVPB	Blood	Urine	Emesis
160	1000	50		250	

Shift 0700–1500 **Date** 8-17-xx ← →

Intake				Output	
Oral	IV	IVPB	Blood	Urine	Emesis
540	1000	150		175	325

Shift 1500–2300 **Date** 8-17-xx ← →

Intake				Output	
Oral	IV	IVPB	Blood	Urine	Emesis
250	500	50	250	475	

TOTALS: **Intake** = 3950 mL **Output** = 1225 mL

The nurse uses clinical decision making to evaluate the patient's intake and output record to determine whether any follow-up action is needed for safe patient care.

CHAPTER 19

Calculating Intake and Output

LEARNING OUTCOMES

Calculate oral intake and output.

Document intake and output.

Identify the equipment used to measure intake.

Identify the equipment used to measure output.

The measurement of **intake** and **output (I & O)** during the shift and within a 24-hour period provides important information about a patient's fluid and electrolyte balance. The health-care provider may order the measurement of intake and output for the patient, or the nurse may independently place the patient on intake and output.

Calculating Oral Intake

Calculating intake is a simple process. The nurse measures the amount of liquid the patient consumes or is given throughout the shift. Oral intake includes the measurement of any food that is liquid or that turns into liquid at room temperature, such as ice cream and gelatin. Intake is recorded in mL; therefore, if the nurse knows the amount of intake in mL then a simple addition is all that is necessary.

Example:

The patient is on I & O. For breakfast, the patient drank 120 mL of juice, 240 mL of coffee, and 375 mL of water.

To calculate the patient's intake for breakfast, the nurse just adds the numbers:

$$
\begin{array}{r}
120 \text{ mL (juice)} \\
240 \text{ mL (milk)} \\
+\ 375 \text{ mL (water)} \\
\hline
735 \text{ mL}
\end{array}
$$

In the clinical setting, the nurse will encounter eating utensils, such as the teaspoons, tablespoons, and standard food containers that are filled to a certain capacity, such as 4 oz, 6 oz, and 8 oz, on a patient's meal tray (Fig. 19-1).

Hospitals, skilled nursing facilities, and other healthcare facilities identify the amount of liquid for the standard containers (cup, glass, soup bowl, etc.) used in their facility. For prepackaged foods such as ice cream, gelatin, and popsicles, the nurse can identify the amount on the package or on the lid of the container.

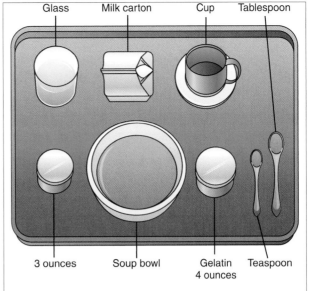

Figure 19-1. Common containers and utensils on a patient's meal tray.

Converting to mL

Because nurses record a patient's intake in mL, household measurements, such as the teaspoon, tablespoon, glass, cup, and ounce, need to be converted to mL. Metric equivalent measurements for common household utensils are identified on Table 19-1.

Knowing the equivalent measurements helps the nurse to accurately convert the units. Although the ratio and proportion and dimensional analysis methods can be used for converting units of measurement, the nurse can calculate the number of mL by simply multiplying the household measurement in the problem by the metric equivalent. Look at the household to metric equivalent problems in Table 19-2. Notice how multiplication is used to convert the numbers.

Table 19-1. Metric Equivalents for Household Measurements

HOUSEHOLD MEASUREMENTS	ABBREVIATION	METRIC EQUIVALENTS
tablespoon	Tbs, tbs, T	15 mL
teaspoon	tsp, Tsp, t	5 mL
ounce	oz	30 mL

Table 19-2. Using the Metric Equivalent Measurements to Calculate Oral Intake

CALCULATING ORAL INTAKE	METRIC EQUIVALENT	MULTIPLY	INTAKE (ML)
The patient drank 3 oz of milk. How many mL of milk did the patient drink?	1 oz = 30 mL	30 mL × 3	90 mL
The patient ate 5 tsp of gelatin. How many mL of gelatin did the patient eat?	1 tsp = 5 mL	5 mL × 5	25 mL
The patient took 7 Tbs of broth. How many mL of broth did the patient take?	1 Tbs = 15 mL	15 mL × 7	105 mL

Memorize these standard metric equivalents commonly used to accurately convert a household amount to mL:

- 1 tsp = 5 mL
- 1 Tbs = 15 mL
- 1 oz = 30 mL

APPLY LEARNED KNOWLEDGE 19-1

Circle "True" if the statement is correct. Circle "False" if the statement is incorrect.

1. For dinner, the patient drank 4 oz of water. This is equivalent to 120 mL.	True	False
2. The patient takes 3 Tbs of ice cream. This is equivalent to 15 mL.	True	False
3. The patient takes 5 tsp of gelatin. This is equivalent to 25 mL.	True	False
4. The patient eats 4 tsp of soup. This is equivalent to 15 mL.	True	False
5. For lunch, the patient drank 8 oz of tea. This is equivalent to 240 mL.	True	False

Calculating Intake for the Shift

The nurse monitors the patient's intake throughout the shift by writing down the patient's liquid intake on a clinical worksheet. At the end of the shift, the nurse adds the intake and records the total in the patient's Intake and Output Record. In the example below, notice how the household units of measurement are converted to the metric equivalent so that recorded amount is in mL in the intake column on the Intake and Output clinical worksheet.

Example:

For the breakfast, the patient drank 4 oz of juice, 90 mL of coffee, and 6 oz of milk. For the lunch, the patient drinks 8 oz of milk and eats 120 mL of ice cream. By the end of the shift, the patient drank 500 mL of water.

MEASURING ICE CHIPS

A patient may request a cup of ice chips or ice chips may be the only oral intake allowed. To calculate intake with ice chips, remember that ice chips melt to approximately one-half of their original volume. Therefore, if you give a patient a 6 ounce cup of ice chips, the ice will melt to approximately 3 ounces of water. The nurse would record 90 mL as the intake.

Name **C. Patient**   MR **49231**   Date **10-2-xx**

Intake and Output Worksheet

Shift	Oral	Other	Urine	Emesis	Other
7-3	120				
	90				
	180				
	240				
	120				
	500				
Total (mL)	1250				

 Patient education is an integral part of patient care. Nurses can assist patients to understand their daily fluid needs and many patients can be taught to keep track of their own fluid intake throughout the day.

FORMULA TUBE FEEDINGS ARE PART OF THE ORAL INTAKE

There are times when a patient is not able to take fluids orally and requires formula feeding through a tube for a period of time. Feeding tubes can be placed in the stomach, **duodenum,** or **jejunum.** The specific nutritional needs for a patient with a feeding tube necessitates the development of a nutritional plan to ensure that the patient receives the appropriate nutrients, calories, and water. Collaboration between the health-care provider who orders the formula, the nutritionist who assesses the patient and develops the nutritional plan, and nurse who implements and monitors the tube feedings helps to assure that the nutritional and fluid needs of the patient are addressed.

The type of formula and the rate of the formula feedings are determined by the health-care provider. The formula tube feeding may be ordered as a **continuous feeding** (Example 1) or the formula feeding may be ordered on an **intermittent feeding** schedule (Example 2).

Example 1:

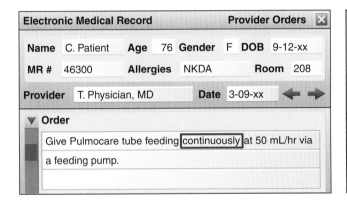

Example 2:

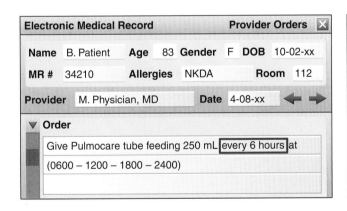

A patient who is receiving formula tube feedings will periodically be given water through the feeding tube. Water can be given after administration of medications, after administration of intermittent formula feedings, or at other times throughout the shift.

The amount of water is measured and recorded as part of the intake for the patient. In the following example, the nurse records the formula tube feedings for the 0700 to 1500 (7 a.m. to 3 p.m.) shift. Notice how the 50 mL of water is added twice for the shift, after the 0800 feeding and after the 1400 feeding, as intake on the worksheet. The total intake for the shift is 500 mL, which includes the water given during the shift. When recording the intake on the electronic medical record, the nurse selects the type of feeding tube from a list provided and enters the total intake.

Example:

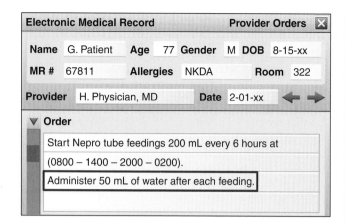

Electronic Medical Record		Provider Orders	☒
Name G. Patient	**Age** 77	**Gender** M **DOB** 8-15-xx	
MR # 67811	**Allergies** NKDA	**Room** 322	
Provider H. Physician, MD		**Date** 2-01-xx ← →	
▼ **Order**			
Start Nepro tube feedings 200 mL every 6 hours at (0800 – 1400 – 2000 – 0200).			
Administer 50 mL of water after each feeding.			

Name G. Patient   MR 67811   Date 2-01-xx

Intake and Output Worksheet

Shift	Oral	Tube	Urine	Emesis	Other
7-3		(Feeding)			
		200			
		50			
		200			
		50			
Total (mL)		500			

APPLY LEARNED KNOWLEDGE 19-2

Read the clinical situation and decide whether the Intake and Output record is correct or incorrect.

1. The nurse documents intake after the patient ate 4 Tbs of gelatin.
   Correct   Incorrect

Intake and Output Worksheet

Shift	Oral	Urine
7-3	20	
Total (mL)		

2. The patient drinks 8 oz of ice chips. The intake is recorded on the I & O form.
   Correct   Incorrect

Intake and Output Worksheet

Shift	Oral	Urine
7-3	240	
Total (mL)		

APPLY LEARNED KNOWLEDGE 19-2—cont'd

3. The patient eats 5 tsp of gelatin. The nurse makes the following documentation.

   Correct   Incorrect

Intake and Output Worksheet		
Shift	**Oral**	**Urine**
7-3	25	
Total (mL)		

4. The nurse gives the patient 180 mL of formula, followed by 100 mL of water through the feeding tube.

   Correct   Incorrect

Intake and Output Worksheet			
Shift	**Oral**	**Tube**	**Urine**
7-3		*(Feeding)* 180 100	
Total (mL)		280	

5. The nurse gives the patient 240 mL of formula at 0800 and 240 mL at 1400 through the feeding tube. The nurse documents intake.

   Correct   Incorrect

Intake and Output Worksheet			
Shift	**Oral**	**Tube**	**Urine**
7-3		*(Feeding)* 240	
Total (mL)		240	

Calculating Output

Measuring output is part of the intake and output. Any liquid drainage produced by the body is counted in the output. Fluid drainage produced by the body and measured as output includes:

- Urine
- *Emesis* (vomitus, vomit)
- Gastric drainage (*nasogastric* tube, *jejunostomy* tube, or *gastric* tube drainage)
- Wound drainage (drainage obtained from wound drainage devices)
- Chest tube drainage
- Diarrhea
- *Colostomy* or *ileostomy* drainage
- Fluid that is removed through special procedures (*thoracentesis* or *paracentesis* drainage)

In the clinical setting, containers for collecting output drainage have calibrations that allow direct measurement of output (Fig. 19-2).

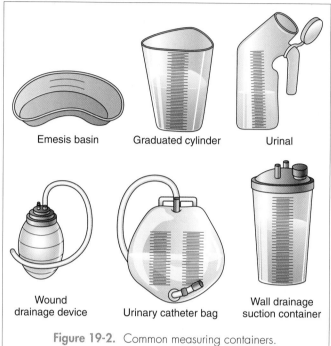

Emesis basin   Graduated cylinder   Urinal

Wound drainage device   Urinary catheter bag   Wall drainage suction container

Figure 19-2. Common measuring containers.

Recording Output

Output is recorded in mL, and is identified under specific categories, such as urine, gastric drainage, emesis, wound drainage, and others. For urine output, the amount measured at each *voiding* is entered in the I & O worksheet and the total is entered in the I & O record at the end of the shift. The same is true each time the patient vomits. Gastric and wound drainage containers are usually emptied and measured at the end of the shift.

When recording the output on the electronic medical record, the nurse selects the category (urine, emesis, gastric drainage, etc.) from a list provided and enters the total output for each category. If using a printed Intake and Output form, the nurse writes in the category if it is not identified on the form.

Example:

The patient **voided** 225 mL at 4 p.m. At 8:00 p.m., he vomited 300 mL of clear fluid and voided 75 mL at 10:00 p.m. The nurse emptied 50 mL from the wound drainage device at the end of the shift.

   The nurse records the amount of output for each category, then adds each type of output to arrive at the total amount for each category.

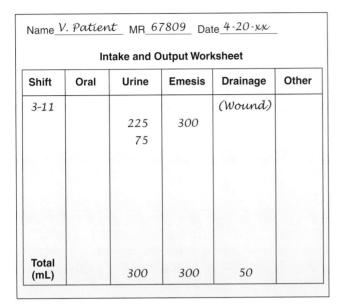

Name _V. Patient_ MR _67809_ Date _4-20-xx_

Intake and Output Worksheet

Shift	Oral	Urine	Emesis	Drainage	Other
3-11		225 75	300	(Wound)	
Total (mL)		300	300	50	

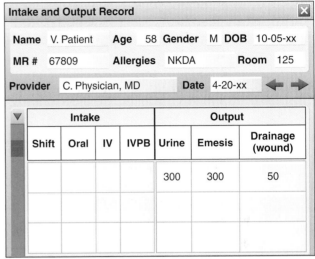

Intake and Output Record

| Name | V. Patient | | Age | 58 | Gender | M | DOB | 10-05-xx |

| MR # | 67809 | | Allergies | NKDA | | Room | 125 |

| Provider | C. Physician, MD | | Date | 4-20-xx |

	Intake			Output		
Shift	Oral	IV	IVPB	Urine	Emesis	Drainage (wound)
				300	300	50

APPLY LEARNED KNOWLEDGE 19-3

Circle "True" if the output recorded and calculated is correct. Circle "False" if the output recorded and calculated is incorrect.

1. The patient has a gastric tube that drained 425 mL during the evening shift. The patient voided 300 mL.

   True   False

Intake and Output Worksheet

Shift	Oral	Urine	Emesis	Drainage	Other
3-11		425		(Gastric) 300	
Total (mL)		425		300	

Continued

APPLY LEARNED KNOWLEDGE 19-3—cont'd

2. The patient voided 75 mL at 1000, 100 mL at 12:00 PM, and vomited 250 mL at 1400. The patient has a nasogastric tube that drained 450 mL for the 7 to 3 shift.

   True   False

Intake and Output Record ✕

Name	G. Patient	Age	68	Gender	M	DOB	7-13-xx
MR #	76321		Allergies	NKDA		Room	202

Provider L. Physician, MD   Date 6-23-xx ← →

Intake			Output		
Oral	IV	IVPB	Urine	Emesis	Drainage (NG)
			175	250	450

3. The patient has a surgical wound device that drained 15 mL during the evening shift. The patient voided 225 mL at 1600 and 300 mL at 10:00 PM.

   True   False

Intake and Output Worksheet

Shift	Oral	Urine	Emesis	Drainage	Other
3-11		225 300		(Wound) 15	
Total (mL)		525		15	

4. The patient's gastric tube drained 375 mL on the evening shift. The patient voided 235 mL at 1700 and 125 mL at 9:00 PM.

   True   False

Intake and Output Worksheet

Shift	Oral	Urine	Emesis	Drainage	Other
3-11		235 125	375	(Gastric)	
Total (mL)		360	375		

APPLY LEARNED KNOWLEDGE 19-3—cont'd

5. The patient had emesis of 325 mL at 0700. A nasogastric (NG) tube drained 350 mL during the shift. The patient voided 250 mL at 0800 and 415 mL at 1400.

True   False

Intake and Output Worksheet

Shift	Oral	Urine	Emesis	Drainage	Other
7-3		250 415	325	(NG)	
Total (mL)		665	325	350	

THE PATIENT WITH BLADDER IRRIGATION

There are times when the physician orders **bladder irrigation** for a patient. Bladder irrigations are ordered for various medical conditions. However, more commonly, bladder irrigations are ordered after prostate or bladder surgery.

Bladder irrigation involves the instillation of a solution or **irrigant** into the bladder through a **urinary catheter.** The urinary catheter is a flexible tube that is inserted into the bladder to allow urine to drain freely into a urinary drainage bag. Patients with continuous bladder irrigations have a specifically designed urinary catheter, known as a 3-way catheter, which has a third opening or **lumen** that allows for the instillation of the irrigant (Fig. 19-3).

The purpose of the irrigation is to minimize small blood clots from forming in the bladder and to wash out blood clots that may obstruct the catheter and block the flow of urine after bladder or prostate surgery. The physician orders the type of irrigant and the rate for instilling the irrigant into the bladder. The bladder irrigation can be ordered as a continuous irrigation or as an intermittent irrigation.

After the instillation of the irrigant into the bladder, the irrigant flows out of the bladder and into the catheter. The irrigant, combined with the urine, drains into the urinary drainage bag (Fig. 19-4).

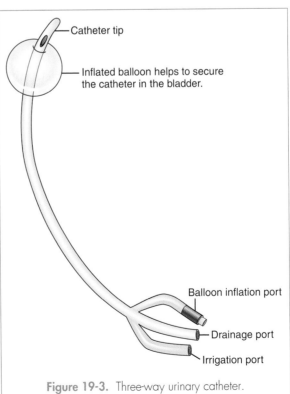

Catheter tip

Inflated balloon helps to secure the catheter in the bladder.

Balloon inflation port

Drainage port

Irrigation port

Figure 19-3. Three-way urinary catheter.

CALCULATING THE URINE OUTPUT FOR A PATIENT WITH CONTINUOUS BLADDER IRRIGATION

In calculating the output for a patient with continuous bladder irrigation, it is important to remember that the drainage that collects in the urinary drainage bag is a combination of urine and irrigant. Therefore, to calculate the actual urine output, the amount of irrigant instilled must be subtracted from the total output collected in the urinary drainage bag.

Example:

The physician orders a continuous bladder irrigation with normal saline to infuse at 50 mL/hr to keep the urine free of clots. The nurse starts the normal saline irrigation at 7:00 a.m. and infuses the normal saline for the entire 8 hour shift. At 3:00 p.m., the nurse empties 925 mL from the urinary drainage bag. What is the patient's output?

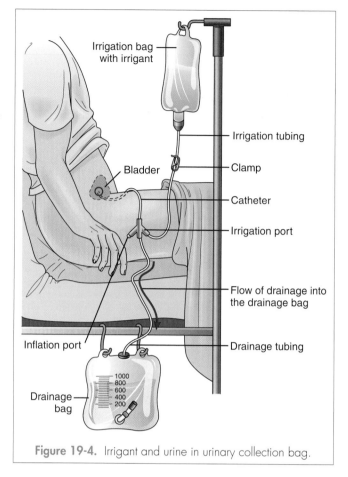

Figure 19-4. Irrigant and urine in urinary collection bag.

■ To calculate the actual urine output, the nurse must subtract the amount of irrigant from the total output. Here are the points to consider:

1. Total amount of drainage obtained from the urinary drainage bag is measured.

2. Total amount of irrigant infused during the shift is calculated.

Actual urine output is calculated by subtracting the total amount of irrigant infused from total output in the urinary drainage bag.

■ Solve: Total amount of drainage from the urinary drainage bag at 3:00 p.m.:   925 mL
Total amount of irrigant infused during the shift (50 mL/hr × 8 hr):   − 400 mL
Actual urine output: 525 mL

 Frequent monitoring and emptying of the urinary drainage bag is necessary when a patient has continuous bladder irrigation. It may be necessary for the nurse to empty the urinary drainage bag several times during the shift.
This will minimize the risk of obstruction and ensure the continuous flow of urine and irrigant into the urinary drainage bag.

APPLY LEARNED KNOWLEDGE 19-4

Circle "True" if the output is calculated correctly. Circle "False" if the output is calculated incorrectly.

1. A continuous bladder irrigation with normal saline was started to infuse at 50 mL/hr at 5:00 p.m. At 11:00 p.m., the nurse emptied 800 mL from the urinary drainage bag.
True   False

Intake and Output Worksheet

Shift	Oral	Urine	Emesis	Drainage	Other
3-11					*(UA catheter)*
Total (mL)					500

2. The patient has a continuous bladder irrigation with normal saline infusing at 30 mL/hr from 3:00 p.m. to 11:00 p.m. The nurse emptied 775 mL at 11:00 p.m. from the urinary drainage bag.
True   False

Intake and Output Worksheet

Shift	Oral	Urine	Emesis	Drainage	Other
3-11					*(UA catheter)*
Total (mL)					240

3. The patient has a continuous bladder irrigation infusing at 75 mL/hr from 10:00 a.m. to 2:00 p.m. At 3:00 p.m., the nurse emptied 850 mL from the urinary drainage bag.
True   False

Intake and Output Worksheet

Shift	Oral	Urine	Emesis	Drainage	Other
7-3					*(UA catheter)*
Total (mL)					550

Continued

APPLY LEARNED KNOWLEDGE 19-4—cont'd

4. The patient has a continuous bladder irrigation infusing at 50 mL/hr from 7:00 a.m. to 10:00 a.m. and again from 12:00 to 3:00 p.m. At 3:00 p.m., the nurse emptied 1,050 mL from the urinary drainage bag.
True   False

Intake and Output Worksheet

Shift	Oral	Urine	Emesis	Drainage	Other
7-3					(UA catheter)
Total (mL)					900

5. The patient has a continuous bladder irrigation infusing at 60 mL/hr from 8:00 a.m. to 2:00 p.m. At 3:00 p.m. the nurse emptied 1,000 mL from the urinary drainage bag.
True   False

Intake and Output Worksheet

Shift	Oral	Urine	Emesis	Drainage	Other
7-3					(UA catheter)
Total (mL)					640

CLINICAL REASONING 19-1

The nurse is caring for a patient who is on I & O. The patient refuses to drink the apple juice and cold water that is at the bedside. During the handoff report at 1500, the day nurse reports the patient's oral intake for the shift was only 200 mL of a homemade tea brought in by a family member. The patient's physician has allowed the family to bring in the tea but wants the patient to drink four glasses (8 ounces each) of tea during the evening shift. How many mL will the nurse ask the patient to drink for the shift?

Patients who are placed on intake and output require careful assessment and ongoing monitoring to ensure that their daily fluid needs are met. Although the addition of a patient's intake and output does not require complex calculations, the monitoring and accurate documentation of the intake and output are an integral part of evaluating the hydration status of the patient.

Developing Competency

Calculate the intake for problems 1 through 5.

1. The patient drank 180 mL of coffee, 6 ounces of orange juice, and 180 mL water. What is the patient's intake?

   _____

2. For lunch, the patient ate 3 oz of ice cream and drank 8 oz of milk and one 6 oz glass of ice chips. What is the patient's intake? _____

3. For breakfast, the patient takes 2 Tbs of gelatin, drinks 240 mL of coffee, and 4 ounces of apple juice. For lunch, the patient drinks 180 mL of milk and 450 mL of water. What is the patient's total intake? _____

4. The patient has formula feedings through a feeding tube. She is given 300 mL every 4 hours (0400, 0800, 1200, 1600, 2000, 2400) around the clock. The nurse gives 100 mL of water after each feeding. How much intake will the patient receive in the 2300 to 0700 (11 to 7) shift? _____

5. The patient has tube feedings. He is given 225 mL every 4 hours (0200, 0600, 1000, 1400, 1800, 2200) around the clock. The nurse gives 50 mL of water after each feeding. An additional 100 mL of water is administered after the medications are given at 1200. How much intake will the patient receive in the 0700 to 1500 (7 to 3) shift? _____

Calculate the output for problems 6 through 10.

6. The patient voided 180 mL at 8:00 AM and 435 at 2:00 PM. Complete the patient's output record.

Intake and Output Worksheet

Shift	Oral	Urine	Emesis	Drainage	Other
7-3					
Total (mL)					

7. The patient had emesis of 200 mL at 10:00 AM and voided 325 at 12:00 PM and 175 at 2:00 PM. Complete the patient's output record.

Intake and Output Worksheet

Shift	Oral	Urine	Emesis	Drainage	Other
7-3					
Total (mL)					

8. The patient has a nasogastric tube connected to suction. The nasogastric tube drained 250 mL of gastric drainage. The patient voided 300 mL at 4:30 PM and 175 mL at 8:00 PM. Complete the patient's output record.

Intake and Output Worksheet					
Shift	Oral	Urine	Emesis	Drainage	Other
3-11				(NG)	
Total (mL)					

9. The patient has a continuous bladder irrigation infusing at 50 mL/hr from 7:00 AM to 12:00 PM. At 3:00 PM, the nurse emptied 925 mL from the urinary drainage bag. Calculate the actual urine output. _____

10. The patient has a continuous bladder irrigation infusing at 75 mL/hr from 3:00 PM to 8:00 PM. At 11:00 PM, the nurse emptied 1,175 mL from the urinary drainage bag. Calculate the actual urine output. _____

Calculate the intake and output for problems 11 through 15.

11. For breakfast, the patient took one 180 mL cup of coffee, 240 mL of milk, and a 4 oz glass of juice. For lunch, the patient took 240 mL of water and 6 oz of tea. The patient has a wound drainage device. At the end of the shift, the nurse emptied 30 mL from the wound drainage device. The patient voided 225 mL at 8:00 AM and 150 mL at 2:00 PM. Use the I & O worksheet to record the patient's intake and output for the 7 to 3 shift.

Intake and Output Worksheet					
Shift	Oral	Urine	Emesis	Drainage	Other
7-3				(Wound)	
Total (mL)					

12. For dinner, the patient drinks 6 oz of tea, 180 mL of broth, 9 oz of soda, and eats two popsicles (3 ounces each). He drank 500 mL of water for the shift. The patient has a continuous bladder irrigation infusing at 25 mL/hr from 4:00 PM to 11:00 PM. At 11:00 PM, the nurse empties 725 mL from the urinary drainage bag. Use the I & O worksheet to record the patient's intake and output for the 7 to 3 shift.

Intake and Output Worksheet

Shift	Oral	Urine	Emesis	Drainage	Other
3-11					(UA catheter)
Total (mL)					

13. The patient has a continuous tube feedings infusing at 75 mL/hr for the 2300 to 0700 shift. The nurse gives 100 mL of water after the administration of medications at 0200. Record the patient's 8 hr intake on I & O worksheet for the 2300 to 0700 (11 to 7) shift.

Intake and Output Worksheet

Shift	Oral	Tube	Urine	Emesis	Other
11-7		(Feeding)			
Total (mL)					

14. For breakfast, the patient drank one 180 mL cup of coffee and a 4 oz glass of juice. For lunch, the patient ate 3 tsp of gelatin and drank 6 oz of tea. The patient voided 525 mL at 8:00 AM and 300 mL at 2:00 PM. The nurse emptied 35 mL of wound drainage for the shift. Record the total intake and output on the electronic record for the 0700 to 1500 (7 to 3) shift.

Intake and Output Record ⊠

| Name | N. Patient | Age | 62 | Gender | F | DOB | 12-07-xx |

MR # 76321 Allergies NKDA Room 401

Provider C. Physician, MD Date 4-20-xx ⬅ ➡

Intake			Output		
Oral	IV	IVPB	Urine	Emesis	Wound

15. For breakfast, the patient drank 6 tsp of milk, 240 mL of coffee, and 3 ounces of juice. For lunch, the patient drank an 8 ounce container of milk and 550 mL of water during the shift. The patient has a continuous bladder irrigation infusing at 60 mL/hr from 10:00 AM to 15:00 PM. At 1500, the nurse emptied 1,025 mL from the urinary drainage bag. Record the total intake and output on electronic record for the 0700 to 1500 (7 to 3) shift.

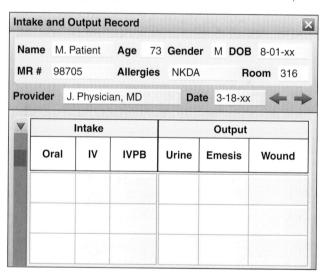

Intake and Output Record ⊠

| Name | M. Patient | Age | 73 | Gender | M | DOB | 8-01-xx |

MR # 98705 Allergies NKDA Room 316

Provider J. Physician, MD Date 3-18-xx ⬅ ➡

Intake			Output		
Oral	IV	IVPB	Urine	Emesis	Wound

CHAPTER 20

Parenteral Intake

LEARNING OUTCOMES

Calculate parenteral intake from a primary IV infusion.

Calculate parenteral intake from an IV piggyback.

Parenteral intake includes any IV fluid that infuses into the patient. Whether the IV fluid is from the primary line, IV piggybacks, or blood products, the intravenous fluid is counted as **parenteral intake.** Parenteral intake is recorded every shift or when the ordered amount of IV fluid has infused. The electronic intake and output record (Fig. 20-1) provides a systematic format for entering the amount of intake from various sources. Notice the columns for recording parenteral intake. The nurse records the amount of parenteral intake throughout the shift so that by the end of the shift a total amount is obtained. Accurate and timely documentation of the intake every shift helps to inform the physician of the daily fluid status of the patient.

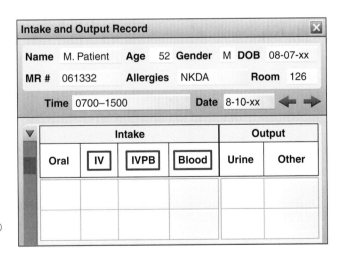

Figure 20-1. Example of an electronic I & O record highlighting parenteral intake.

Documenting Primary IV Intake

Accurate calculation of the amount of IV fluid infused during the shift is necessary for recording and reporting the IV intake for the shift. Most commonly, the primary IV fluid intake is recorded 1 hour prior to the end of the shift. Any primary IV fluid that infuses after the parenteral intake has been recorded will become part of the parenteral intake for the oncoming shift (Table 20-1).

Table 20-1. Sample Documentation Times of IV Fluid Intake in Clinical Practice

	8 HOUR SHIFT	RECORDING OF IV FLUID INTAKE
Day shift	**0700 to 1500** **7:00 AM to 3:00 PM**	The nurse for this shift calculates the IV fluid intake starting at **0600** and ending at **1400.**
Evening shift	**1500 to 2300** **3:00 PM to 11:00 PM**	The nurse for this shift calculates the IV fluid intake starting at **1400** and ending at **2200.**
Night shift	**2300 to 0700** **11:00 PM to 7:00 AM**	The nurse for this shift calculates the IV fluid intake starting at **2200** and ending at **0600.**

Because shift times vary in heathcare settings (i.e., 8 vs. 12 hour shifts), it is imperative that the nurse understands how parenteral intake for each shift is recorded in the specific clinical facility to minimize errors in documentation.

Calculating Parenteral Intake From a Primary IV Infusion

Primary IVs may infuse during all or part of the shift; therefore, the nurse must know the hourly rate (mL/hr) of the IV and the number of hours the IV infused during the shift. When calculating the parenteral intake, the nurse simply multiplies:

Hourly IV rate × Number of hours the IV fluid infused = IV intake

The nurse will calculate the parental intake 1 hour before the end of the shift, at which time the intake is "closed" for the shift. Table 20-2 demonstrates the 24 hour parenteral intake for a continuous primary IV for every shift.

Table 20-2. Documenting primary IV intake every shift.

CLINICAL SITUATION

7 to 3 shift:

An IV of 1,000 mL 0.9 % NaCl is started at 7:00 AM to infuse at 50 mL/hr.

The nurse calculates parenteral intake 1 hour before the end of the shift.

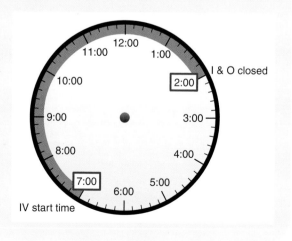

Table 20-2. Documenting primary IV intake every shift—cont'd

CLINICAL SITUATION

Multiply:

Hourly IV rate :	50 mL/hr
Number of hours infused :	× 7 hr
Total IV intake :	350 mL

Record:

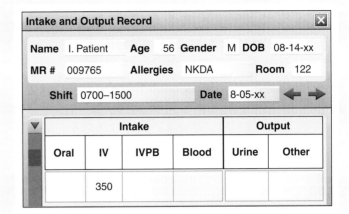

3 to 11 shift:

The day shift nurse reports that the patient has a continuous IV of 0.9% NaCl infusing at 50 mL/hr. IV intake for the evening shift is 400 mL.

The nurse calculates parenteral intake 1 hour before the end of the shift.

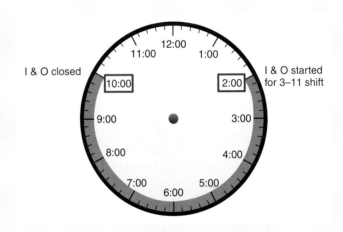

Multiply:

Hourly IV rate :	50 mL/hr
Number of hours infused :	× 8 hr
Total IV intake :	400 mL

Record:

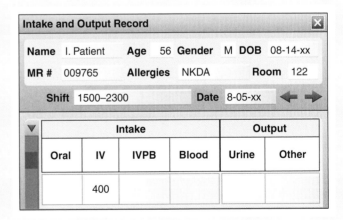

Continued

Table 20-2. Documenting primary IV intake every shift—cont'd

CLINICAL SITUATION

11 to 7 shift:

The evening shift nurse reports that the patient
has a continuous IV of 0.9% NaCl infusing at
50 mL/hr. IV intake for the shift is 400 mL.

The nurse calculates parenteral intake 1 hour
before the end of the shift.

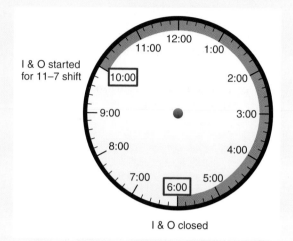

I & O closed

Multiply:

Hourly IV rate :	50 mL/hr
Number of hours infused :	× 8 hr
Total IV intake :	400 mL

Record:

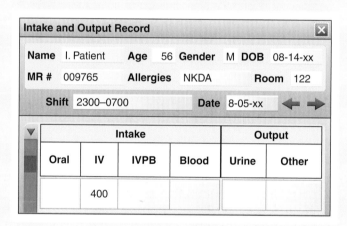

	Intake			Output	
Oral	IV	IVPB	Blood	Urine	Other
	400				

Use of Military Time

Military time is commonly used in electronic medical records to indicate the time of day.
Unlike clock time, which uses a.m. and p.m. to represent morning or night hours, military
time uses four digits. The first two digits represent the hours and the last two digits
represent the minutes. Military time is based on the number of hours in a day (0000 to
1100 representing morning hours, and 1200 to 2400 representing afternoon and evening
hours). Military time is discussed in Chapter 15, Calculating Infusion and Completion
Time. Table 20-3 shows the calculation of parenteral intake for the 0700 to 1500 shift
using military time.

Table 20-3. Military Time Use With Parenteral Intake.

CLINICAL SITUATION

0700 to 1500 shift

The physician orders 1,000 mL of D_5/0.9% NaCl at 125 mL/hr. The nurse starts the IV at 1100. What is the parenteral intake for the 0700 to 1500 shift?

The nurse calculates parenteral intake 1 hour before the end of the shift.

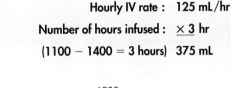

Hourly IV rate :   125 mL/hr

Number of hours infused :   × 3 hr

(1100 − 1400 = 3 hours)   375 mL

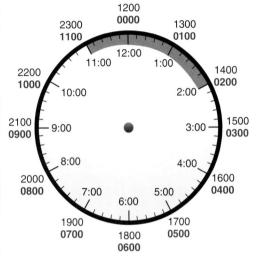

Interruption of the Continuous Flow of IV Fluid

Although the administration of a primary IV fluid is intended to be continuous, there are times when the continuous flow of the IV is interrupted. This interruption may be due to the *infiltration* of the IV, accidental removal of the IV catheter, or problems with maintaining the ordered number of mL/hr. The period of time necessary for restarting the IV may be just a few minutes or may be longer. During this time, the IV fluid is not infusing into the patient. Therefore, when calculating the IV intake, the nurse needs to calculate the IV intake based on the number of hours the IV fluid actually infused during the shift. Look at the following example.

Example:

IV fluid stopped and restarted during the shift.

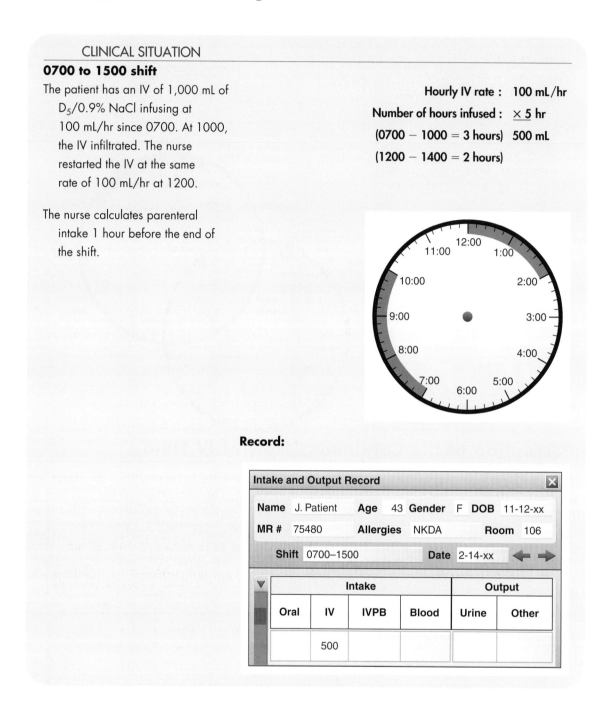

CLINICAL SITUATION

0700 to 1500 shift

The patient has an IV of 1,000 mL of D₅/0.9% NaCl infusing at 100 mL/hr since 0700. At 1000, the IV infiltrated. The nurse restarted the IV at the same rate of 100 mL/hr at 1200.

The nurse calculates parenteral intake 1 hour before the end of the shift.

Hourly IV rate :   100 mL/hr
Number of hours infused :   × 5 hr
(0700 − 1000 = 3 hours)   500 mL
(1200 − 1400 = 2 hours)

Record:

Intake and Output Record						☒
Name J. Patient	**Age** 43	**Gender** F	**DOB** 11-12-xx			
MR # 75480	**Allergies** NKDA		**Room** 106			
Shift 0700–1500		**Date** 2-14-xx	← →			

	Intake			Output	
Oral	IV	IVPB	Blood	Urine	Other
	500				

Change in Hourly Rate During the Shift

When the physician writes a new IV order that either increases or decreases the number of mL/hr during the shift, the nurse calculates the IV intake for each of the hourly infusion rates: the starting hourly rate and the new hourly rate. Look at how the IV intake is calculated in the following example.

Example:

Change in the hourly rate (mL/hr) of the primary IV per physician's order.

CLINICAL SITUATION

2300 to 0700 shift

The patient's IV of 1,000 mL of D₅W infusing at 75 mL/hr was started at 2300. At 0300, the MD increases the IV hourly rate to 100 mL/hr.

The nurse calculates parenteral intake 1 hour before the end of the shift.

Hourly IV rate : 75 mL/hr
Number of hours infused : × 4 hr
(2300 − 0300 = 4 hours) 300 mL

New hourly IV rate : 100 mL/hr
Number of hours infused : × 3 hr
(0300 − 0600 = 3 hours) 300 mL

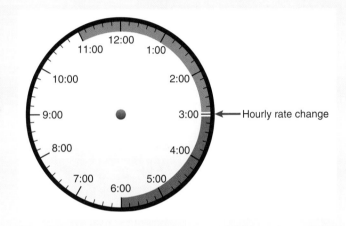

Record:

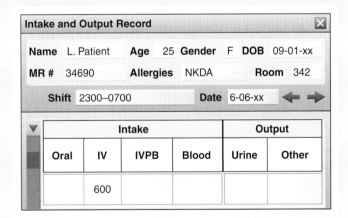

APPLY LEARNED KNOWLEDGE 20-1

Calculate the IV intake for the following problems.

1. The nurse begins 500 mL of 0.9% NaCl at 0800 to infuse at 50 mL/hr. Parenteral intake is closed at 1400. Calculate the IV intake for the 0700 to 1500 shift. _____

2. An IV of 1,000 mL of 0.45% NaCl is started at 1700 to infuse at 125 mL/hr. Parenteral intake is closed at 2200. Calculate the IV intake for the 1500 to 2300 shift. _____

Continued

APPLY LEARNED KNOWLEDGE 20-1—cont'd

3. A liter of 0.45% NaCl is started at 1600 to infuse at 75 mL/hr. At 2000, the IV hourly rate is increased to 100 mL/hr per MD order. Parenteral intake is closed at 2200. Calculate the IV intake for the 1500 to 2300 shift. _____

4. The nurse starts 500 mL of D_5/NS at 100 mL/hr at 0100. At 0200, the hourly rate is decreased to 50 mL/hr per MD order. Parenteral intake is closed at 0600. Calculate the IV intake for the 2300 to 0700 shift. _____

5. The nurse hangs 1 liter of D_5W at 1500 to infuse at 83 mL/hr. Parenteral intake is closed at 2200. Calculate the IV intake for the 1500 to 2300 shift. _____

The IV Piggyback (IVPB)

The IVPB is used as a method of delivering intravenous medications to the patient. The physician's order for the administration of an IVPB includes the name of the medication, the dose, the route, and the time or frequency of administration. The IVPB medication is diluted in a specific volume of intravenous fluid as recommended by the drug manufacturer. In premixed IVPBs, detailed information related to the medication dose and volume is identified on the label (Fig. 20-2).

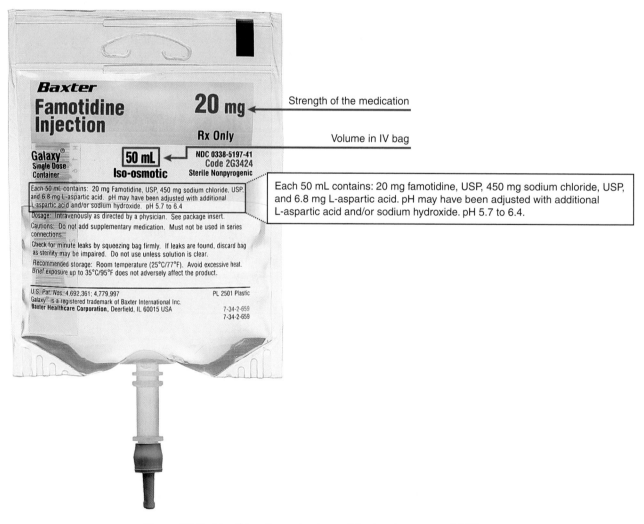

Figure 20-2. Identifying the total volume of fluid in the premixed IVPB.

Depending on the medication and the dose ordered by the physician, each IVPB medication may be mixed in a different amount of volume. The nurse must be careful to identify and record accurately the IV fluid volume from each IVPB administered.

In Figure 20-3, the total volume listed in the premixed vancomycin 1 g IVPB is 200 mL. Notice the detailed information in regards to the medication dose and volume: "Each 100 mL contains: Vancomycin Hydrochloride, USP equivalent to 500 mg vancomycin . . ." Although this information indicates 500 mg in each 100 mL, this is not the dosage strength for this IVPB. The Vancomycin drug label has the strength of the medication (1 g) listed separately from the form of the drug (200 mL). Together, these prominent numbers indicate the dosage strength of 1 g/200 mL for this IVPB. If the physician ordered Vancomycin 500 mg, the nurse must use a different IVPB that contains only 500 mg of the drug.

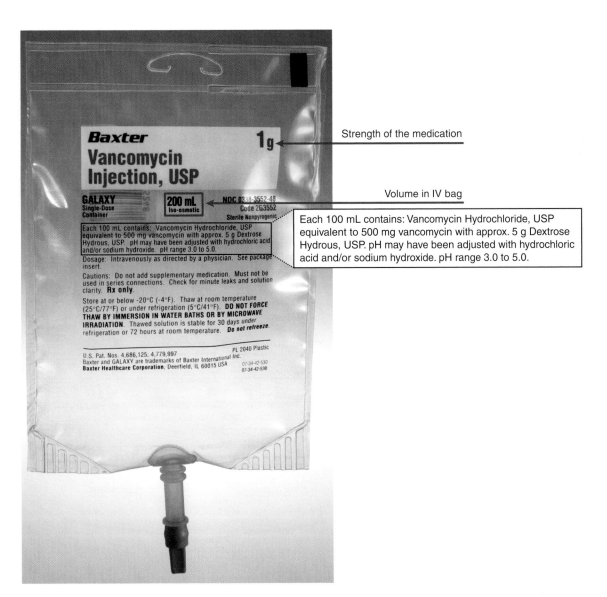

Figure 20-3. Vancomycin 1 g IVPB.

After administration of an IVPB, the nurse documents the volume in the IVPB as parenteral fluid in the I & O record and records the administration of the medication in the medication record.

 The nurse's role as patient advocate and the Six Rights of Medication Administration require that the nurse seek clarification on any drug information that is unfamiliar or is presented in a different format.

Calculating the IVPB Intake

Patients may receive one or several IVPBs during the shift. Each IVPB administered during the shift is part of the parenteral intake. Once the IVPB has been administered, the volume of fluid in the IVPB is recorded. Look at the following two examples of how the IVPB intake is recorded for different shifts.

Example 1:

IVPB administration for the 0700 to 1500 shift.

CLINICAL SITUATION	PHARMACY SENDS	IVPB ADMINISTRATION FOR THE 0700 TO 1500 SHIFT
The patient receives Cefazolin 500 mg IVPB q.6h at 0800, 1400, 2000, and 0200.	Cefazolin 500 mg in 100 mL 0.9% NaCl	The nurse will administer one dose of cefazolin at 0800 and another dose at 1400.

Intake and Output Record ☒

Shift 0700–1500   Date 2-05-xx ← →

	Intake				Output	
Oral	IV	IVPB	Blood	Urine	Other
		100			
		100			

Example 2:

IVPB administration for the 2300 to 0700 shift.

CLINICAL SITUATION	PHARMACY SENDS	IVPB ADMINISTRATION FOR THE 2300 TO 0700 SHIFT
The patient receives the following IVPBs: Cefepime 0.5 g IVPB q.12h at 0100 and 1300. Famotidine 20 mg IVPB q.12h at 0900 and 2100.	Cefepime 0.5 g in 100 mL 0.9% NaCl Famotidine 20 mg in 50 mL 0.9% NaCl	The nurse will administer one dose of cefepime at 0100. The nurse will not give famotidine during the 2300 to 0700 shift.

Intake and Output Record ☒

Shift 2300–0700   Date 2-05-xx ← →

	Intake				Output	
Oral	IV	IVPB	Blood	Urine	Other
		100			

APPLY LEARNED KNOWLEDGE 20-2

Calculate the total IVPB intake for the shift indicated.

1. The patient receives the following IVPB: Cefazolin 1 g in 100 mL D_5W IVPB q.8h at 0900–1700–0100.
   A. What is the IVPB intake for the 0700 to 1500 shift? _____

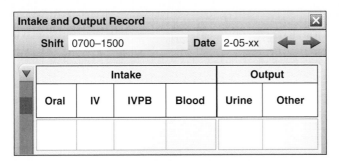

   B. What is the IVPB intake for the 1500 to 2300 shift? _____

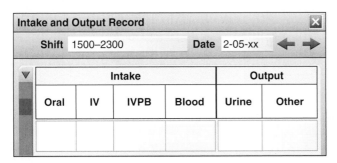

2. The patient receives the following IVPBs: Metronidazole 0.5 g in 100 mL D_5W IVPB q.12h at 0800–2000 and Potassium chloride 20 mEq in 250 mL D_5W IVPB at 1300.
   A. What is the IVPB intake for the 0700 to 1500 shift? _____

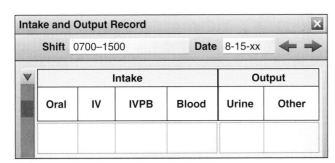

   B. What is the IVPB intake for the 1500 to 2300 shift? _____

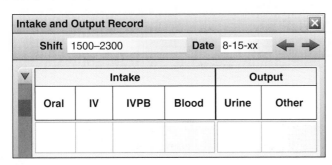

Continued

APPLY LEARNED KNOWLEDGE 20-2—cont'd

3. The following IVPBs are on the medication administration record for the patient: Cimetidine 300 mg in 50 mL 0.9% NaCl IVPB q.6h at 0800 – 1400 – 2000 – 0200 and Vancomycin 0.5 g in 100 mL D$_5$W IVPB at 1000.

A. What is the IVPB intake for the 1500 to 2300 shift? _____

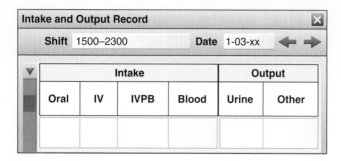

Intake and Output Record   ☒

Shift 1500–2300   **Date** 1-03-xx ⬅ ➡

	Intake			Output	
Oral	IV	IVPB	Blood	Urine	Other

B. What is the IVPB intake for the 2300 to 0700 shift? _____

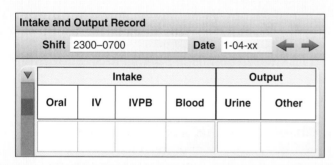

Intake and Output Record

Shift 2300–0700   **Date** 1-04-xx ⬅ ➡

	Intake			Output	
Oral	IV	IVPB	Blood	Urine	Other

4. Based on the medication record, the IVPB intake for the 1500 to 2300 shift will be:

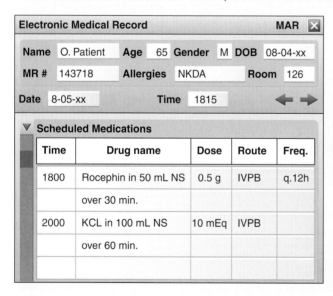

Electronic Medical Record   **MAR** ☒

Name O. Patient	**Age** 65	**Gender** M	**DOB** 08-04-xx
MR # 143718	**Allergies** NKDA		**Room** 126
Date 8-05-xx		**Time** 1815	⬅ ➡

▼ Scheduled Medications

Time	Drug name	Dose	Route	Freq.
1800	Rocephin in 50 mL NS	0.5 g	IVPB	q.12h
	over 30 min.			
2000	KCL in 100 mL NS	10 mEq	IVPB	
	over 60 min.			

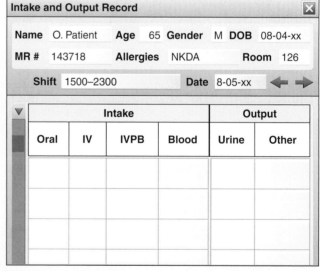

Intake and Output Record   ☒

Name O. Patient	**Age** 65	**Gender** M	**DOB** 08-04-xx
MR # 143718	**Allergies** NKDA		**Room** 126
Shift 1500–2300		**Date** 8-05-xx	⬅ ➡

	Intake			Output	
Oral	IV	IVPB	Blood	Urine	Other

APPLY LEARNED KNOWLEDGE 20-2—cont'd

5. Based on the medication record, the IVPB intake for the 2300 to 0700 shift will be:

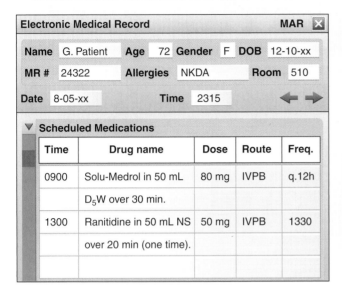

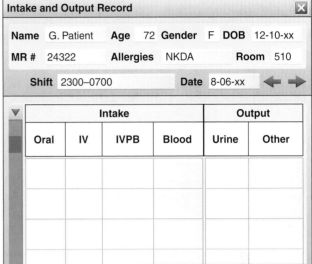

The 24 Hour Parenteral Intake

Parenteral intake is a major component of a patient's intake and is critical in monitoring the fluid balance of the patient. The 24 hour intake and output record provides an overview of a patient's 24 hour fluid balance and serves as a tool to further assess the fluid needs of a patient. A review of the 24 hour intake and output record (Fig. 20-4), helps to distinguish the amount of intake and output for every shift and further provides information regarding the intake from various sources. Accurate documentation is necessary to help the physician determine the daily parenteral fluid needs of a patient.

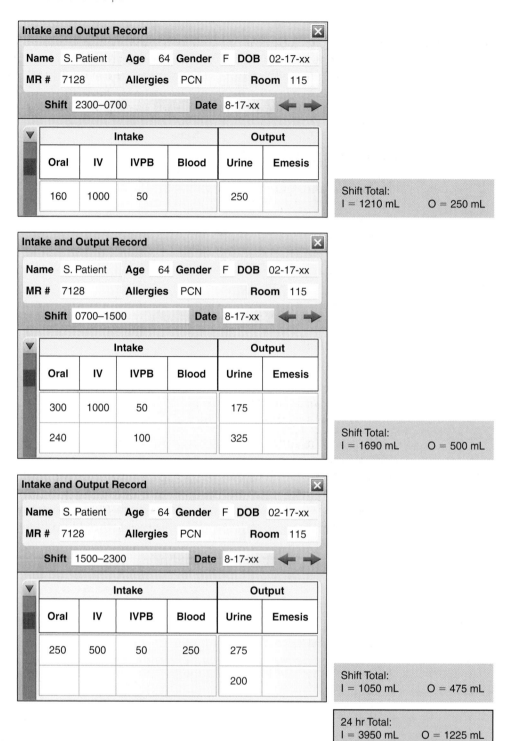

Figure 20-4. Sample electronic intake and output record with 24 hour totals.

CLINICAL REASONING 20-1

At the handoff report, the 1500 to 2300 shift nurse is informed that the patient has a primary IV of 0.9% NaCL at 50 mL/hr started at 1000. The primary IV was stopped at 1100 and the patient received one unit (225 mL) of whole blood from 1100 to 1300. The primary IV of 0.9% NaCL was restarted at the same rate (50 mL/hr) at 1300. The I & O record is closed at 1400, 1 hour prior to the end of the shift. In reviewing the parenteral intake for the 0700 to 1500 shift, the nurse finds the following:

Intake and Output Record ☒

Shift 0700–1500   **Date** 3-06-xx ← →

Intake				Output	
Oral	IV	IVPB	Blood	Urine	Other
400	100	225		250	
100				175	

The nurse is most correct initially to:

A. clarify the primary IV intake for the shift.
B. clarify the documentation of the whole blood.
C. report a 0700 to 1500 parenteral intake of 375 mL.
D. review the IVPBs ordered for the patient.

The safe care of patients mandates timely communication between physicians, nurses, and ancillary health-care providers. Accuracy in the documentation of the parenteral intake every shift with 24 hour totals communicates information in regards to a patient's fluid status. This information is used to further assess and evaluate the patient. The nurse, who is at the patient's bedside throughout the shift, is central to the process of monitoring, documenting, and communicating a patient's fluid intake and overall fluid balance.

Developing Competency

Calculate the parenteral intake for the following problems.

1. On the 7 to 3 shift, the patient has an IV of D_5/0.9% NaCL started at 1100 to infuse at 150 mL/hr. The I & O record is closed at 1400, 1 hour prior to the end of the shift. Calculate the parenteral intake. _____

2. An IV of 1,000 mL of 0.45% NaCl is started at 1600 to infuse at 125 mL/hr. The I & O record is closed at 2200, 1 hour prior to the end of the shift. Calculate the parenteral intake for the 1500 to 2300 shift. _____

3. A liter of D_5/0.45% NS is started at 0200 to infuse at 75 mL/hr. The IV flow rate is increased at 0400 to 100 mL/hr per M.D. order. The I & O record is closed at 0600, 1 hour prior to the end of the shift. Calculate the parenteral intake for the 2300 to 0700 shift. _____

4. A liter of lactated Ringer's is started at 0700 to infuse at 150 mL/hr. The IV flow rate is decreased at 1100 to 100 mL/hr per MD order. The I & O record is closed at 1400, 1 hour prior to the end of the shift. Calculate the parenteral intake for the 0700 to 1500 shift. _____

5. A liter of 0.9% NaCl is started at 1700 to infuse at 100 mL/hr. The IV infiltrates at 2000 and is restarted at 2200 at the same IV rate. The I & O record is closed at 2200, 1 hour prior to the end of the shift. Calculate the parenteral intake for the 1500 to 2300 shift. _____

6. 500 mL of 0.9% NaCl is started at 0900 to infuse at 75 mL/hr. The patient pulls out the IV at 1200. The nurse restarts the IV at 1300 at the same IV rate. The I & O record is closed at 1400, 1 hour prior to the end of the shift. Calculate the parenteral intake for the 0700 to 1500 shift. _____

7. The patient receives the following IVPBs: Cefazolin 1 g in 100 mL D$_5$W IVPB q.8h at 0900 – 1700 – 0100 and Ondansetron 10 mg in 50 mL 0.9% NaCl at 1000.
   (A) What is the IVPB intake for the 0700 to 1500 shift? _____
   (B) What is the IVPB intake for the 1500 to 2300 shift? _____

8. The patient receives the following IVPBs: Furosemide 20 mg in 50 mL 0.9% NaCl IVPB at 1300 and Phenytoin 50 mg in 50 mL 0.9% NaCl IVPB at 1600.
   (A) What is the IVPB intake for the 0700 to 1500 shift? _____
   (B) What is the IVPB intake for the 1500 to 2300 shift? _____

9. The patient receives the following IVPBs: Naficillin 0.5 g in 50 mL D$_5$W IVPB q.4h at 0900 – 1300 – 1700 – 2100 – 0100 – 0500 and Famotidine 20 mg IVPB in 50 mL 0.9% NaCl q.12h at 0800 and 2000.
   A. What is the IVPB intake for the 0700 to 1500 shift? _____
   B. What is the IVPB intake for the 1500 to 2300 shift? _____
   C. What is the IVPB intake for the 2300 to 0700 shift? _____

10. The nurse is reviewing the patient's electronic medication record and administers the ordered IVPB for the 3 to 11 shift. Record the IVPB intake on the intake and output record.

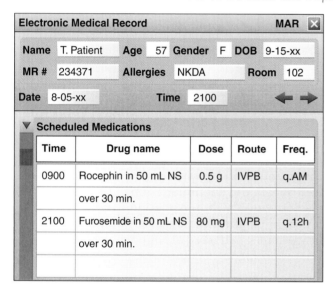

11. The patient has an IV of D$_5$/NS started at 0800 to infuse at 100 mL/hr continuously. The I & O record is closed at 1400, 1 hour prior to the end of the shift. Select the correct parenteral intake for the 0700 to 1500 shift.
   a. 600 mL
   b. 700 mL
   c. 800 Ml

12. The patient receives the following IVPBs: Tobramycin 50 mg in 100 mL D$_5$W IVPB q.AM at 0900 and Famotidine 20 mg IVPB in 100 mL 0.9% NaCl q.12h at 0800 and 2000. The nurse calculated that the patient received 450 mL of IV fluid from the primary line for the 1500 to 2300 shift. Select the correct parenteral intake for the 1500 to 2300 shift.
   a. 450 mL
   b. 550 mL
   c. 650 mL

13. The patient receives the following IVPBs: Tobramycin 50 mg in 100 mL D$_5$W IVPB q.AM at 0900 and Famotidine 20 mg IVPB in 100 mL 0.9% NaCl q.12h at 0800 and 2000. The nurse calculated that the patient received 1,000 mL of IV fluid from the primary line for the 2300 to 0700 shift. Select the correct parenteral intake for the 2300 to 0700 shift.
   a. 875 mL
   b. 975 mL
   c. 1000 mL

14. The patient has an IV of D$_5$/NS started at 0100 to infuse at 150 mL/hr for the first 3 hours and then the rate is decreased to 75 mL/hr. The I & O record is closed at 0600, 1 hour prior to the end of the shift. Select the correct parenteral intake for the 2300 to 0700 shift.
   a. 600 mL
   b. 700 mL
   c. 800 mL

15. The patient has an IV of lactated Ringer's started at 1700 to infuse at 125 mL/hr for the first 4 hours and then the rate is decreased to 75 mL/hr. The I & O record is closed at 2200, 1 hour prior to the end of the shift. Select the correct parenteral intake for the 1500 to 2300 shift.
   a. 500 mL
   b. 575 mL
   c. 650 mL

Intake and Output

Unit Review—Evaluate for Clinical Decision Making

For each question, use your clinical judgment to determine whether the nurse's decision is **Correct** *or* **Incorrect**. *For incorrect problems, write the correct answer.*

1. For breakfast, the patient drank 6 oz of juice, 180 mL of coffee, and 2 oz of milk. For lunch, the patient drinks 4 oz of milk and eats 120 mL of ice cream. The patient drank 300 mL of water by the end of the 0700 to 1500 shift. The patient urinated 325 mL at 0800 and 250 at 1300.

Name *X. Patient*   Age *64*   MR # *765776*   Room *23-A*

Intake and Output Worksheet

Shift	Oral	Other	Urine	Emesis	Other
7-3	*180*		*325*		
	180		*250*		
	60				
	120				
	120				
	300				
Total (mL)	*960*		*575*		

The day shift RN is reviewing the worksheet before recording the patient's intake and output in the electronic medical record. The RN determines that the calculated I & O is:

Correct	Incorrect	Answer: _____

2. The patient had surgery 2 days ago. He has a naso-gastric tube for suction and a wound drainage device. At the end of the evening shift, the nurse emptied 475 mL from the nasogastric suction and 75 mL from the wound drainage device. The patient urinated 225 mL at 1600 and 100 at 2200.

Name _B. Patient_ Age _72_ MR # _912488_ Room _10_

Intake and Output Worksheet

Shift	Oral	Urine	Emesis	Drainage	Other
3-11		225 100	475	(Wound)	
Total (mL)		325	475	75	

The day shift RN is reviewing the worksheet before recording the patient's intake and output in the electronic medical record. The RN determines that the information on the I & O worksheet is:

Correct	Incorrect	Answer: _____

3.

Electronic Medical Record		**Provider Orders**	✕

Name H. Patient   **Age** 78 **Gender** M **DOB** 5-15-xx

MR # 81121   **Allergies** NKDA   **Room** 123

Provider H. Physician, MD   **Date** 2-01-xx ⬅ ➡

▼ **Order**

Start Nepro tube feedings 250 mL every six hours at

(0800–1400–2000–0200).

Administer 100 mL of water after each feeding.

The nurse calculates that the 24 hour intake for this patient would be 1,000 mL. The nurse's 24 hour calculation is:

Correct	Incorrect	Answer: _____

4.

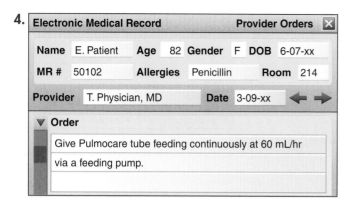

Electronic Medical Record					Provider Orders	☒

Name E. Patient   **Age** 82 **Gender** F **DOB** 6-07-xx

MR # 50102   **Allergies** Penicillin   **Room** 214

Provider T. Physician, MD   **Date** 3-09-xx ⬅ ➡

▼ **Order**

Give Pulmocare tube feeding continuously at 60 mL/hr
via a feeding pump.

The nurse calculates that the 8 hour intake for this
patient would be 480 mL.
The nurse's 8 hour calculation is:

Correct	Incorrect	Answer: _____

5. For dinner the patient drank 6 oz of coffee and 180 mL
of broth, and ate one 3 oz popsicle. He consumed an
8 oz glass of ice chips in the morning. The patient has
a continuous bladder irrigation infusing at 60 mL/hr
from 8:00 AM to 2:00 PM. At 2:00 PM, the nurse
emptied 975 mL from the urinary drainage bag.

Intake and Output Record						☒

Name I. Patient   **Age** 63 **Gender** M **DOB** 11-01-xx

MR # 47321   **Allergies** NKDA   **Room** 234

Provider H. Physician, MD   **Date** 2-17-xx ⬅ ➡

	Intake			Output		
	Oral	IV	IVPB	Urine	Emesis	UA Catheter
	690					735

The nurse calculates the 8 hour intake and output for
the 7 to 3 shift and records it in the electronic medical
record. The nurse's 8 hour calculation is:

Correct	Incorrect	Answer: _____

6. The nurse hangs 1 liter of D_5W at 0800 to infuse at
75 mL/hr. The parenteral intake is closed at 1400,
1 hour prior to the end of the shift. The nurse calculates
a parenteral intake for the 0700 to 1500 shift of
450 mL.
The parenteral intake is:

Correct	Incorrect	Answer: _____

7. A liter of 0.45% NaCl is started at 0100 to infuse at 100 mL/hr. At 0300, the IV hourly rate is increased to 150 mL/hr per MD order. The parenteral intake is closed at 0600, 1 hour prior to the end of the shift. The nurse calculates a parenteral intake for the 2300 to 0700 shift of 550 mL.
The parenteral intake is:

Correct	Incorrect	Answer: _____

8. The IV order is 1,000 mL of 0.9% NaCl q.8h. The nurse starts the IV at 0800. At 1200, the patient pulls out the IV. The nurse restarts the IV at 1300 at the same IV rate. The I & O record is closed at 1400, 1 hour prior to the end of the shift. The nurse calculates a parenteral intake for the 0700 to 1500 shift of 500 mL.
The parenteral intake is:

Correct	Incorrect	Answer: _____

9. The patient receives the following IVPBs: Tobramycin 50 mg in 100 mL D_5W IVPB q.AM at 0900 and Famotidine 20 mg IVPB in 100 mL 0.9% NaCl q. 12h. at 0800 and 2000. The patient has a primary IV of D_5W 1,000 mL started at 0100 at 125 mL/hr. The I & O record is closed at 0600, 1 hour prior to the end of the shift. The nurse calculates a parenteral intake for the 2300 to 0700 shift of 625 mL.
The parenteral intake is:

Correct	Incorrect	Answer: _____

10. The patient receives the following IVPB: Naficillin 0.5 g in 50 mL D_5W IVPB q.6h. at 1000 – 1600 – 2200 – 0400. The patient has a primary IV of lactated Ringer's 1,000 mL started at 1200 to infuse over 10 hours. The I & O record is closed at 1400, 1 hour prior to the end of the shift. The nurse calculates a parenteral intake for the 0700 to 1500 shift of 250 mL.
The parenteral intake is:

Correct	Incorrect	Answer: _____

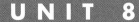
Dosages for Pediatric and Elderly Populations

C hildren and older adults require the nurse to take into account factors such as age, weight, and specific diseases when calculating drug dosages. This unit emphasizes how to identify drug reference information related to these special populations, and includes the administration and calculation of enteral nutrition and replacement IV fluid therapy.

 APPLICATION TO NURSING PRACTICE

Drug references provide the nurse with information specific to the pediatric and older adult populations.

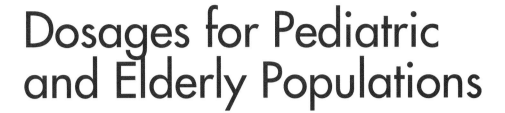

phenytoin (fen-i-toyn)
Dilantin, Phenytek, ✽Tremytoine

Classification
Therapeutic: antiarrhythmics (group IB), anticonvulsants
Pharmacologic: hydantoins

Pregnancy Category D

Indications
Treatment/prevention of tonic-clonic (grand mal) seizures and complex partial seizures...

Route/Dosage
Anticonvulsant

PO (Children 10–16 yr): 6–7 mg/kg/day in 2–3...
PO (Children 7–9 yr): 7–8 mg/kg/day in 2–3...
PO (Children 4–6 yr): 7.5–9 mg/kg/day in 2–3...

Antiarrhythmic
IV (Children): 1.25 mg/kg q 5 min, may repeat up to total loading dose of 15 mg/kg...

LORazepam (lor-az-e-pam)
Ativan

Classification
Therapeutic: anesthetic adjuncts, antianxiety agents, sedative/hypnotics
Pharmacologic: benzodiazepines

Schedule IV

Pregnancy Category D

Indications
Anxiety disorder (oral). Preoperative sedation (injection). Decreases preoperative anxiety and provides amnesia...

Use Cautiously in:... Geri: Lower doses recommended for geriatrics or debilitated patients. Hypnotic use should be short-term.

Route/Dosage

PO (Geriatric or Debilitated Patients)
Anxiety—0.5–2 mg/day in divided doses initially.
Insomnia—0.25–1 mg initially, ↑ as needed...

The nurse selects relevant information from the drug reference when calculating the appropriate dosage for a specific patient.

CHAPTER 21

Considerations for the Pediatric Population

LEARNING OUTCOMES

Identify best practices in the administration of oral and parenteral medications for children.

Calculate and verify safe dose for pediatric medications based on body weight.

Discuss the importance of replacement fluid therapy.

Calculate replacement fluid therapy.

Children present critical challenges for the nurse both in the calculation of drug dosages and in the administration of medications. The pediatric population includes children from birth to the age of 18 years. This age span encompasses several stages including neonates, infants, children, adolescents, and young adults. In each of these stages, differences in physical size, organ development, body fat, and gastric function affect the pharmacokinetic processes of absorption, metabolism, distribution, and excretion of drugs. When administering medication to children, the nurse must be aware that the unique factors of age, weight, height, organ development, and medical condition are important in determining the dose of medication to be administered. Because these factors are variable and unique to each child, it is not possible for the drug manufacturer to accurately identify a standard drug dose as is frequently seen for the adult patient. Therefore, medications for children are ordered based on the physical size and weight of the child. For the older adolescent and the young adult, medication dosages may be based on weight or on the standard dose depending on such factors as the child's physical size and weight, the drug, and the child's medical condition.

Administration of Medications to Children by the Oral Route

Unlike the administration of oral medication to adults, the administration and preparation of oral medications for children necessitate that the nurse consider the child's developmental stage, the form of the drug (solid or liquid), and the most age-appropriate dosage delivery device to administer the drug. Because oral medications for infants and young children are ordered and administered in liquid form, the nurse must select a dosage delivery device that is calibrated to accurately measure the ordered dose and also appropriate for the developmental age of the child. This helps to ensure safety in administration and to facilitate the administration of the entire dose of medication.

Oral medications in solid form (tablets, capsules) may be ordered for the older child and the adolescent. Safety in medication administration requires the nurse to take into account the size of the tablet or capsule and the child's clinical condition. Large tablets or capsules may be difficult to swallow and thereby increase the risk of choking and asphyxiation. Easy-to-swallow drug forms, such as chewable tablets, fast melt tablets, or disintegrating tablets, may be available for some drugs. Regardless of the form of the drug, the nurse must carefully assess the child's ability to swallow prior to the administration of any oral medication.

The oral route for the administration of medications is preferred over the administration of injections in children. However, with oral medications as well as those given by other routes, the child's cooperation is essential to ensure that the full dose of medication is administered. Therefore, as part of the medication administration process to children, the nurse must plan and include thoughtful, nonthreatening interventions to gain the child's cooperation.

LIQUID DOSAGE DELIVERY DEVICES SPECIFIC TO THE ORAL ROUTE

Oral dosage delivery devices are medication administration devices that are calibrated and marked with metric and/or household units of measurement for accurate measurement of liquid doses of medication. Using the appropriate dosage delivery device helps to minimize the risk of accidental overdose. Table 21-1 identifies oral dosage delivery devices available for the administration of liquid medications to children by the oral route.

Table 21-1. Oral Route: Dosage Delivery Devices for Liquid Medications

ORAL ROUTE	USEFUL INFORMATION
Cylindrical dosing spoon	• The dosing spoon provides a more accurate measurement of the liquid medication than a regular household spoon. • Notice the calibrations on the measuring device and the end shape facilitating the administration of liquid medications.
Oral syringe	• The oral syringe is available in various sizes ranging from 1 mL to 10 mL capacity. • The barrel of the syringe may be clear or amber, and the special tip design prevents the attachment of a needle. • Notice the tip of the syringe is designed to allow small amounts the liquid medication to be squirted into the child's mouth. • The oral syringe may come prefilled with medication and capped. The cap is removed prior to the administration of the medication.

Continued

Table 21-1. Oral Route: Dosage Delivery Devices for Liquid Medications—cont'd

ORAL ROUTE	USEFUL INFORMATION
Calibrated dropper 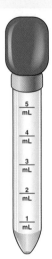	• The dropper is calibrated to hold a certain amount of medication, usually 1 mL to 5 mL. • When using a dropper, the nurse needs to ensure that all medication is administered, because the dropper may pull back medication when the pressure is released from the top of the dropper.
Nipple dispenser measuring device/medicine dispensing bottle/pacifier 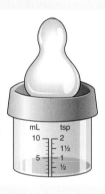	• These infant medication dispensing devices are calibrated to measure a certain amount of medication, usually from 1 tsp to 3 tsp. • Devices are designed to facilitate the delivery of the full dose of medication to infants and young children.

Administration of Medications to Children by the Parenteral Route

The administration of medications by injection to children employs interventions that promote safe practice for all patients such as:

■ Right drug, dose, time, route, and patient

■ Using correct technique in the administration of the drug

■ Using gloves to adhere to standard precautions

In the administration of injections to children, consideration must be given to the child's developmental stage and muscle mass. The nurse must keep in mind that safety recommendations in the selection of injection sites, needle length, and maximum volume per injection site are made based on the muscle mass of the growing child. For example, when administering an IM injection to an infant or a young toddler, the nurse is aware that the infant has reduced muscle mass in comparison with the muscle mass of an older child. Therefore, the **vastus lateralis** muscle, located in the middle one-third of the anterolateral thigh, is the recommended site as it has adequate muscle mass and is free of major blood vessels minimizing the risk of harm. The ***ventrogluteal*** muscle, located between the

greater trochanter and the ***anterior iliac crest,*** is also an appropriate injection site for the older infant and child. The nurse must be aware that complications, such as nerve damage and ***tissue necrosis,*** can occur with injections. Therefore, careful assessment of the injection site and selection of the appropriate needle length are critical decisions in the administration of the injection. Table 21-2 provides an example of how the selection of needle length for an IM injection and maximum volume is influenced by the developmental stage and muscle mass of the growing child.

Table 21-2. IM Injection: Needle Length and Maximum Volume per Injection Site

AGE	NEEDLE LENGTH CONSIDERATIONS*	MAXIMUM VOLUME PER INJECTION
Newborn	5/8" needle length	0.5 mL
Infant or toddler	5/8" to 1" needle length	1 mL
Young child	1" to 1½" needle length	2 mL
Adolescent	1" to 1½" needle length	2 mL to 2.5 mL

*For IM injection in the anterolateral thigh based on muscle mass

It is important for the nurse to stay up to date with current research and evaluate the specific needs of every child to minimize the risk of harm and promote safe drug delivery and absorption.

 The World Health Organization in its 2010 publication WHO Best Practices for Injections and Related Procedures Toolkit *indicates that "a safe injection is one that does not harm the recipient, does not expose the provider to any avoidable risks and does not result in waste that is dangerous for the community."*
(http://whqlibdoc.who.int/publications/2010/9789241599252_eng.pdf).

Administration of Intravenous Fluids to Children

When intravenous fluids are ordered for a child, the nurse must initiate and implement interventions that minimize the risk of harm. From the consideration of the appropriate venipuncture site for the developmental stage of the child, to the initiation of interventions that prevent fluid overload, safety in the administration of IV fluids to children necessitates:

■ the administration of IV fluids at lower infusion rates (mL/hr).

■ use of safety equipment to minimize accidental overinfusion of IV fluid.

■ daily weight.

Because of the differences in body weight, the amount of fluid lost during illness, and the medical condition of the child, the fluid needs of each child vary. The nurse must be acutely aware that complications affecting the fluid status of children can occur rapidly. Therefore, monitoring the IV infusion and assessing the child for complications related to fluid overload and electrolyte disturbances are priority nursing interventions. In the administration of IV therapy, interventions that help to regulate, monitor, and minimize the risk of harm during the administration of the IV fluid include the use of:

■ Electronic IV infusion devices, such as smart pumps and syringe pumps
  • Smart pumps help to reduce medication infusion errors and provide accuracy in the delivery of IV fluids at the correct infusion rate.
  • Syringe pumps provide accuracy in the delivery of very small doses of medications over a preset period of time.
■ Buretrol or volume control fluid chamber devices (Fig. 21-1)
  • Volume control fluid chamber devices assist the nurse to limit the amount of fluid that is allowed to infuse into the patient, therefore minimizing the risk of accidental

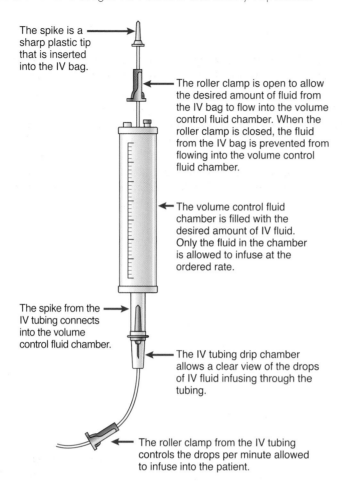

The spike is a sharp plastic tip that is inserted into the IV bag.

The roller clamp is open to allow the desired amount of fluid from the IV bag to flow into the volume control fluid chamber. When the roller clamp is closed, the fluid from the IV bag is prevented from flowing into the volume control fluid chamber.

The volume control fluid chamber is filled with the desired amount of IV fluid. Only the fluid in the chamber is allowed to infuse at the ordered rate.

The spike from the IV tubing connects into the volume control fluid chamber.

The IV tubing drip chamber allows a clear view of the drops of IV fluid infusing through the tubing.

The roller clamp from the IV tubing controls the drops per minute allowed to infuse into the patient.

Figure 21-1. Example of a volume chamber device.

infusion of a large volume of IV fluid. These volume control fluid chamber devices are designed to connect onto the IV tubing, between the IV bag and the primary IV tubing (see Fig. 21-1). The volume control fluid chamber is filled with a small amount of IV fluid from the IV bag (i.e., 50 mL to 150 mL). In some health-care institutions, electronic IV infusion pumps are minimizing or eliminating the use of the volume control fluid chamber devices.

■ Small-volume IV bags (25 mL, 50 mL, 100 mL, 250 mL, 500 mL)

- Small-volume IV bags limit the amount IV fluid that may accidentally infuse into the child from an IV bag.

■ Microdrop tubing for infusion of gravity IVs

- Microdrop tubing delivers less volume per mL (60 gtt/mL) than the standard macro-drop tubing (10, 15, or 20 gtt/mL), minimizing accidental infusion of a large volume of IV fluid.

■ Intake and output records

- Accurate documentation of fluid intake, fluid losses (drainage, emesis, diarrhea, etc.) and urine output helps the physician to assess the child's changing IV fluid requirements.

Electronic devices require the nurses to use skills such as entering data, interpreting the information displayed on the device, responding to safety alerts, and demonstrating proficiency in the use of electronic device features. It is important for the nurse to remember that the electronic device is a tool and not a substitute for clinical expertise. Human errors may still occur with the use of any device. Therefore, having another nurse double-check the medication, the dose, and the infusion rates of pediatric medications always constitutes safe practice.

Weight-Based Dosing Used to Verify Safe Dose in Children

The use of weight to calculate a drug dose is known as ***weight-based dosing.*** The nurse uses the recommended weight-based dose information from the drug reference to verify that the ordered dose is a safe dose for the child. The calculation of safe dose including weight-based dosing calculation is covered in Chapter 17, Verifying Safe Dose.

Drug references provide extensive weight-based dosing information and identify the recommended weight-based dose specific to the clinical use, age range, weight, and route(s) of administration. Because weight is the primary factor in the calculation, it is important for the nurse to use the child's current weight in kilograms. Because manufacturers may list information in various formats, nurses must become familiar in gathering the correct weight-based dosing information specific to the clinical use or symptoms (Fig. 21-2).

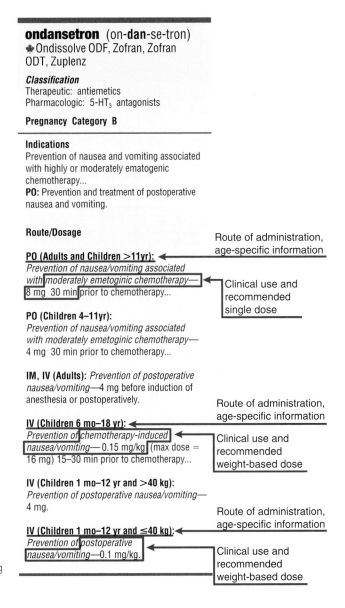

Figure 21-2. Information found in a drug reference.

The mathematical symbols ">" and "≥" ("greater than" and "greater than or equal to") and "<" and "≤" ("less than" and "less than or equal to") are seen in drug references and other sources. In communicating medical information, such as in writing and transcribing medications, the Institute of Safe Medication Practices recommends that these symbols not be used because they can be misinterpreted and lead to medication errors.

To work effectively with the recommended weight-based dose, the nurse must use critical thinking skills to:

- interpret and correlate the drug reference information with specific patient data.
- accurately calculate the recommended weight-based dose.
- make a clinical decision regarding the safety of the ordered dose.

These skills are applied prior to administering the drug to the child. Although this critical thinking process may be considered a routine part of working with drug reference information, the careful application of this process with children is fundamental to the administration of a safe dose. Figure 21-3 provides an example of how the nurse gathers and correlates specific patient data to the weight-based dosing information from a drug reference.

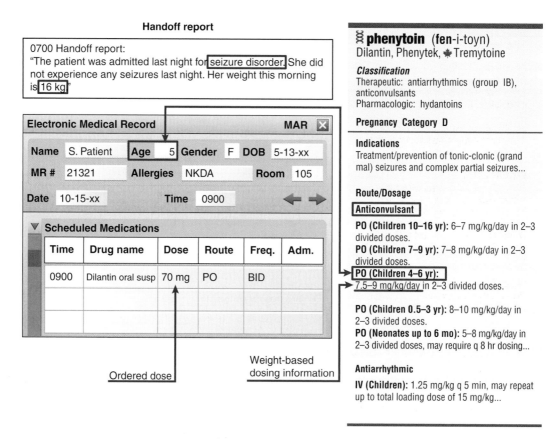

Figure 21-3. Correlation of specific patient data and drug reference information.

After calculating the recommended weight-based dose, the nurse will compare the recommended dose with the ordered dose and make a clinical decision regarding the safe dose. Weight-based dosing is common practice in the administration of medications to children. Accurate interpretation of weight-based dosing is critical in verifying safe dose.

APPLY LEARNED KNOWLEDGE 21-1

Use the drug reference information to determine whether the answer is True or False.

ondansetron (on-**dan**-se-tron)
✤ Ondissolve ODF, Zofran, Zofran
ODT, Zuplenz

Classification
Therapeutic: antiemetics
Pharmacologic: 5-HT$_3$ antagonists

Pregnancy Category B

Indications
Prevention of nausea and vomiting associated
with highly or moderately emetogenic
chemotherapy...
PO: Prevention and treatment of postoperative
nausea and vomiting.

Route/Dosage

PO (Adults and Children >11yr):
*Prevention of nausea/vomiting associated
with moderately emetoginic chemotherapy—*
8 mg 30 min prior to chemotherapy...

PO (Children 4–11yr):
*Prevention of nausea/vomiting associated
with moderately emetoginic chemotherapy—*
4 mg 30 min prior to chemotherapy...

IM, IV (Adults): *Prevention of postoperative
nausea/vomiting—*4 mg before induction of
anesthesia or postoperatively.

IV (Children 6 mo–18 yr):
*Prevention of chemotherapy-induced
nausea/vomiting—* 0.15 mg/kg (max dose =
16 mg) 15–30 min prior to chemotherapy...

IV (Children 1 mo–12 yr and >40 kg):
Prevention of postoperative nausea/vomiting—
4 mg.

IV (Children 1 mo–12 yr and ≤40 kg):
*Prevention of postoperative
nausea/vomiting—*0.1 mg/kg.

1. The PO dose of Zofran for adults and children older than age 11 years is the same.   True   False

2. The PO dose of Zofran for children 4 to 11 years is considered weight-based dosing.   True   False

3. The IV dose of Zofran 4 mg may be used for all children with nausea.   True   False

4. The IV weight-based dose of 0.1 mg/kg is recommended for children heavier   True   False
than 40 kg.

5. The weight-based dose of Zofran IV for children 6 months to 18 years is specific for   True   False
chemotherapy-induced nausea and vomiting.

Replacement Fluid Therapy

Children who are ill are more vulnerable to alterations in fluid and electrolyte balance. Water imbalances as well as electrolyte imbalances can occur more frequently and more rapidly in infants and children than in adults. A child who is unable to take fluids orally will require **maintenance IV fluids** to help restore fluid losses that occur from normal processes such as breathing, sweating, and urine and stool output. However, a child who has fever or is experiencing persistent diarrhea, vomiting, or loss of fluid through drainage such as nasogastric suction has an additional ongoing loss of fluids and electrolytes. A child experiencing these fluid losses will require additional intravenous fluids or **replacement IV fluid therapy.** The amount of replacement fluid is usually based on the amount of fluid loss that occurred over a specific period of time. The physician may order additional IV fluid that replaces the fluid loss **"mL for mL"** to maintain adequate hydration. For example, if the child had a fluid loss of 300 mL from nasogastric drainage on the 2300 to 0700 shift, the nurse will infuse 300 mL of replacement IV fluid during the 0700 to 1500 shift.

THE PHYSICIAN'S ORDER FOR REPLACEMENT FLUID THERAPY

It is important to recognize that replacement fluid therapy is ordered in addition to the maintenance intravenous fluids. When a child is on IV replacement fluid therapy, the physician's order will include:

- A primary IV order
- A replacement IV fluid order
- The maximum hourly IV rate (mL/hr)

Figure 21-4 provides an example of a replacement fluid IV order. Notice how the order indicates to replace the amount of drainage "mL for mL".

To implement the order "Replace NG drainage mL for mL q.8h with the replacement IV of 500 mL D^5/0.45 NS," the nurse must first know the amount of NG drainage from the previous 8 hours. The nurse may obtain this information from the end of shift handoff report or from the intake and output record. In clinical practice, the start of the replacement IV fluid therapy is a priority nursing intervention because it helps to restore the child's fluid balance. This is especially true if the child is continuing to lose fluid.

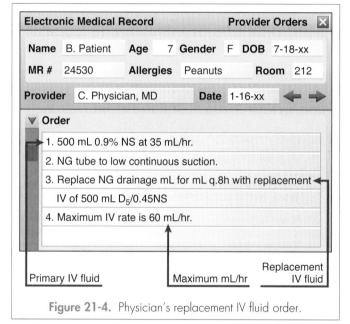

Figure 21-4. Physician's replacement IV fluid order.

After identifying the amount of fluid loss from the previous shift, the nurse needs to know the maximum IV rate (mL/hr) that the child may receive. It is important to keep in mind that the primary IV will continue to infuse simultaneously with the replacement IV for the length of time necessary to replace the fluid loss. During this time, the primary IV will infuse at the ordered rate, so the nurse needs to calculate how much additional IV fluid may be given so that the maximum mL/hr is not exceeded.

Using the physician's order in Figure 21-5, look at how the replacement IV fluid rate is calculated based on the ordered maximum mL/hr in the following example.

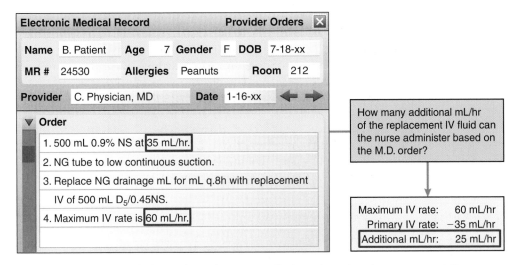

Figure 21-5. Calculating the replacement IV fluid rate based on the maximum mL/hr.

To prevent exceeding the maximum mL/hr as ordered, the nurse will infuse the replacement IV fluid at 25 mL/hr. To help in the planning of care, administration of other medications, and reporting patient status, it is necessary for the nurse to know how long it will take to infuse the replacement IV fluid and at what time it will be completed. A thorough explanation of calculating infusion time and completion time is found in Chapter 15, Calculating Infusion and Completion Time. However, the following example shows how infusion and completion time is calculated for the replacement IV fluid (Fig. 21-6).

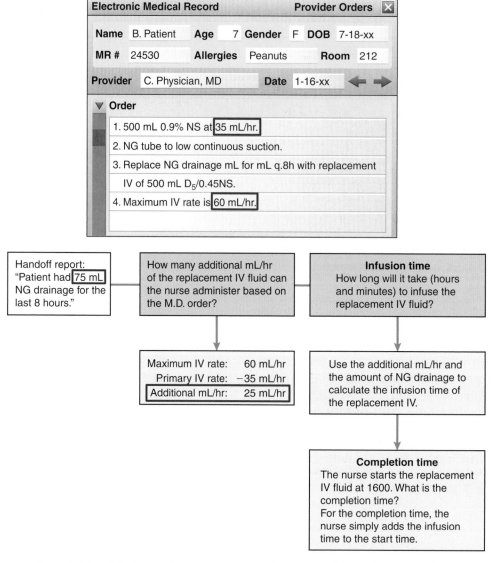

Figure 21-6. Calculating infusion time and completion time of the replacement IV fluid.

In dimensional analysis, the set up begins with the amount of drainage rather than the ordered amount, and the replacement IV fluid rate (mL/hr) is the conversion factor.

The formula method $\dfrac{D}{H} \times Q = x$ cannot be used for fluid replacement problems. Instead, the formula for infusion time can be used:

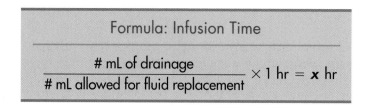

Formula: Infusion Time

$$\frac{\# \text{ mL of drainage}}{\# \text{ mL allowed for fluid replacement}} \times 1 \text{ hr} = \textbf{x} \text{ hr}$$

Linear Ratio & Proportion

Known :: Unknown

Infusion Time

25 mL : 1 hr :: 75 mL : x hr

$$25x = 75$$

$$\frac{25x}{25} = \frac{75}{25}$$

$$x = 3 \text{ hr}$$

Completion Time

$$
\begin{array}{r}
1600 \\
+\ 0300 \\
\hline
1900
\end{array}
$$

Dimensional Analysis

$$\frac{\text{Drainage}}{\text{Amount}} \times \frac{\text{Conversion}}{\text{Factor}} = \frac{\text{Desired}}{\text{Amount}}$$

Infusion Time

$$\frac{75 \text{ mL}}{1} \times \frac{1 \text{ hr}}{25 \text{ mL}} = x \text{ hr}$$

$$\frac{75 \times 1 \text{ hr}}{1 \times 25} = \frac{75}{25} = 3 \text{ hr}$$

Completion Time

$$
\begin{array}{r}
1600 \\
+\ 0300 \\
\hline
1900
\end{array}
$$

Fractional Ratio & Proportion

Known = Unknown

Infusion Time

$$\frac{25 \text{ mL}}{1 \text{ hr}} \quad \frac{75 \text{ mL}}{x \text{ hr}}$$

$$25x = 1 \times 75$$

$$\frac{25x}{25} = \frac{75}{25}$$

$$x = 3 \text{ hr}$$

Completion Time

$$
\begin{array}{r}
1600 \\
+\ 0300 \\
\hline
1900
\end{array}
$$

Formula: Infusion Time

$$\frac{\# \text{mL of drainage}}{\# \text{mL allowed for fluid replacement}} \times 1 \text{ hr} = x \text{ hr}$$

$$\frac{75 \text{ mL}}{25 \text{ mL}} \times 1 \text{ hr} = x \text{ hr}$$

$$\frac{3}{1} \times 1 \text{ hr} = x \text{ hr}$$

$$x = 3 \text{ hr}$$

Completion Time

$$
\begin{array}{r}
1600 \\
+\ 0300 \\
\hline
1900
\end{array}
$$

Based on the 75 mL of output and the replacement IV infusing at 25 mL/hr, the infusion time is 3 hours. The completion time of 1900 was calculated using the initial start time of 1600 for the replacement IV fluid and adding the infusion time of 3 hours. The nurse can monitor the hourly rate and plan on discontinuing or stopping the replacement IV fluid at 1900.

APPLY LEARNED KNOWLEDGE 21-2

Use the physician's orders and the handoff report to answer the following questions.

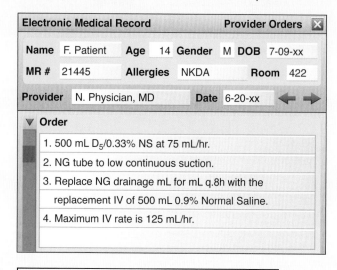

Electronic Medical Record		Provider Orders ⊠
Name F. Patient	**Age** 14 **Gender** M **DOB** 7-09-xx	
MR # 21445	**Allergies** NKDA	**Room** 422
Provider N. Physician, MD	**Date** 6-20-xx ← →	

▼ Order

1. 500 mL D$_5$/0.33% NS at 75 mL/hr.
2. NG tube to low continuous suction.
3. Replace NG drainage mL for mL q.8h with the
   replacement IV of 500 mL 0.9% Normal Saline.
4. Maximum IV rate is 125 mL/hr.

Handoff report:
"Patient had 225 mL NG drainage for the last 8 hours."

1. Identify the mL/hr of the primary IV fluid. _____

2. Identify the replacement IV fluid. _____

3. Calculate the additional mL/hr allowed for the replacement IV fluid. _____

4. How many mL will the nurse need to replace for the previous 8 hours? _____

5. What is the infusion time for the replacement IV fluid? _____

CLINICAL REASONING 21-1

At 0800, the nurse admits a 10-year-old child who is experiencing symptoms of asthma. The physician orders medications, including prednisone 5 mg PO at 0900, 1500, 2100, 0300. The drug reference includes the following information:

> *PO (Children): Asthma exacerbation – 1 mg/kg q.6hr for 48 hr, then 1 to 2 mg/kg/day (maximum 60 mg/day) in divided doses twice daily.*

> *In preparing to administer the 0900 dose of medication, which action by the nurse should be done first?*

> *A. Verify safe dose after the initial administration of prednisone 5 mg.*
> *B. Clarify the frequency of administration with the physician.*
> *C. Question the frequency of administration.*
> *D. Obtain the current weight of the child.*

Care of the pediatric patient necessitates an understanding of the specific needs associated with the developmental stage of the child. When administering medications to children, the nurse must use critical thinking skills to correlate and interpret pertinent patient data with the information found in the drug reference. Vigilance in monitoring the administration of IV fluids is required to promote safe practice and prevent patient harm.

Developing Competency

Use the drug reference information for diphenhydramine (Benadryl) to answer questions 1 through 6.

diphenhydrAMINE (oral, parenteral)
(dye-fen-**hye**-dra-meen)

Banophen, Benadryl Dye-Free Allergy, Benadryl Allergy, Benadryl, ✳Benylin, ✳Calmex, Compoz, Compoz Nighttime Sleep Aid, Nytol, Scot-Tussin Allergy DM, Siladril, Silphen, Sleep-Eze 3, Sleepwell 2-night, Sominex, Snooze Fast, Sominex, Tusstat, Twilite, Unisom Nighttime Sleep-Aid

Classification
Therapeutic: allergy, cold, and cough remedies, antihistamines, antitussives

Pregnancy Category B

Indications
Relief of allergic symptoms...Mild nighttime sedation. Prevention of motion sickness...

Route/Dosage

PO (Adults and Children >12yr):
Antihistamine/antiemetic/antivertiginic—25–50 mg q 4-6 hr, not to exceed 300 mg/day. *Antitussive*—25 mg q 4 hr as needed, not to exceed 150 mg/day. *Antidyskinetic*—25-50 mg q 4 hr (not to exceed 400 mg/day). *Sedative/hypnotic*—50 mg 20–30 min before bedtime.

PO (Children 6–12yr):
Antihistamine/antiemetic/antivertiginic—12.5–25 mg q 4-6 hr (not exceed 150 mg/day). *Antidyskinetic*—1–1.5 mg/kg q 6–8 hr as needed (not to exceed 300 mg/day). *Antitussive*—12.5 mg q 4 hr (not to exceed 75 mg/day). *Sedative/hypnotic*—1 mg/kg/dose 20–30 min before bedtime (not to exceed 50 mg).

PO (Children 2–6yr):
Antihistamine/antiemetic/antivertiginic—6.25–12.5 mg q 4–6 hr...(not to exceed 37.5 mg/day)...*Antitussive*—6.25 mg q 4 hr (not to exceed 37.5 mg/24 hr). *Sedative/hypnotic*—1 mg/kg/dose 20–30 min before bedtime (not to exceed 50 mg).

IM, IV (Adults): 25–50 mg q 4 hr as needed (may need up to 100 mg dose, not to exceed 400 mg/day).

IM, IV (Children): 1.25 mg/kg (37.5 mg/m^2) 4 times daily (not to exceed 300 mg/day).

1. For children under 12 years of age, the PO dose of Benadryl for antiemetic use must be calculated based on the weight of the child.

True   False

2. For children under 12 years of age, the PO dose of Benadryl for sedative use must be calculated based on the weight of the child.
True   False

3. An 8-year-old child may receive a total of 6 doses of 6.25 mg Benadryl PO for antitussive use in a day.
True   False

4. The recommended weight-based dose for children is the same for the IM and IV routes of administration.
True   False

5. For children greater than age 12 years, the PO antiemetic dosage range is 25 to 50 mg.
True   False

6. The PO antitussive maximum dose for children greater than age 12 years is 300 mg/day.
True   False

Use the drug reference information for clonidine to answer questions 7 through 10.

cloNIDine (klon-i-deen)
Catapres, Catapres-TTS, ✹Dixarit, Duraclon, Kapvay

Classification
Therapeutic: antihypertensives
Pharmacologic: adrenergics (centrally acting)

Pregnancy Category C

Indications

PO, Transdermal: Mild to moderate hypertension...

Route/Dosage

PO (Adults and Adolescents ≥12 yr): *Hypertension (immediate release)*—100 mcg (0.1 mg) BID, ↑ by 100-200 mcg (0.1–0.2 mg)/day q 2–4 days...

PO (Geriatric Patients): *Hypertension (immediate release)*—100 mcg (0.1 mg) at bedtime initially, ↑ as needed.

PO (Children): *Hypertension (immediate release)*—Initial 5–10 mcg/kg/day divided BID-TID, then ↑ gradually to 5–25 mcg/kg/day in divided doses q 6 hr; maximum dose: 0.9 mg/day. *ADHD (Kapvay-extended release) (children >6yr)* 0.1 mg once daily at bedtime; after 1 wk, ↑ dose to 0.1 mg in AM and at bedtime; after 1 wk, ↑ dose to 0.1 mg in AM and 0.2 mg at bedtime; after 1 wk, ↑ dose to 0.2 mg in AM and at bedtime (max dose = 0.4 mg/day)...*Neuropathic pain (immediate release)*—2 mcg/kg/dose q 4–6 hr then ↑ gradually over days up to 4 mcg/kg/dose q 4–6 hr.

7. The initial PO dose of cloNIDine for children with hypertension is 5 to 25 mcg/kg/day in divided doses.
True   False

8. The maximum PO dose of cloNIDine for children with hypertension is 0.9 mg/day.
True   False

9. The maximum PO dose for children with ADHD is 0.4 mg/day.
True   False

10. The PO dose for children with neuropathic pain is based on weight-based dosing.
True   False

Use the following physician's order to answer questions 11 through 15.

Electronic Medical Record   **Provider Orders** ☒

Name T. Patient   **Age** 12 **Gender** F **DOB** 5-23-xx

MR # 25672   **Allergies** NKDA   **Room** 323

Provider F. Physician, MD   **Date** 10-21-xx ⬅ ➡

▼ **Order**

1. 500 mL 0.9% NS at 50 mL/hr.

2. NG tube to low continuous suction.

3. Replace NG drainage mL for mL q.8h with
   replacement IV of 500 mL D_5/0.45NS.

4. Maximum IV rate is 100 mL/hr.

Handoff report:
"Patient had 150 mL NG drainage for the last 8 hours."

11. Identify the mL/hr of the primary IV fluid. _____

12. Identify the replacement IV fluid. _____

13. Calculate the additional mL/hr allowed for the replacement IV fluid. _____

14. How many mL will the nurse need to replace from the previous 8 hours? _____

15. What is the infusion time for the replacement IV fluid? _____

Use the following physician's order to answer questions 16 through 20.

Electronic Medical Record   **Provider Orders** ☒

Name R. Patient   **Age** 15 **Gender** M **DOB** 2-11-xx

MR # 301223   **Allergies** NKDA   **Room** 403

Provider S. Physician, MD   **Date** 5-09-xx ⬅ ➡

▼ **Order**

1. 500 mL 0.9% NS at 75 mL/hr.

2. NG tube to low continuous suction.

3. Replace NG drainage mL for mL q.8h with
   replacement IV of 500 mL D_5/0.45NS.

4. Maximum IV rate is 125 mL/hr.

Handoff report:
"Patient had 300 mL NG drainage for the last 8 hours."

16. Identify the mL/hr of the primary IV fluid. _____

17. Identify the primary IV fluid. _____

18. Calculate the additional mL/hr allowed for the replacement IV fluid. _____

19. What is the infusion time for the replacement IV fluid? _____

20. What is the completion time of the replacement IV if the nurse starts the replacement IV fluid at 1500?
_____

CHAPTER 22

Considerations for the Older Adult Population

LEARNING OUTCOMES

Identify factors that increase the older adult's risk for medication-related problems.

Implement a vigilant process for the administration of medications to the older adult.

Calculate the dilution of formula tube feedings.

The growing **geriatric** population presents a unique challenge for healthcare professionals to provide individualized care that will promote a better quality of life. As individuals get older, age-related changes lead to the development of acute and chronic conditions (i.e., heart disease, diabetes mellitus, hypertension, respiratory problems) and require a variety of medications to control or to alleviate the symptoms. It is not uncommon for the older adult with a chronic condition to take five or more drugs per day.

The benefits of drug therapy are numerous. However, age-related changes contribute to a decline in the body's ability to effectively absorb, metabolize, distribute, and excrete drugs, thereby increasing the older adult's risk for medication-related problems. As with all medications, safety involves the application of the Six Rights of Medication Administration, but in caring for the older adult, the nurse needs to be critically vigilant of the following factors:

- **Polypharmacy:** polypharmacy refers to the use of multiple medications, including prescription medications, over-the-counter medications, vitamins, and herbal preparations. The older adult frequently takes several prescription and nonprescription drugs daily.

- **Drug-drug interactions:** the combination of drugs (prescription and nonprescription drugs) may affect a drug's action, so that the desired effects may be increased, decreased, or chemically altered. Polypharmacy contributes to an increased risk for drug-drug interactions

- **Drug-nutrient/drug-natural product interactions:** several nutrients and natural products are known to interfere with the action of certain drugs. The effect on the drug may lead to an increase or a decrease in the absorption, metabolism, distribution, or excretion of the drug.

- **Potentially inappropriate medications (PIMs):** In 2012, the American Geriatrics Society in conjunction with a panel of experts produced a list of drugs that may be inappropriate for use in the older adult because of the age-related changes that affect the drug's effectiveness and increase its potential for toxicity. This list of potentially inappropriate medications (PIMs), known as the Beers list, brings attention to drugs that should be used with caution or avoided in the older adult (Table 22-1). Drug references may identify a PIM by including wording such as "Appears on Beers list" or "On Beers list" as part of the drug information. Some PIMs may also be on the High Alert Medications list published by the Institute for Safe Medication Practices (ISMP). Go to the Safe Dosage Resources on DavisPlus for the 2012 PIM list by the American Geriatrics Society and the ISMP High Alert Medications list.

Table 22-1. Potentially Inappropriate Medications for the Older Adult

GENERIC NAME	TRADE NAME
carisoprodol	Soma
diazepam	Valium
flurazepam	Dalmane
hydroxyzine	Vistaril, Atarax
ketorolac	Toradol
lorazepam	Ativan
meperidine	Demerol
meprobamate	Equagesic
secobarbital	Seconal

For a complete listing, see the 2012 *American Geriatrics Society Updated Beers Criteria for Potentially Inappropriate Medication use in Older Adults* at http://www.americangeriatrics.org/files/documents/beers/PrintableBeers PocketCard.pdf

■ **Adverse drug reaction (ADR):** an ADR is an unintended and harmful response to a drug.

■ **Adverse drug event (ADE):** an ADE refers to injury that occurs from a drug. This may be a result of the adverse drug reaction, a medication error, or effects from a drug that lead to injury. The injury may include physical harm, mental harm, or loss of function.

Careful consideration of these factors in the administration of medications prompts the nurse to do a more in-depth research of the pharmacological interactions of drugs and to maintain a comprehensive approach in reviewing the drug therapy of the older adult.

 It is recommended by the American Geriatrics Society, as well as other geriatric-focused healthcare organizations, that drugs on the Beers list be used with caution in the older adult. The physician determines the therapeutic benefits and risks in prescribing a PIM to an older adult based on the older adult's medical condition and diagnosis. The nurse can assist the older adult and the physician by purposefully monitoring for and reporting early signs and symptoms that may indicate an adverse drug reaction.

Medication Administration and the Older Adult

The medication order for the older adult is written the same as any drug order prescribed by the physician. Solving for the dosage to administer can be done using one of the methods of calculation (Fig. 22-1).

M.D. order:

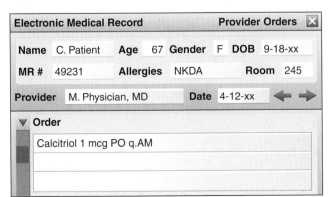

Pharmacy sends:

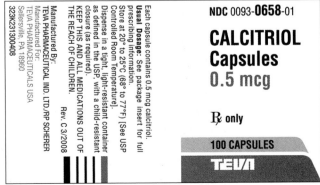

Figure 22-1. Drug order for an older adult.

How many capsules will the nurse administer?

Linear Ratio & Proportion

Known   ::   Unknown

$$0.5 \text{ mcg} : 1 \text{ cap} :: 1 \text{ mcg} : x \text{ cap}$$

$$0.5x = 1$$

$$\frac{0.5x}{0.5} = \frac{1}{0.5}$$

$$x = 2 \text{ cap}$$

Dimensional Analysis

$$\frac{\text{Ordered}}{\text{Amount}} \times \frac{\text{Dosage}}{\text{Strength}} = \frac{\text{Desired}}{\text{Amount}}$$

$$\frac{1 \text{ mcg}}{1} \times \frac{1 \text{ cap}}{0.5 \text{ mcg}} = x \text{ cap}$$

$$\frac{1 \times 1 \text{ cap}}{1 \times 0.5} = \frac{1}{0.5} = 2 \text{ cap}$$

Fractional Ratio & Proportion

Known   ::   Unknown

$$\frac{0.5 \text{ mcg}}{1 \text{ cap}} \quad \frac{1 \text{ mcg}}{x \text{ cap}}$$

$$0.5x = 1$$

$$\frac{0.5x}{0.5} = \frac{1}{0.5}$$

$$x = 2 \text{ cap}$$

Formula Method

$$\frac{D}{H} \times Q = x$$

$$\frac{1 \text{ mcg}}{0.5 \text{ mcg}} \times 1 \text{ cap} = x \text{ cap}$$

$$2 \times 1 \text{ cap} = 2 \text{ cap}$$

The nurse would administer 2 capsules.

In addition to calculating the drug dosage, medication administration in the older adult warrants a broader discussion. Safe medication administration includes the use of critical thinking to assist in correlating the purpose and use of the drug, assessing and monitoring for side effects and desired outcomes, and clear, thorough patient education. In the administration of medication to the older adult, the nurse must also be mindful of the factors (polypharmacy, drug-drug interactions, etc.) that place the older adult at a high risk.

The Vigilant Process for Medication Administration

The authors recommend the application of a "Vigilant Process" or a systematic step-by-step approach for addressing the factors associated with medication use in the older adult. The Vigilant Process presents a template that guides the nurse to focus on geriatric considerations related to the use of a specific drug. The Vigilant Process includes a three-step approach:

Step 1: Gathering information about the drug with a focus on the older adult.

Step 2: Correlation of data, including assessing, monitoring, and evaluating for desired and undesired effects of the drug.

Step 3: Teaching relevant drug information to the older adult and family.

STEP 1 OF THE VIGILANT PROCESS

Drug references and reliable Internet resources provide valuable information pertinent to drug therapy. When gathering information, the nurse should particularly consider information that has implications for the older adult, such as:

- Usual dose for the older adult vs. ordered dose
- Indications for use with correlation of drug to disease process or condition
- Adverse reactions/side effects/precautions specific for the older adult
- Pharmacological drug class: drug-drug interactions; drug-nutrient/drug-natural products interactions
- IV medications with special instructions for the older adult related to
  - dilution of IV medications
  - rate of administration of IV drugs

Figure 22-2 shows pertinent drug information for lorazepam PO from a drug reference.

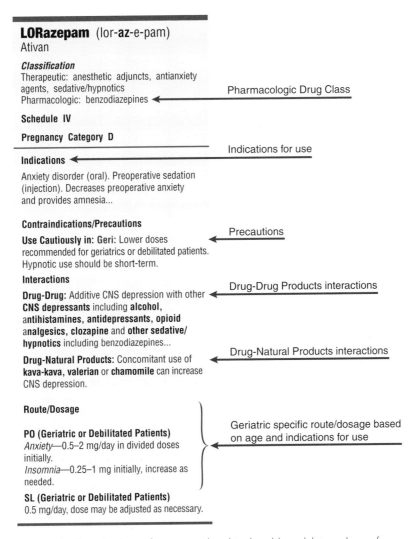

Figure 22-2. Sample drug information related to the older adult in a drug reference.

 Because new research findings are continuously being published, it is important for the nurse to use supplemental drug references, seek current up-to-date information, and ensure implementation of best practices.

In applying Step 1 of the Vigilant Process, the nurse identifies specific information related to the ordered drug and then proceeds to use the questions listed in "Older Adult Considerations" column as a guide to help focus on pertinent drug information. Table 22-2 shows the template for Step 1 of the Vigilant Process.

Table 22-2. Template: Step 1: Information Gathering With Older Adult Considerations

ORDERED DRUG	GUIDE FOR DRUG INFORMATION GATHERING AND THE OLDER ADULT
Name:	• Is ordered dose within the usual dose?
	• Is there a potential for drug-drug/drug–natural product interaction?
Drug Class:	• Why is this drug ordered for older adults?
PIM?	• What is the desired patient outcome after the administration of this drug?
High Alert?	• Any current drug research recommendations?

 Older adults may be more sensitive to the effects of a drug, so a lower than the usual dose of a drug may be prescribed.

STEP 2 OF THE VIGILANT PROCESS

After the nurse completes Step 1 of the Vigilant Process, the nurse researches the recommended follow-up assessment information and purposefully assesses, monitors, and evaluates for the effects of the drug. This step also includes the correlation of acute and chronic illnesses present in the older adult, as well as prescriptions and over-the-counter medications that may alter or enhance the drug-drug interactions. Table 22-3 presents the template for Step 2 of the Vigilant Process.

Table 22-3. Template: Step 2: Correlating Data for Assessing, Monitoring, and Evalutating for Desired and Undesired Drug Effects

DRUG REFERENCE RECOMMENDATIONS FOR ASSESSING/MONITORING/EVALUATING	GUIDE TO CORRELATING DATA
Assessment considerations: • Geri:	• What specific signs and symptoms will the nurse assess and monitor? When will the effects of the drug be seen?
Monitor: • Pertinent lab tests • Drug effects	• What lab tests need to be monitored? • What physical signs/symptoms indicate undesired effects of the drug? • What nursing actions will the nurse implement to promote patient safety while on this drug?
Evaluation: • Drug-drug interactions	• What prescription and over-the-counter medications may enhance or alter the therapeutic effects of this drug?

STEP 3 OF THE VIGILANT PROCESS

Patient teaching is a critical part of all nurse-patient interactions. By addressing the factors that may increase the risk for adverse drug reactions, Step 3 of the Vigilant Process broadens the scope of teaching to include a greater understanding of the patient's drug therapy and its relationship to the disease process, interactions with other drugs, foods, and other natural products (Table 22-4).

Table 22-4. Template: Step 3: Teaching Relevant Drug Information to the Older Adult and Family

DRUG REFERENCE INFORMATION FOR TEACHING THE OLDER ADULTS/FAMILY TEACHING	ASSESSMENT FOR PATIENT TEACHING—FOCUS ON THE SPECIFIC NEEDS OF THE OLDER ADULT
Polypharmacy considerations: • Drug-drug • Drug-nutrition • Drug–natural products	• What prescription drugs are you currently taking? • Do you take any vitamin or herbal supplements or over-the-counter drugs? • Do you drink/eat (check for specific drug-food interactions). Inquire about cultural foods that may contribute to drug-food interactions.
Teaching: • Safety considerations related to drug effects • Follow-up	• This drug may cause you to . . . • This drug is best taken (i.e., with meals, at bedtime).

Although the three-step Vigilant Process may be used in the administration of medications to all patients, it is of particular importance in patients who take multiple medications (polypharmacy).

APPLY LEARNED KNOWLEDGE 22-1

Use the physician's orders and a drug reference or the 2012 American Geriatrics Society Beers Criteria for Potentially Inappropriate Medication Use in Older Adults to answer the questions.

1.
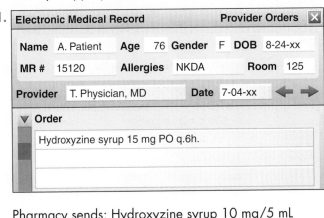

Pharmacy sends: Hydroxyzine syrup 10 mg/5 mL

(A) The nurse will administer _____

(B) Is hydroxyzine considered a PIM drug?   ☐ Yes   ☐ No

Continued

APPLY LEARNED KNOWLEDGE 22-1—cont'd

2.

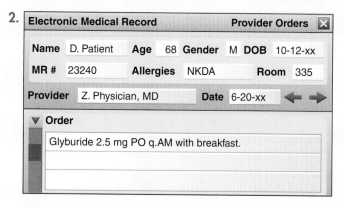

Electronic Medical Record			Provider Orders		☒
Name D. Patient	**Age** 68	**Gender** M	**DOB** 10-12-xx		
MR # 23240	**Allergies** NKDA		**Room** 335		
Provider Z. Physician, MD		**Date** 6-20-xx	← →		

▼ **Order**

Glyburide 2.5 mg PO q.AM with breakfast.

Pharmacy sends: Glyburide 1.25 mg tablets
(A) The nurse will administer _____
(B) Is glyburide considered a PIM drug? ☐ Yes ☐ No

3.

Electronic Medical Record			Provider Orders		☒
Name M. Patient	**Age** 69	**Gender** M	**DOB** 5-15-xx		
MR # 54480	**Allergies** NKDA		**Room** 112		
Provider M. Physician, MD		**Date** 4-28-xx	← →		

▼ **Order**

Meperidine 20 mg IM STAT

Available: Meperidine 25 mg/1 mL
(A) The nurse will administer _____
(B) Is meperidine considered a PIM drug? ☐ Yes ☐ No

4.

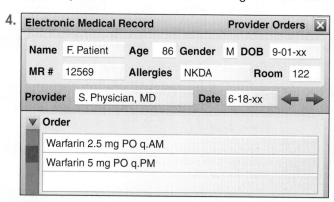

Electronic Medical Record			Provider Orders		☒
Name F. Patient	**Age** 86	**Gender** M	**DOB** 9-01-xx		
MR # 12569	**Allergies** NKDA		**Room** 122		
Provider S. Physician, MD		**Date** 6-18-xx	← →		

▼ **Order**

Warfarin 2.5 mg PO q.AM

Warfarin 5 mg PO q.PM

Pharmacy sends: Warfarin 5 mg scored tablets.
(A) For the AM dose, the nurse will administer: _____

APPLY LEARNED KNOWLEDGE 22-1—cont'd

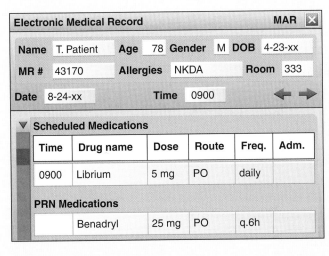

HIGH ALERT

℀ warfarin (war-fa-rin)
Coumadin, Jantoven

Classification
Therapeutic: anticoagulants
Pharmacologic: coumarins

Pregnancy Category X

Indications

Drug-Natural Products:
St. John's wort decreases effect. Increased bleeding risk with anise, arnica, chamomile, clove, dong quai, fenugreek, feverfew, garlic, ginger, ginkgo biloba, Panax ginseng, licorice, and others.

Drug-Food:
Ingestion of large quantities of foods high in vitamin K content...may antagonize the anticoagulant effect of warfarin.

(B) Use the drug reference above to list three herbal supplements that may increase the effects of warfarin. _____

5. The nurse is reviewing the MAR of the older adult patient experiencing anxiety. Select all statements that are correct.

HIGH ALERT

chlordiazePOXIDE
(klor-dye-az-e-**pox**-ide)
~~Libritabs~~, Librium

Classification
Therapeutic: antianxiety agents, sedative/hypnotics
Pharmacologic: benzodiazepines

Schedule IV

Pregnancy Category D

Use Cautiously in: ...Geri: Long-acting benzodiazepines cause prolonged sedation in the elderly. Appears on Beers list and is associated with increased risk of falls (decrease dose required or consider short-acting benzodiazepine); Debilitated patients (initial dose reduction required).

Route/Dosage

PO (Geriatric or Debilitated Patients):
Anxiety—5 mg 2–4 times daily initially, increase as needed.

Electronic Medical Record | **MAR** ☒

| Name | T. Patient | Age | 78 | Gender | M | DOB | 4-23-xx |

| MR # | 43170 | Allergies | NKDA | | Room | 333 |

| Date | 8-24-xx | | Time | 0900 | ← → |

▼ Scheduled Medications

Time	Drug name	Dose	Route	Freq.	Adm.
0900	Librium	5 mg	PO	daily	

PRN Medications

| | Benadryl | 25 mg | PO | q.6h | |

a. Benadryl is a PIM drug.

b. The ordered dose of Librium is less than the usual dose stated in the drug reference.

c. Potential for side effect or adverse drug reaction is decreased because the Librium dose is a lower than usual dose.

Enteral Nutrition and Formula Tube Feedings

The nurse will frequently care for older adults who are unable to eat by mouth due to conditions such as malnutrition and stroke. When a patient is unable to take in oral nutrition, the physician may order the administration of **enteral nutrition.** Enteral nutrition is a method of providing nutrients into the gastrointestinal system through a feeding tube.

There are several types of feeding tubes that are used to administer enteral nutrition (Table 22-5). Feeding tubes are available in various lengths and diameters. The diameter or opening of a tube is measured in French units (each French unit is equal to 0.33 mm) and is abbreviated "Fr." The number identified on the tube, for example, 22 Fr, indicates the size of the diameter of the tube. The bigger the number, the greater is the diameter of the tube. Feeding tubes identified as large bore have an opening with a diameter generally 12 Fr or larger. Feeding tubes identified as small bore have an opening with a diameter of less than 12 Fr.

Table 22-5. Common Enteral Feeding Tubes

ENTERAL FEEDING TUBE	DESCRIPTION	PLACEMENT
NG (nasogastric) tube	An NG tube is inserted through one of the nostrils, down the nasopharynx and the esophagus, and into the stomach. **Purpose:** NG tubes are used for short-term feeding in patients who have intact gag and cough reflexes, and adequate gastric emptying.	
PEG (percutaneous endoscopic gastrostomy) tube **G-tube (gastrostomy tube)**	A PEG or G-tube is inserted through a small surgical incision in the abdominal wall, directly into the stomach. **Purpose:** These feeding tubes are used for the administration of long-term nutrition (usually more than 6 to 8 weeks).	
J-tube (jejunostomy tube)	A J-tube is inserted through a small surgical incision in the abdominal wall directly into the jejunum. **Purpose:** A J-tube is used for the administration of long-term nutrition (usually more than 6 to 8 weeks) in patients who require feeding into the small intestine.	

Commercially Prepared Formulas

Once the feeding tube has been inserted, the physician will order a commercially prepared formula that meets the nutritional needs of the patient. There are many types of commercially prepared formulas. Each type is made to provide a certain number of calories and nutrients, and some formulas are made for disease-specific conditions.

Figure 22-3 gives an example of a commercially prepared formula. In reading the Jevity 1.2 Cal formula label, it is important not to confuse the number of calories listed on the label with the volume (mL) of formula in the container. Depending on the system of fluid measure used (U.S. fluid ounce, imperial fluid ounce, etc.) and the equivalent measurements, the volume in an ounce will vary slightly.

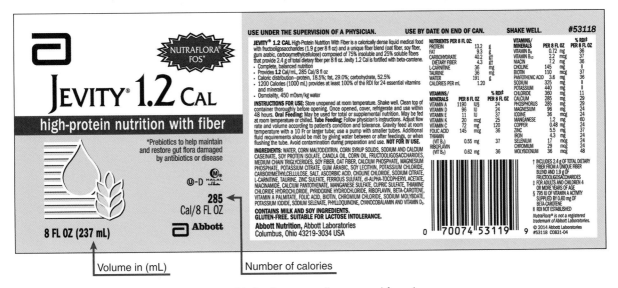

Figure 22-3. Commercially prepared formula.

Commercially prepared formula is also available in prefilled 1,000 mL ready-to-hang containers (Fig. 22-4). These prefilled containers are used for the administration of continuous tube feedings and are administered through an enteral feeding pump. The nurse must change the prefilled ready-to-hang container and tubing according to manufacturer guidelines and healthcare facility protocol.

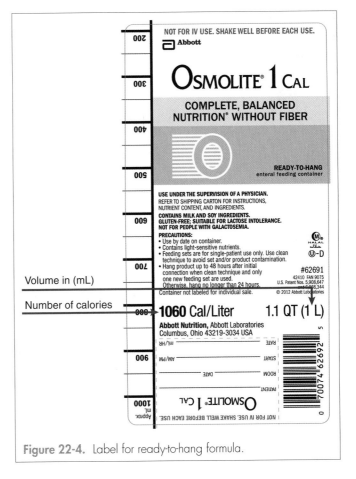

Figure 22-4. Label for ready-to-hang formula.

The Physician's Order for a Tube Feeding

The physician's order provides the necessary information for the administration of enteral nutrition to the patient. To minimize errors in the interpretation and administration of enteral nutrition, the American Society for Parenteral and Enteral Nutrition (A.S.P.E.N.), a professional society of physicians, nurses, dietitians, pharmacists, and allied health professionals recommend that the enteral nutrition order include the following (Fig. 22-5):

■ Patient identifier information

■ Formula type

■ Delivery device (enteral tube, i.e., NG, PEG, J-tube)

■ Rate and administration method (bolus, gravity, enteral feeding pump, etc.)

The nurse uses this information to verify and double-check the enteral nutrition order.

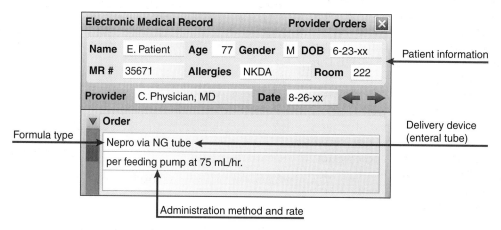

Figure 22-5. Components of an enteral nutrition order.

Methods of Administering Formula Tube Feedings

The method for the administration of the tube feeding will be ordered by the physician. The administration method will depend on the feeding tube placement (stomach, jejunum, etc.), the size of the feeding tube, and the type of enteral formula ordered for the patient. Common methods for the administration of the tube feeding include the following:

■ *Intermittent:* these feedings are given at specific rates and times throughout the day and include:

• bolus administration using a 50 or 60 mL syringe to deliver the volume of formula over 15 to 20 minutes

• gravity administration using a feeding tube bag to deliver the volume of formula over 30 to 60 minutes.

■ *Continuous:* the ordered mL/hr of formula are continuously given through an enteral feeding pump

■ *Cyclic:* this type of feeding is similar to the administration of a continuous feeding but the formula is administered during a defined period of time, such as overnight.

Strength of the Formula

The strength of the formula is based on the patient's physiological condition and nutritional needs.

Formula feedings are generally ordered to be given either:

■ Full-strength (recommended)

■ Diluted to a lesser strength

Regardless of the strength of the formula ordered, the nurse must always verify the type and strength of formula, rate of administration, enteral tube and site, and patency of the feeding tube prior to the administration of the formula feeding.

FULL-STRENGTH FORMULA TUBE FEEDING

When a formula is ordered full strength, the nurse administers the volume of formula according to the method and frequency of administration ordered by the physician. The use of full strength formula is recommended to ensure the patient receives the required nutrients and calories.

DILUTION OF A FORMULA TUBE FEEDING

Dilution of a formula tube feeding is not common practice because the mixing and handling of the formula increase the risk of infection. However, an occasional order for the dilution of a tube feeding may still be encountered. When the formula is ordered to be diluted, the physician will generally order the strength of the formula in a fractional format. Look at the following physician's order (Fig. 22-6).

To prepare the ordered strength of the formula, the nurse must first understand what the fraction means. The numerator and denominator of the fraction each have a separate meaning:

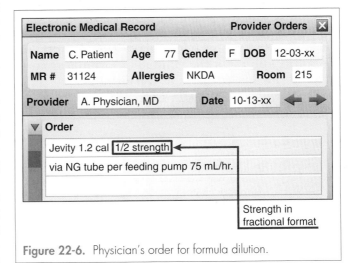

Figure 22-6. Physician's order for formula dilution.

■ The numerator refers to the part of the mixture that is the commercial formula.

■ The denominator refers to the total number of parts (water + formula) or the volume in the feeding bag.

Example:

DILUTED FORMULA	REPRESENTS:
Ordered strength:	
$\frac{1}{2}$	$\frac{1}{}$ = the part of the mixture that is the commercial formula
	$\frac{}{2}$ = the total number of parts: 1 part is the formula
	$\frac{1}{}$ part is the water
	$\frac{}{2}$ parts together make up the volume in the feeding bag
Ordered strength:	
$\frac{1}{3}$	$\frac{1}{}$ = the part of the mixture that is the commercial formula
	$\frac{}{3}$ = the total number of parts: 1 part is the formula
	$\frac{2}{}$ parts are the water
	$\frac{}{3}$ parts together make up the volume in the feeding bag
Ordered strength:	
$\frac{3}{4}$	$\frac{3}{}$ = the part of the mixture that is the commercial formula
	$\frac{}{4}$ = the total number of parts: 3 parts are the formula
	$\frac{1}{}$ part is the water
	$\frac{}{4}$ parts together make up the volume in the feeding bag

CALCULATING THE VOLUME OF WATER TO ADD TO MAKE A DILUTE TUBE FEEDING

When the nurse has an order to dilute the tube feeding, the question that needs to be answered is, "How much water needs to be added to make the ordered strength?" This calculation may be done using a specific formula or using the linear or fractional ratio and proportion methods. Dimensional analysis and the formula $\dfrac{D}{H} \times Q = x$ cannot be used to solve for the dilution of the formula tube feeding.

Formula for Dilution of a Tube Feeding

In working with the formula for dilution of a tube feeding, the nurse uses the volume (mL) of formula in the can and the ordered strength to set up and solve for the total volume in the feeding bag (water + formula). Once the total volume in the feeding bag is calculated, the nurse subtracts the volume of formula from the total volume in the feeding bag to arrive at the answer. Look at the formula:

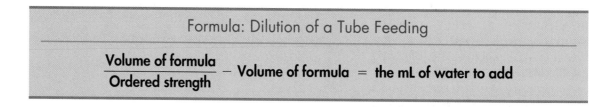

Formula: Dilution of a Tube Feeding

$$\frac{\text{Volume of formula}}{\text{Ordered strength}} - \text{Volume of formula} = \text{the mL of water to add}$$

The formula for dilution of the tube feeding provides a convenient method for calculating the number of mL of water to add to dilute the tube feeding. Example #1 demonstrates the use of the formula.

Example 1:

Using the formula for dilution of a tube feeding

M.D. order: Commercial formula available:

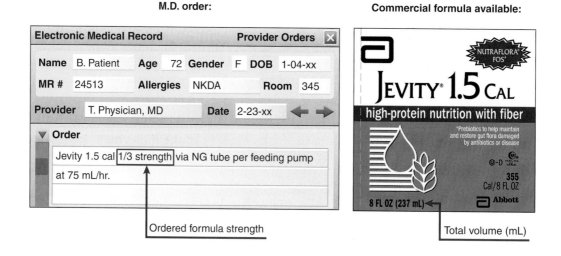

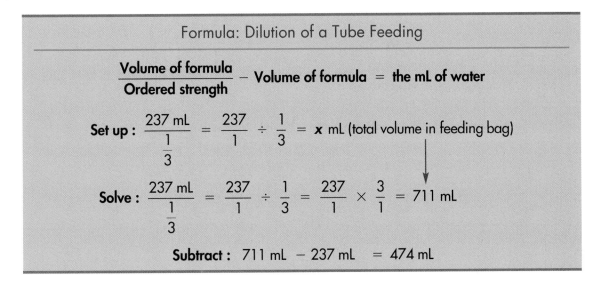

Formula: Dilution of a Tube Feeding

$$\frac{\text{Volume of formula}}{\text{Ordered strength}} - \text{Volume of formula} = \text{the mL of water}$$

Set up : $\dfrac{237 \text{ mL}}{\frac{1}{3}} = \dfrac{237}{1} \div \dfrac{1}{3} = x$ mL (total volume in feeding bag)

Solve : $\dfrac{237 \text{ mL}}{\frac{1}{3}} = \dfrac{237}{1} \div \dfrac{1}{3} = \dfrac{237}{1} \times \dfrac{3}{1} = 711 \text{ mL}$

Subtract : $711 \text{ mL} - 237 \text{ mL} = 474 \text{ mL}$

The nurse adds 474 mL of water to the formula feeding bag to make the 1/3 ordered strength.

Any ordered strength for dilution of a tube feeding can be solved by using this formula. Look at Example 2.

Example 2:

Formula: dilution of a tube feeding

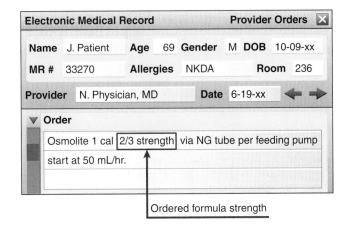

Available: Osmolite 1 cal in 250 mL cans.
Calculate the total mL of water to add to the formula to make the ordered strength.

Formula: Dilution of a Tube Feeding

$$\frac{\text{Volume of formula}}{\text{Ordered strength}} - \text{Volume of formula} = \text{the mL of water}$$

Set up : $\dfrac{250 \text{ mL}}{\frac{2}{3}} = \dfrac{250}{1} \div \dfrac{2}{3} = x \text{ mL (total volume in feeding bag)}$

Solve : $\dfrac{250 \text{ mL}}{\frac{2}{3}} = \dfrac{250}{1} \div \dfrac{2}{3} = \dfrac{250}{1} \times \dfrac{3}{2} = 375 \text{ mL}$

Subtract : $375 \text{ mL} - 250 \text{ mL} = 125 \text{ mL}$

To dilute this tube feeding, the nurse adds 125 mL of water to the formula feeding bag to make the 2/3 ordered strength.

Linear Ratio and Proportion Method and Fractional Ratio and Proportion Method

The ratio and proportion method can also be used to solve for the number of mL of water to add to make the diluted formula. Using the ratio and proportion method (linear or fractional) requires two steps:

■ Step 1: calculate the volume (water +formula) that will be in the formula feeding bag.
■ Step 2: calculate the number of mL of water to add to make the ordered strength.

Using the physician's order and the volume of formula in the can in the following example, look at how the ratio and proportion method is used.

Example 1:

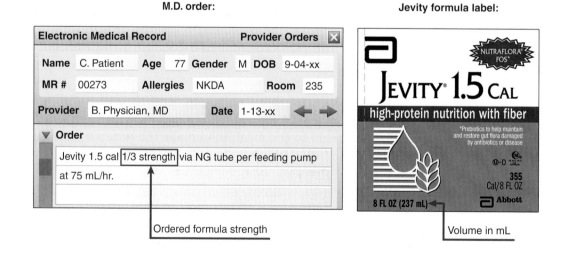

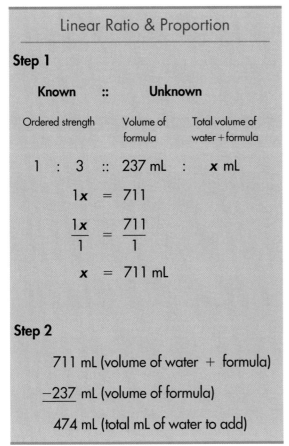

The nurse will add 474 mL of water to the formula feeding bag to make the $\frac{1}{3}$ ordered strength.

In the following example all three methods: ratio and proportion (linear and fractional) and the formula for dilution of a tube feeding are used to calculate the amount of water to add.

Example 2:

MD order:

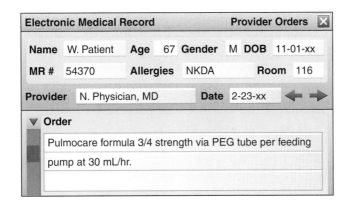

Available: Pulmocare formula in 240 mL cans.
Calculate the total mL of water to add to the formula to make the ordered strength.

Linear Ratio & Proportion

Step 1

Known	::	Unknown

Ordered strength · Volume of formula · Total volume of water + formula

$$3 : 4 :: 240\ \text{mL} : x\ \text{mL}$$

$$3x = 4 \times 240$$

$$\frac{3x}{3} = \frac{960}{3}$$

$$x = 320\ \text{mL}$$

Step 2

320 mL (volume of water + formula)

−240 mL (volume of formula)

80 mL (total mL of water to add)

Dimensional Analysis

Dimensional analysis cannot be used to solve the dilution of enteral feeding problems.

Fractional Ratio & Proportion

Step 1

Known = Unknown

Ordered strength

$$\frac{3}{4} \quad \underset{\diagdown}{\overset{\diagup}{\diagup\diagdown}} \quad \frac{240\ \text{mL}}{x\ \text{mL}} \quad \begin{array}{l}\text{(Volume of formula)}\\ \text{(Total volume of}\\ \text{water + formula)}\end{array}$$

$$3x = 4 \times 240$$

$$\frac{3x}{3} = \frac{960}{3}$$

$$x = 320\ \text{mL}$$

Step 2

320 mL (volume of water + formula)

−240 mL (volume of formula)

80 mL (total mL of water to add)

Formula: Dilution of a Tube Feeding

$$\frac{\text{Volume of formula}}{\text{Ordered strength}} - \text{Volume of formula}$$

$$= \text{the mL of water}$$

Set up : $\dfrac{240\ \text{mL}}{\dfrac{3}{4}} = \dfrac{240}{1} \div \dfrac{3}{4} = x\ \text{mL}$

Solve :

$$\frac{240\ \text{mL}}{\dfrac{3}{4}} = \frac{240}{1} \div \frac{3}{4} =$$

$$\frac{240}{1} \times \frac{4}{3} = 320\ \text{mL}$$

Subtract : 320 mL − 240 mL = 80 mL

When using the ratio and proportion method, it is important to remember that the answer in Step 1 is not the final answer. The answer in Step 1 identifies the total volume of formula and water that will be in the formula feeding bag. The nurse must remember to apply Step 2 in order to calculate the amount of water to add to dilute the formula.

APPLY LEARNED KNOWLEDGE 22-2

Use the physician's orders and the available formula to calculate the ordered strength of formula.

1.

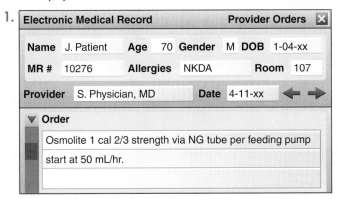

Electronic Medical Record **Provider Orders** ☒

Name J. Patient **Age** 70 **Gender** M **DOB** 1-04-xx

MR # 10276 **Allergies** NKDA **Room** 107

Provider S. Physician, MD **Date** 4-11-xx ⬅ ➡

▼ **Order**

Osmolite 1 cal 2/3 strength via NG tube per feeding pump

start at 50 mL/hr.

Available: Osmolite 1 cal in 240 mL cans.

Calculate the volume of water to add to make the ordered strength. _____

2.

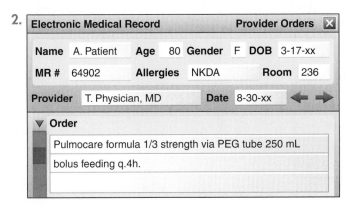

Electronic Medical Record **Provider Orders** ☒

Name A. Patient **Age** 80 **Gender** F **DOB** 3-17-xx

MR # 64902 **Allergies** NKDA **Room** 236

Provider T. Physician, MD **Date** 8-30-xx ⬅ ➡

▼ **Order**

Pulmocare formula 1/3 strength via PEG tube 250 mL

bolus feeding q.4h.

Available: Pulmocare formula in 240 mL cans.

Calculate the volume of water to add to make the ordered strength. _____

3.

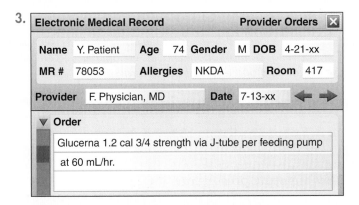

Electronic Medical Record **Provider Orders** ☒

Name Y. Patient **Age** 74 **Gender** M **DOB** 4-21-xx

MR # 78053 **Allergies** NKDA **Room** 417

Provider F. Physician, MD **Date** 7-13-xx ⬅ ➡

▼ **Order**

Glucerna 1.2 cal 3/4 strength via J-tube per feeding pump

at 60 mL/hr.

Available: Glucerna 1.2 cal in 180 mL cans.

Calculate the volume of water to add to make the ordered strength. _____

Continued

APPLY LEARNED KNOWLEDGE 22-2—cont'd

4.
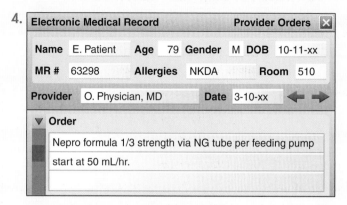

Electronic Medical Record			Provider Orders ☒
Name E. Patient	**Age** 79	**Gender** M **DOB** 10-11-xx	
MR # 63298	**Allergies** NKDA	**Room** 510	
Provider O. Physician, MD	**Date** 3-10-xx ← →		

▼ **Order**

Nepro formula 1/3 strength via NG tube per feeding pump start at 50 mL/hr.

Available: 200 mL Nepro formula.
Calculate the volume of water to add to make the ordered strength. _____

5.
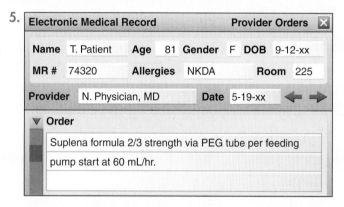

Electronic Medical Record			Provider Orders ☒
Name T. Patient	**Age** 81	**Gender** F **DOB** 9-12-xx	
MR # 74320	**Allergies** NKDA	**Room** 225	
Provider N. Physician, MD	**Date** 5-19-xx ← →		

▼ **Order**

Suplena formula 2/3 strength via PEG tube per feeding pump start at 60 mL/hr.

Available: 200 mL Suplena formula.
Calculate the volume of water to add to make the ordered strength. _____

 The tube feeding has been started; the nurse continuously monitors the patient for gastrointestinal complications (i.e., diarrhea, nausea, vomiting, cramps, abdominal distention, delayed emptying) that may indicate a need to change the formula or the rate of administration.

Labeling of Formula Tube Feeding Container

The American Society for Parenteral & Enteral Nutrition (A.S.P.E.N.) recommends that formula feeding bags and containers be clearly labeled with specific information to avoid any misinterpretations and potential for misconnections (Fig. 22-7). It is recommended by A.S.P.E.N. that healthcare facilities institute precautions (i.e., staff education, special labels on containers, use of colored-coded tubings or connectors) to ensure safety in the administration of enteral feedings. Health-care professionals must possess the knowledge to continuously implement safety measures at the patient's bedside, such as understanding the purpose of all tubes, assessing all tubing from the container to the point of entry into the patient, and accurately labeling all tubes and containers to prevent misconnections.

```
┌─────────────────────────────────────────────────────────────┐
│                     ENTERAL USE ONLY                        │
│         Institution and Department Name—Contact Information  │
│                                                             │
│   Patient Name _____  Patient ID _____     │
│   Room Number _____                                       │
├─────────────────────────────────────────────────────────────┤
│                 Generic (Brand) Formula Name                │
│                                                             │
│   Formula: _____                  │
│                     _____grams of protein/_____kcal/container │
│                     _____mL/container                      │
│   Prepared by:_____  Date:_____  Time:_____    │
├─────────────────────────────────────────────────────────────┤
│                      Delivery Site                          │
│                                                             │
│   Route of Delivery:_____  Enteral Access Site:_____ │
│  (JW)─────────────────────────────────────────────────(JW) │
│                      Administration                         │
│   Method of Administration:   Bolus   Intermittent   Continuous │
│   Rate of Administration:_____mL/hr             │
│                                                             │
│   Formula Hung by:_____, Nurse Date:_____ Time:_____ │
│   Expiration vs Beyond Use Date:_____ Time:_____ │
└─────────────────────────────────────────────────────────────┘
```

Figure 22-7. Recommended enteral feeding label from A.S.P.E.N. (Bankhead, R., Boullata, J., Brantley, S., Corkins, M., Guenter, P., Krenitsky, J., . . . Wessel, J. (2009). A.S.P.E.N. Enteral Nutrition Practice Recommendations. *JPEN: Journal of Parenteral and Enteral Nutrition, 33*(2), 122–167. first published January 26, 2009; doi:10.1177/0148607108330314. Reprinted by Permission of SAGE Publications.)

CLINICAL REASONING 22-1

The nurse is preparing the 0900 dose of 125 mcg of digoxin PO for the older adult patient. Prior to administering the medication, the nurse reads the following information from the drug reference:

HIGH ALERT

digoxin (di-**jox**-in)
Lanoxin, ✽Toloxin

Classification
Therapeutic: antiarrhythmics, inotropics
Pharmacologic: digitalis glycosides

Pregnancy Category C

Indications
Heart failure. Atrial fibrillation and atrial flutter (slows ventricular rate)...

Route/Dosage
PO (Geriatric Patients): Initial daily dosage should not exceed 0.125 mg.

Assessment
Geri: Digoxin has been asociated with an increased risk for falls in the elderly...

Toxicity and Overdosage:
Geri: Older adults are at increased risk for toxic effects of digoxin (appears on Beers list) due to age-related decreased renal clearance... Digoxin requirements in the older adult may change and a formerly therapeutic dose can become toxic.

Based on the 0900 medication and the drug reference, select the correct statement(s) (select all that apply).

A. The ordered dose is within the usual daily dose.
B. The drug should not be prescribed for the older adult.
C. The ordered dose has a low risk of toxicity for this patient.
D. The ordered dose should be prescribed in milligrams not micrograms.
E. High alert drugs have an increased risk of causing serious injury or death.

The increasing number of older adults with acute and chronic illnesses will require the nurse to take a more active role in providing individualized care to improve the quality of life for a vulnerable population. Nurses must apply a purposeful approach for gathering drug information, correlating information, monitoring drug dosages and drug interactions, and seeking up-to-date information that will help promote safe patient outcomes for the older adult. Implementing the use of the recommended Vigilant Process will promote an awareness of the factors that increase the older adult's risk for adverse drug reactions.

Developing Competency

Use the drug reference information to answer questions 1 through 10 related to drug therapy in the older adult.

⁑ doxepin (dox-e-pin)
Silenor, ✽SINEquan, Zonalon

Classification
Therapeutic: antianxiety agents, antidepressants, antihistamines (topical), sedative/hypnotics
Pharmacologic: tricyclic antidepressants

Pregnancy Category C

Indications: PO: Management of Depression, Insomnia.

Contraindications/Precautions

Use Cautiously in: Geri: Pre-existing cardiovascular disease (increased risk of adverse reactions); Prostatic enlargement (more susceptible to urinary retention); Seizures;...

Geri: Appears on *Beers list* and is associated with increased falls risk for secondary to anticholinergic and sedative effects. Geriatric patients should have initial dosage reduction.

Route/Dosage

PO (Geriatric Patients): *Antidepressant* 25–50 mg/day initially, may be increased as needed.
Insomnia
3 mg at bedtime, may be increased as needed to 6 mg at bedtime (should not exceed 3 mg/day if concurrently taking cimetidime).

Implementation
• **PO:** Administer medication with or immediately following a meal to minimize gastric irritation. ...
• Oral concentrate must be diluted in at least 120 mL of water, milk, ...Do not mix with carbonated beverages or grape juice. Use calibrated measuring device to ensure accurate amount.

Patient/Family Teaching
• **PO:** Instruct patient to take medication as directed. Take missed doses as soon as possible unless almost time for next dose... Abrupt discontinuation may cause nausea, vomiting, diarrhea, headache, trouble sleeping with vivid dreams, and irritability.

MD order: Doxepin 25 mg oral concentrate PO daily for depression.

1. Is the ordered dose within the usual recommended dose?
   ☐ Yes   ☐ No
   Pharmacy sends: Doxepin oral concentrate 10 mg/mL.

2. How many mL with the nurse administer per dose? _____

3. How many ounces of water will the nurse use to dilute the oral concentrate? _____

4. The nurse may instruct the family to dilute the oral concentrate in 120 mL of the patient's favorite soda.
   ☐ Yes   ☐ No

5. The nurse may instruct the patient/family to stop the medication once the patient feels better and is less depressed.
   ☐ Yes   ☐ No

---

temazepam (tem-az-a-pam)
Restoril

Classification
Therapeutic: sedative/hypnotics
Pharmacologic: benzodiazepines

Schedule IV

Pregnancy Category X

Indications: Short-term management of insomnia (less than 4 weeks).

Contraindications/Precautions

Use Cautiously in: Geri: Elderly patients have increased sensitivity to benzodiazepines. Appears on the _Beers list_ and is associated with increased risk of falls (decreased dose required).

Route/Dosage

PO (Adults): 15–30 mg at bedtime initially if needed; some patients may require only 7.5 mg.
PO (Geriatric Patients or Debilitated Patients): 7.5 mg at bedtime.

Assessment
• Assess mental status (orientation, mood, behavior) and potential for abuse prior to administering medication. ...
• **Geri:** Assess CNS effects and risk of falls. Institute falls prevention strategies.

Implementation
• Supervise ambulation and transfer of patients after administration. Remove cigarettes. Side rails should be raised and call bell within reach at all times.
• **PO:** Administer with food if GI irritation becomes a problem.

Patient/Family Teaching
• Instruct patient to take temazepam as directed...
• May cause daytime drowsiness or dizziness. Caution patient to avoid driving or other activities requiring alertness... **Geri:** Instruct patient and family how to reduce falls risk at home.
• Advise patient to avoid the use of alcohol and other CNS depressants and to consult healthcare professional before using OTC preparations that contain antihistamines or alcohol.

MD order: Temazepam 7.5 mg one capsule at hour of sleep every night.

6. Is the ordered dose within usual recommended dose for the older adult?

☐ Yes   ☐ No

7. Ordered dose is low, so the older adult will not experience dizziness or drowsiness.

☐ Yes   ☐ No

8. Temazepam may be administered with food.

☐ Yes   ☐ No

9. The following medications are taken by the older adult. Which drug would the nurse initially caution the patient about taking while on temazepam?
   a. aspirin (anti-inflammatory, antithrombotic)
   b. diphenhydramine (antihistamine)
   c. ibuprophen (nonsteroidal anti-inflammatory)
   d. atorvastatin (lipid-lowering)

10. The effects of temazepam may last longer than eight hours.

☐ Yes   ☐ No

Use the physician's order to answer questions 11 through 20.

11.

Electronic Medical Record	Provider Orders ☒

Name	G. Patient	**Age**	78	**Gender**	F	**DOB**	8-15-xx

MR # 63010   **Allergies** NKDA   **Room** 105

Provider M. Physician, MD   **Date** 5-08-xx ⬅ ➡

▼ **Order**

Suplena formula 1/3 strength via PEG tube per feeding

pump start at 60 mL/hr.

Available: Suplena formula in 240 mL cans. Select the answer that indicates the volume of water to add to make the ordered strength.

a. 240 mL   b. 480 mL   c. 720 mL

12.

Electronic Medical Record	Provider Orders ☒

Name S. Patient   **Age** 82   **Gender** M   **DOB** 7-02-xx

MR # 31210   **Allergies** NKDA   **Room** 333

Provider V. Physician, MD   **Date** 4-19-xx ⬅ ➡

▼ **Order**

Isocal formula 1/3 strength give 250 mL bolus feeding q.4h.

Available: 180 mL of Isocal formula. Calculate the volume of water to add to make the ordered strength.

_____

13.

Electronic Medical Record	Provider Orders ☒

Name H. Patient   **Age** 75   **Gender** F   **DOB** 10-15-xx

MR # 04590   **Allergies** NKDA   **Room** 216

Provider N. Physician, MD   **Date** 3-06-xx ⬅ ➡

▼ **Order**

Jevity 1.2 Cal formula 2/3 strength administer 300 mL

gravity feeding q.6h.

Available: 180 mL of Jevity 1.2 Cal. Calculate the volume of water to add to make the ordered strength.

_____

14.

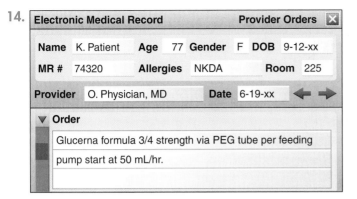

Available: 240 mL Glucerna formula. Calculate the volume of water to add to make the ordered strength.

_____

15.

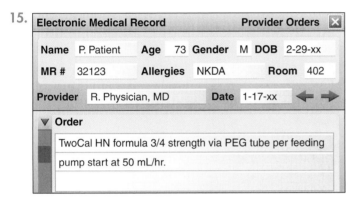

Available:

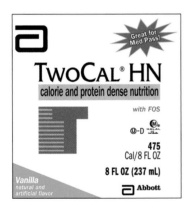

Calculate the volume of water to add to make the ordered strength. _____

16.

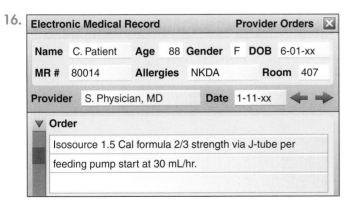

Available: Isosource 1.5 Cal in 250 mL cans. Select the answer that indicates volume of water to add to make the ordered strength.

a. 125 mL   b. 250 mL   c. 375 mL

17.

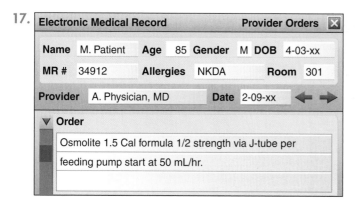

Available: Osmolite 1.2 Cal in 200 mL cans. Select the answer that indicates volume of water to add to make the ordered strength.

a. 100 mL   b. 150 mL   c. 200 mL

18.

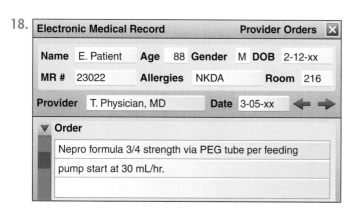

Available: Nepro formula in 240 mL cans. Calculate the volume of water to add to make the ordered strength.

_____

19.

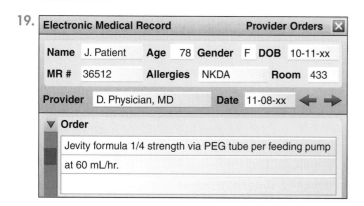

Available: Jevity formula in 240 mL cans. Calculate the volume of water to add to make the desired strength.

_____

20.

Electronic Medical Record	Provider Orders ☒

Name L. Patient   **Age** 82 **Gender** F **DOB** 3-08-xx

MR # 11235   **Allergies** NKDA   **Room** 325

Provider Z. Physician, MD   **Date** 7-01-xx ⬅ ➡

▼ **Order**

Glucerna 1.2 Cal formula 1/2 strength via PEG tube per feeding pump at 50 mL/hr.

Available:

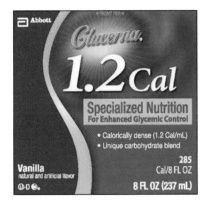

Calculate the volume of water to add to make the desired strength. _____

Dosages for Pediatric and Elderly Populations

Unit Review—Evaluate for Clinical Decision Making

*For each question, use your clinical judgment to determine whether the nurse's decision is **Correct** or **Incorrect**. For incorrect problems, write the correct answer.*

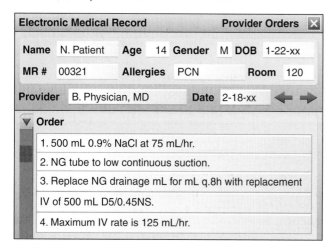

Electronic Medical Record	Provider Orders ⊠
Name N. Patient **Age** 14 **Gender** M **DOB** 1-22-xx	
MR # 00321 **Allergies** PCN **Room** 120	
Provider B. Physician, MD **Date** 2-18-xx ⬅ ➡	

▼ **Order**

1. 500 mL 0.9% NaCl at 75 mL/hr.
2. NG tube to low continuous suction.
3. Replace NG drainage mL for mL q.8h with replacement IV of 500 mL D5/0.45NS.
4. Maximum IV rate is 125 mL/hr.

1. The nurse calculates that the replacement IV fluid is 50 mL/hr.
The calculated mL/hr of the replacement IV fluid is:

Correct	Incorrect	Answer: _____

Electronic Medical Record	Provider Orders ⊠
Name W. Patient **Age** 12 **Gender** F **DOB** 3-05-xx	
MR # 22680 **Allergies** Sulfa **Room** 212	
Provider X. Physician, MD **Date** 4-10-xx ⬅ ➡	

▼ **Order**

1. 500 mL 0.9% NaCl at 50 mL/hr.
2. NG tube to low continuous suction.
3. Replace NG drainage mL for mL q.8h with replacement IV of 500 mL D5/0.45NS.
4. Maximum IV rate is 80 mL/hr.

Handoff report:
"Patient had 160 mL NG drainage for the last 8 hours"

2. The nurse calculates that the infusion time for the replacement IV fluid is 2 hours.
The calculated infusion time of the replacement IV fluid is:

Correct	Incorrect	Answer: _____

3. The nurse starts the replacement IV fluid at 0725 and reports a completion time of 1245.
The reported completion time of the IV is:

Correct	Incorrect	Answer: _____

Electronic Medical Record	Provider Orders ⊠
Name H. Patient **Age** 75 **Gender** F **DOB** 10-15-xx	
MR # 04590 **Allergies** NKDA **Room** 216	
Provider N. Physician, MD **Date** 3-06-xx ⬅ ➡	

▼ **Order**

Jevity 1.2 Cal formula 2/3 strength 300 mL gravity feeding q.6h.

4. Available: 280 mL of Jevity 1.2 Cal. The nurse adds 140 mL of water to the 280 mL of formula.
The amount of water added is:

Correct	Incorrect	Answer: _____

midazolam (mid-ay-zoe-lam)
~~Versed~~

Classification
Therapeutic: antianxiety agents, sedative/hypnotics
Pharmacologic: benzodiazepines

Schedule IV

Pregnancy Category D

Indications
PO: Preprocedural sedation and anxiolysis in pediatric patients. **IM, IV:** Preoperative sedation/anxiolysis/amnesia. **IV:** Provides sedation/anxiolysis/amnesia during therapeutic, diagnostic, or radiographic procedures (conscious sedation)...

Route/Dosage
Dose must be individualized, taking caution to reduce dose in geriatric patients and in those who are already sedated.

Preoperative Sedation/Anxiolysis/Amnesia
PO (Children 6 mo–16 yr): 0.25–0.5 mg/kg, may require up to 1 mg/kg (dose should not exceed 20 mg); *patients with cardiac/respiratory compromise or concurrent CNS depressants—0.25 mg/kg.*
IM (Adults Otherwise Healthy and <60 yr): 0.07–0.08 mg/kg 1 hr before surgery (usual dose 5 mg).
IM (Adults ≥60 yr, Debilitated or Chronically Ill): 0.02–0.03 mg/kg 1 hr before surgery (usual dose 1–3 mg).
IM (Children): 0.1–0.15 mg/kg up to 0.5 mg/kg 30–60 min prior to procedure; not to exceed 10 mg/dose.
Conscious Sedation for Short Procedures IV: (Adults and Children Otherwise Healthy >12 yr and <60 yr): 1–2.5 mg initially; dosage may be ↑ further as needed. Total doses >5 mg are rarely needed. (↓ dose by 50% if other CNS depressants are used)...
IV (Children 6–12 yr): 0.025–0.05 mg/kg initially, then titrate dose carefully, may need up to 0.4 mg/kg total, maximum dose 10 mg.
IV (Children 6 mo–5 yr): 0.05 mg/kg initially, then titrate dose carefully, may need up to 0.6 mg/kg total, maximum dose 6 mg.
IV (Geriatric Patients ≥60 yr, Debilitated or Chronically Ill): 1–1.5 mg initially; dose may be ↑ further as needed. Total doses >3.5 mg are rarely needed. (↓ dose by 30% if other CNS depressants are used)...

Status Epilepticus
IV (Children >2 mo): 0.15 mg/kg load followed by a continuous infusion of 1 mcg/kg/min. Titrate dose upward q 5 min until seizure controlled, range: 1–18 mcg/kg/min.

5. The midazolam order for a 10-year-old child scheduled for a procedure today is 2 mg IM. The nurse uses the recommended weight-based dose range of 0.025 to 0.05 mg/kg to verify the safe dose.
The nurse's decision is:

Correct	Incorrect	Answer: _____

6. The midazolam order for a 14-year-old child scheduled for a procedure today is 10 mg PO. The nurse concludes that the ordered dose is within the safe dose recommended for children.
The nurse's decision is:

Correct	Incorrect	Answer: _____

7. The preoperative sedation midazolam order for a 58-year-old adult without any chronic illness is 3 mg IM. The nurse concludes that the ordered dose is less than the usual dose and does not administer the ordered dose until the order is clarified with the physician.
The nurse's decision is:

Correct	Incorrect	Answer: _____

8. The midazolam order for a 72-year-old adult scheduled for a procedure under conscious sedation is 1 mg IV. The nurse concludes that this dose is within the recommended dose range for the patient.
The nurse's decision is:

Correct	Incorrect	Answer: _____

9. The nurse concludes that the titrated dose of midazolam continuous IV for a 6-year-old child experiencing status epilepticus must be verified using the child's current weight in kg.
The nurse's decision is:

Correct	Incorrect	Answer: _____

10. The nurse is aware that midazolam is a benzodiazepine. Using the Beers list, the nurse concludes that midazolam may be potentially inappropriate in the treatment of agitation in the older adult.
The nurse's decision is:

Correct	Incorrect	Answer: _____

Answer Key

Answers to chapter exercises will be found in the following order: Apply Learned Knowledge, Clinical Reasoning, and Developing Competency. Answers to Unit Tests follow the chapter answers.

ANSWERS TO CHAPTER QUESTIONS

Chapter 1

CLINICAL REASONING 1.1 (P. 12)

A, C, D, and E are correct.
B is incorrect. The route of administration is ordered by the health-care provider and not determined by the nurse.

DEVELOPING COMPETENCY (P. 12)

1. **b.** The medication order has a dangerous symbol.

2. **b.** The ordered dose has a trailing zero.
   c. The nurse is correct to question the ordered dose.

3. **a.** The medication order is written incorrectly.

4. **b.** The dose should be written as 1.2 million.
   c. Units (u) should not be abbreviated.

5. **b.** "ml" should be written as "mL".

6. **b.** check the MD order to verify dose.

7. **d.** first check the MD order to verify the route.

8. **a.** administer the Benadryl at 2100.

9. **c.** note no 0700-1500 meds ordered.

10. **a.** interpret that the 0900 medication was given.

11. True

12. False. A Black box warning is included in specific medications and not in all prescription medications.

13. True

14. False. Promoting a culture of safety is the responsibility of all health-care staff not just the physicians.

15. True

Chapter 2: The Drug Label

APPLY LEARNED KNOWLEDGE 2.1 (P. 18)

1. False. The generic name refers to the chemical or pharmacological name of the drug.

2. False. Tall man lettering is used to distinguish between look-alike or sound-alike drugs.

3. True

4. True

5. True

APPLY LEARNED KNOWLEDGE 2.2 (P. 23)

1. **Generic;** Dosage form: sterile liquid preparation; Dosage strength: 2 mg/mL; Route(s) of administration: IM use or IV use

2. **Generic and Brand;** Dosage form: solid oral preparation (tablet); Dosage strength: 750 mg per tablet; Route(s) of administration: oral

3. **Generic and Brand;** Dosage form: solid oral preparation (tablet); Dosage strength: 5 mg per tablet; Route(s) of administration: oral

4. **Generic and Brand;** Dosage form: sterile liquid preparation; Dosage strength: 1 mg/10 mL or 0.1 mg/mL; Route(s) of administration: IV

5. **Generic and Brand;** Dosage form: solid oral preparation (tablet); Dosage strength: 125 mcg per tablet or 0.125 mg per tablet; Route(s) of administration: oral

APPLY LEARNED KNOWLEDGE 2.3 (P. 27)

1. CII on a drug label: CII indicates that the drug is a controlled substance. The drug is identified as being under the controlled substance schedule category II.

2. Usual dosage: The typical dosage that is normally prescribed to treat a particular disorder or disease.

3. Expiration date: The timeframe in which the drug may be dispensed and used.

4. Reconstitution: The mixing of a powdered drug with a liquid, thus converting it into liquid form.

5. Dosage form: The solid or liquid form that holds the strength of medication.

CLINICAL REASONING 2.1 (P. 30)

No, the dose of the new prescription is a fixed combination drug of irbesartan and hydrochlorothiazide 300 mg/12.5 mg PO daily. Taking two pills from the previous prescription will double the dose of both drugs. The hydrochlorothiazide dose of the new prescription is 12.5 mg. Taking two tablets will increase the dose of hydrochlorothiazide to 25 mg. The patient should fill the new prescription and take the new medication as ordered.

DEVELOPING COMPETENCY (P. 31)

1. Correct.
2. Correct.
3. Incorrect. *Tall man lettering consists of a mixed combination lowercase and uppercase letters in the name of the drug.*
4. Incorrect. *This is a single-dose vial indicating that the vial must be discarded even if the entire contents have not been used.*
5. Correct.
6. Incorrect. *The ordered route of administration is IM and the available drug is in tablet form.*

7. Correct. *The Lanoxin drug label indicates that the tablet is scored.*
8. Correct.
9. Correct.
10. Incorrect. *The dosage strength is made up of two parts: the strength of the medication with the unit of measurement and the dosage form. For this drug the dosage form is mL. The dosage strength is written as 100 mcg/1 mL or 0.1 mg/1 mL.*
11. **b.** Multi-dose; **d.** Total amount is 5 mL; **e.** Tall man lettering
12. **b.** Dosage strength: 0.5 mcg in each capsule; **c.** Oral route of administration; **d.** Generic name
13. **b.** Total amount: 1 mL; **d.** Generic name; **f.** Controlled substance
14. **a.** Dosage strength: 5 mg/mL; **b.** Dosage strength: 25 mg/5 mL; **d.** Generic name; **e.** Storage information
15. **d.** Controlled substance; **f.** Storage information

Chapter 3: The Metric System

APPLY LEARNED KNOWLEDGE 3.1 (P. 43)

1. False
2. False
3. True
4. False
5. True

APPLY LEARNED KNOWLEDGE 3.2 (P. 44)

1. False
2. False
3. False
4. True
5. True

APPLY LEARNED KNOWLEDGE 3.3 (P. 49)

1. *Starting place:* m   *Desired place:* mc   *Answer:* 400 mcg
2. *Starting place:* m   *Desired place:* k   *Answer:* 0.001 km
3. *Starting place:* k   *Desired place:* da   *Answer:* 30 dag
4. *Starting place:* d   *Desired place:* m   *Answer:* 15 mL
5. *Starting place:* m   *Desired place:* L   *Answer:* 0.55 L

APPLY LEARNED KNOWLEDGE 3.4 (P. 50)

1. Correct
2. Incorrect. 0.75 g
3. Correct.
4. Incorrect. 250 km
5. Incorrect. 60 mcg
6. Incorrect. 15 L

CLINICAL REASONING 3.1 (P. 50)

The nurse has provided the patient with the correct information. Using the metric line, the nurse has correctly identified that 500 mcg is equivalent to 0.5 mg.

DEVELOPING COMPETENCY (P. 50)

1. 0.02 hg
2. 250 m
3. 0.5 m
4. 6.5 dL
5. 0.7 mg
6. 0.025 g
7. 0.75 mg
8. 1,500 mL

9. 2 L

10. 10 cL

11. 0.00004 cg

12. 1,000 mL

13. 0.1 km

14. 1 daL

15. 0.1 hg

16. *Metric notation error:* Trailing zero; *Corrected Notation:* 0.1 mL

17. *Metric notation error:* Use decimal fractions; *Corrected Notation:* 0.5 mg

18. *Metric notation error:* Use singular form; *Corrected Notation:* 15 mL

19. *Metric notation error:* Put a space between the quantity & metric unit; *Corrected Notation:* 5 cm

20. *Metric notation error:* Quantity before unit; *Corrected Notation:* 3 m

Chapter 4: The Household System

APPLY LEARNED KNOWLEDGE 4.1 (P. 54)

1. *Standard Abbreviation(s):* oz

   Household Equivalent Measurement: 6 tsp, 2 Tbs

   Metric Equivalent Measurement: 30 mL

2. *Standard Abbreviation(s):* gtt

   Household Equivalent Measurement: none

   Metric Equivalent Measurement: none

3. *Standard Abbreviation(s):* Tbs

   Household Equivalent Measurement: 3 tsp

   Metric Equivalent Measurement: 15 mL

4. *Standard Abbreviation(s):* tsp

   Household Equivalent Measurement: none

   Metric Equivalent Measurement: 5 mL

5. *Standard Abbreviation(s):* none

   Household Equivalent Measurement: none

   Metric Equivalent Measurement: 240 mL

6. *Standard Abbreviation(s):* none

   Household Equivalent Measurement: none

   Metric Equivalent Measurement: 180 mL

CLINICAL REASONING 4.1 (P. 54)

The nurse has incorrectly instructed the patient on the amount to take for each dose, 2 tsp is equal to 10 mL not 1 oz, 2 Tbs is equal to 1 oz.

DEVELOPING COMPETENCY (P. 55)

1. a. 2 Tbs equals 30 mL; c. 1 Tbs equals 15 mL

2. b. 6 tsp equals 30 mL; c. 1 tsp equals 5 mL

3. c. 1 oz equals 30 mL

4. b. 1 oz equals 30 mL

5. b. 1 oz equals 30 mL

6. a. 5 mL equals 1 tsp; b. 15 mL equals 3 tsp

7. b. 15 mL equals 1 Tbs; c. 1 Tbs equals 15 mL

8. a. 15 mL equals 1 Tbs

9. d. 1 oz equals 2 Tbs

10. a. 1 oz equals 30 mL

Chapter 5: Linear Ratio and Proportion

APPLY LEARNED KNOWLEDGE 5.1 (P. 63)

1. 10 mg : 1 tablet

2. 250 mg : 5 mL

3. 12.5 mg : 1 tablet

4. 25 mg : 1 mL or 50 mg : 2 mL

5. 25 mg : 5 mL

APPLY LEARNED KNOWLEDGE 5.2 (P. 67)

1. b. 4 mg : 1 drop :: 16 mg : x drop, x = 4 drop

2. b. 650 gram : 1 mL :: 500 gram : x mL, x = 0.77 mL

3. a. 20 mg : 1 tablet :: x mg : 0.5 tablet, x = 10 mg

4. b. 2.5 mg : 0.5 mL :: 5 mg : x mL, x = 1 mL

5. a. 4 mg : 1 dose :: x mg : 6 dose, x = 24 mg

APPLY LEARNED KNOWLEDGE 5.3 (P. 70)

1. 0.5 pill

2. 0.25 mL

3. 3 capsules

4. 2.5 tsp

5. 1.6 ounces

CLINICAL REASONING 5.1 (P. 76)

The patient is taking the correct amount of medication. The label on the Griseofulvin Oral Suspension bottle gives two dosage strengths: 125 mg/5 mL and 125 mg/1 teaspoonful. Either of these equivalent dosage strengths can be used to set up the problem. The metric line is used to convert g to mg (0.375 g = 375 mg). In addition, a conversion between tsp and Tbs is required to solve the problem.

DEVELOPING COMPETENCY (P. 76)

1. 5 mg : 1 tablet

2. 750 mg : 1 tablet

3. 125 mcg : 1 tablet or 0.125 mg : 1 tablet

4. Yes, even though the x is in an unusual place, the units match and the proportion is set up correctly.

5. No, the nurse has not chosen the correct dosage strength. The correct proportion is: 350 g : 1 tablet :: 700 g : x tablet

6. The nurse will give 0.5 tablet. (0.25 g : 1 tablet :: 0.125 g : x tablet)

7. The nurse will give 3.5 mL. (2.5 mg : 1 mL :: 8.75 mg : x mL)

8. The nurse will give 2.5 pills. (0.05 mg : 1 pill :: 0.125 mg : x pill)

9. 600 mg

10. 2 tsp

11. 0.75 mL

12. 4.5 mL

13. 0.7 ounce

14. 2 tablets

15. 5 bottles

16. 3 capsules

17. 4 tablets each day

18. 3 tsp

19. 0.75 mL

20. 0.5 oz

Chapter 6: Fractional Ratio and Proportion

APPLY LEARNED KNOWLEDGE 6.1 (P. 84)

1. $\dfrac{10\ mg}{1\ tablet}$

2. $\dfrac{250\ mg}{5\ mL}$

3. $\dfrac{12.5\ mg}{1\ tablet}$

4. $\dfrac{25\ mg}{1\ mL}$ or $\dfrac{50\ mg}{2\ mL}$

5. $\dfrac{25\ mg}{5\ mL}$

APPLY LEARNED KNOWLEDGE 6.2 (P. 88)

1. b. $\dfrac{4\ mg}{1\ drop} = \dfrac{16\ mg}{x\ drop}$, **x** = 4 drop

2. b. $\dfrac{650\ gram}{1\ mL} = \dfrac{500\ gram}{x\ mL}$, **x** = 0.77 mL

3. a. $\dfrac{20\ mg}{1\ tablet} = \dfrac{x\ mg}{0.5\ tablet}$, **x** = 10 mg

4. b. $\dfrac{2.5\ mg}{0.5\ mL} = \dfrac{5\ mg}{x\ mL}$, **x** = 1 mL

5. a. $\dfrac{4\ mg}{1\ dose} = \dfrac{x\ mg}{6\ dose}$, **x** = 24 mg

APPLY LEARNED KNOWLEDGE 6.3 (P. 91)

1. ½ pill

2. 0.25 mL

3. 3 capsules

4. 2.5 tsp

5. 1.6 ounces

CLINICAL REASONING 6.1 (P. 98)

The patient is taking the correct amount of medication. The label on the Griseofulvin Oral Suspension bottle gives two dosage strengths: $\dfrac{125\ mg}{5\ mL}$ and $\dfrac{125\ mg}{1\ teaspoon}$. Either of these equivalent dosage strengths can be used to set up the problem. The metric line is used to convert g to mg (0.375 g = 375 mg). In addition, a conversion between tsp and Tbs is required to solve the problem.

DEVELOPING COMPETENCY (P. 99)

1. $\dfrac{5 \text{ mg}}{1 \text{ tablet}}$

2. $\dfrac{750 \text{ mg}}{1 \text{ tablet}}$

3. $\dfrac{125 \text{ mcg}}{1 \text{ tablet}}$ or $\dfrac{0.125 \text{ mg}}{1 \text{ tablet}}$

4. Yes, even though the *x* is in an unusual place, the units match and the proportion is set up correctly.

5. No, the nurse has not chosen the correct dosage strength. The correct proportion is: $\dfrac{350 \text{ g}}{1 \text{ tablet}} = \dfrac{700 \text{ g}}{x \text{ tablet}}$

6. The nurse will give 0.5 tablet. $\dfrac{0.25 \text{ g}}{1 \text{ tablet}} = \dfrac{0.125 \text{ g}}{x \text{ tablet}}$

7. The nurse will give 3.5 mL. $\dfrac{2.5 \text{ mg}}{1 \text{ mL}} = \dfrac{8.75 \text{ mg}}{x \text{ mL}}$

8. The nurse will give 2.5 pills. $\dfrac{0.05 \text{ mg}}{1 \text{ pill}} = \dfrac{0.125 \text{ mg}}{x \text{ pill}}$

9. 600 mg

10. 2 tsp

11. 0.75 mL

12. 4.5 mL

13. 0.7 ounce

14. 2 tablets

15. 5 bottles

16. 3 capsules

17. 4 tablets each day

18. 3 tsp

19. 0.75 mL

20. 0.5 oz

Chapter 7: Dimensional Analysis

APPLY LEARNED KNOWLEDGE 7.1 (P. 108)

1. $\dfrac{1 \text{ tablet}}{10 \text{ mg}}$ Administer 0.5 tablet.

2. $\dfrac{5 \text{ mL}}{250 \text{ mg}}$ Administer 6 mL.

3. $\dfrac{1 \text{ tablet}}{12.5 \text{ mg}}$ Administer 2 tablets.

4. $\dfrac{1 \text{ mL}}{25 \text{ mg}}$ or $\dfrac{2 \text{ mL}}{50 \text{ mg}}$ Administer 1.6 mL.

5. $\dfrac{5 \text{ mL}}{25 \text{ mg}}$ Administer 40 mL.

APPLY LEARNED KNOWLEDGE 7.2 (P. 111)

1. $\dfrac{1,000 \text{ mg}}{1 \text{ g}}$ Administer 0.5 pill.

2. $\dfrac{1,000 \text{ mg}}{1 \text{ g}}$ Administer 25 mL.

3. $\dfrac{1,000 \text{ mcg}}{1 \text{ mg}}$ Administer 3 capsules.

4. $\dfrac{1 \text{ g}}{1,000 \text{ mg}}$ Administer 2.5 tsp.

5. $\dfrac{1 \text{ g}}{1,000 \text{ mg}}$ Administer 1.6 ounces.

APPLY LEARNED KNOWLEDGE 7.3 (P. 117)

1. *Conversion factor:* $\dfrac{1 \text{ mg}}{1,000 \text{ mcg}}$ *Administer:* 0.2 mL

2. *Dosage Strength:* $\dfrac{5 \text{ mL}}{200 \text{ mg}}$ *Conversion factor:* $\dfrac{1000 \text{ mg}}{1 \text{ g}}$
   Administer: 25 mL

3. *Conversion factor:* $\dfrac{1 \text{ g}}{1,000 \text{ mg}}$ *Conversion factor:* $\dfrac{1 \text{ Tbs}}{15 \text{ mL}}$
   Administer: 0.5 Tbs

4. *Dosage Strength:* $\dfrac{5 \text{ mL}}{0.5 \text{ mg}}$ *Conversion factor:* $\dfrac{1 \text{ mg}}{1,000 \text{ mcg}}$
   Administer: 0.75 mL

5. *Conversion factor:* $\dfrac{1 \text{ g}}{1,000 \text{ mg}}$ *Conversion factor:* $\dfrac{30 \text{ mL}}{1 \text{ oz}}$
   Administer: 6 mL

CLINICAL REASONING 7.1 (P. 118)

The patient is taking the correct amount of medication. The label on the Griseofulvin Oral Suspension bottle gives two dosage strengths: 125 mg/5 mL and 125 mg/1 teaspoon. Either of these equivalent dosage strengths can be used as conversion factors to set up the problem. The metric equivalent measurement 1 g = 1,000 mg, and the household equivalent measurement 3 tsp = 1 Tbs are also used as conversion factors in the problem.

DEVELOPING COMPETENCY (P. 119)

1. $\dfrac{5 \text{ mg}}{1 \text{ tablet}}$ or $\dfrac{1 \text{ tablet}}{5 \text{ mg}}$

2. $\dfrac{750 \text{ mg}}{1 \text{ tablet}}$ or $\dfrac{1 \text{ tablet}}{750 \text{ mg}}$

3. $\dfrac{125 \text{ mcg}}{1 \text{ tablet}}$ or $\dfrac{1 \text{ tablet}}{125 \text{ mcg}}$ or $\dfrac{0.125 \text{ mg}}{1 \text{ tablet}}$ or $\dfrac{1 \text{ tablet}}{0.125 \text{ mg}}$

4. Yes, the setup is correct.

5. No, the setup is not correct. The unnecessary units of measurement, g, do not cancel. The correct setup is:

$$\dfrac{700 \text{ g}}{1} \times \dfrac{1 \text{ tablet}}{350 \text{ g}} = x \text{ tablet}$$

6. $\dfrac{0.125 \text{ g}}{1} \times \dfrac{1 \text{ tablet}}{0.25 \text{ g}} = x \text{ tablet}$
The nurse will give 0.5 tablet.

7. $\dfrac{8.75 \text{ mg}}{1} \times \dfrac{1 \text{ mL}}{2.5 \text{ mg}} = x \text{ mL}$
The nurse will give 3.5 mL.

8. $\dfrac{0.125 \text{ mg}}{1} \times \dfrac{1 \text{ pill}}{0.05 \text{ mg}} = x \text{ pill}$
The nurse will give 2.5 pills.

9. 600 mg

10. 2 tsp

11. 0.75 mL

12. 4.5 mL

13. 0.7 ounce

14. 2 tablets

15. 5 bottles

16. 3 capsules

17. 4 tablets each day

18. 3 tsp

19. 0.75 mL

20. 0.5 oz

Chapter 8: The Formula Method

APPLY LEARNED KNOWLEDGE 8.1 (P. 126)

1. Dosage strength =
$\dfrac{10 \text{ mg}}{1 \text{ tablet}}$ H = 10 mg   Q = 1 tablet

2. Dosage strength =
$\dfrac{250 \text{ mg}}{5 \text{ mL}}$ H = 250 mg   Q = 5 mL

3. Dosage strength =
$\dfrac{12.5 \text{ mg}}{1 \text{ tablet}}$ H = 12.5 mg   Q = 1 tablet

4. Dosage strength =
$\dfrac{25 \text{ mg}}{1 \text{ mL}}$ or $\dfrac{50 \text{ mg}}{2 \text{ mL}}$ H = 25 mg   Q = 1 mL   or
H = 50 mg   Q = 2 mL

5. Dosage strength =
$\dfrac{25 \text{ mg}}{5 \text{ mL}}$ H = 25 mg   Q = 5 mL

APPLY LEARNED KNOWLEDGE 8.2 (P. 130)

1. $\dfrac{50 \text{ mg}}{25 \text{ mg}} \times 1 \text{ tablet} = x \text{ tablet}$ Administer 2 tablets.

2. $\dfrac{750 \text{ mg}}{250 \text{ mg}} \times 5 \text{ mL} = x \text{ mL}$ Administer 15 mL.

3. $\dfrac{25 \text{ mg}}{12.5 \text{ mg}} \times 1 \text{ tablet} = x \text{ tablet}$ Administer 2 tablets.

4. $\dfrac{0.6 \text{ mg}}{1 \text{ mg}} \times 4 \text{ mL} = x \text{ mL}$ or $\dfrac{0.6 \text{ mg}}{0.25 \text{ mg}} \times 1 \text{ mL} = x \text{ mL}$
Administer 2.4 mL.

5. $\dfrac{200 \text{ mg}}{25 \text{ mg}} \times 5 \text{ mL} = x \text{ mL}$ Administer 40 mL.

APPLY LEARNED KNOWLEDGE 8.3 (P. 135)

1. Administer 0.5 pill.

2. Administer 25 mL.

3. Administer 3 capsules.

4. Administer 2.5 tsp.

5. Administer 1.6 ounces.

APPLY LEARNED KNOWLEDGE 8.4 (P. 138)

1. Setup: $\dfrac{500 \text{ mcg}}{2.5 \text{ mg}} \times 1 \text{ mL} = x \text{ mL}$ Administer 0.2 mL.

2. Setup: $\dfrac{1 \text{ g}}{200 \text{ mg}} \times 5 \text{ mL} = x \text{ mL}$ Administer 25 mL.

3. Setup: $\dfrac{750 \text{ mg}}{0.5 \text{ g}} \times 15 \text{ mL} = x \text{ Tbs}$ Administer 1.5 Tbs.

4. Setup: $\dfrac{75 \text{ mcg}}{0.5 \text{ mg}} \times 5 \text{ mL} = x \text{ mL}$ Administer 0.75 mL.

5. Setup: $\dfrac{80 \text{ mg}}{0.4 \text{ g}} \times 1 \text{ oz} = x \text{ mL}$ Administer 6 mL.

CLINICAL REASONING 8.1 (P. 139)

The patient is taking the correct amount of medication. The label on the Griseofulvin Oral Suspension bottle gives two dosage strengths: $\dfrac{125 \text{ mg}}{5 \text{ mL}}$ and $\dfrac{125 \text{ mg}}{1 \text{ teaspoon}}$. Either of these equivalent dosage strengths can be used to set up the problem. Conversions are needed to change the following measurements: tsp to mL and tsp to Tbs.

DEVELOPING COMPETENCY (P. 140)

1. 5 mg/tablet $\dfrac{\overset{\text{ordered}}{\underset{\boxed{5 \text{ mg}}}{\text{amount}}}}{} \times \boxed{1 \text{ tablet}} = x \text{ tablet}$

2. 750 mg/tablet $\dfrac{\overset{\text{ordered}}{\underset{\boxed{750 \text{ mg}}}{\text{amount}}}}{} \times \boxed{1 \text{ tablet}} = x \text{ tablet}$

3. 125 mcg/tablet or 0.125 mg/tablet

$\dfrac{\overset{\text{ordered}}{\underset{\boxed{\substack{125 \text{ mcg} \\ \text{or} \\ 0.125 \text{ mg}}}}{\text{amount}}}}{} \times \boxed{1 \text{ tablet}} = x \text{ tablet}$

4. Yes, the setup is correct.

5. No, the setup is not correct. The D and the H are not in the correct place in the formula. The correct setup is:

$\dfrac{700 \text{ g}}{350 \text{ g}} \times 1 \text{ tablet} = x \text{ tablet}$

6. $\dfrac{0.125 \text{ g}}{0.25 \text{ g}} \times 1 \text{ tablet} = x \text{ tablet}$

The nurse will give 0.5 tablet.

7. $\dfrac{8.75 \text{ mg}}{2.5 \text{ mg}} \times \text{ mL} = x \text{ mL}$ The nurse will give 3.5 mL.

8. $\dfrac{0.125 \text{ mg}}{0.05 \text{ mg}} \times 1 \text{ pill} = x \text{ pill}$

The nurse will give 2.5 pills.

9. 600 mg

10. 2 tsp

11. 0.75 mL

12. 4.5 mL

13. 0.7 ounce

14. 2 tablets

15. 5 bottles

16. 3 capsules

17. 4 tablets each day

18. 3 tsp

19. 0.75 mL

20. 0.5 oz

Chapter 9: Calculating Oral Medication Doses

APPLY LEARNED KNOWLEDGE 9.1 (P. 156)

1. a, b, e, f

2. f

3. a

4. b

5. c, d

APPLY LEARNED KNOWLEDGE 9.2 (P. 161)

1. 4 tablets

2. 10 mL

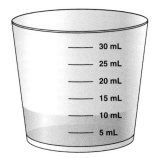

3. 1.5 tablets

4. 1.5 tablets

5. 2 tablets

APPLY LEARNED KNOWLEDGE 9.3 (P. 165)

1. Yes

2. One-half tablet

3. 10 mL

4.

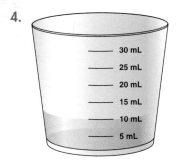

5. 10 mL

APPLY LEARNED KNOWLEDGE 9.4 (P. 169)

1. 1 tablespoon

2. 0.5 ounce

3.

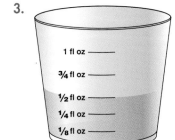

4. 6 tsp

5. 1 ounce

CLINICAL REASONING 9.1 (P. 173)

No, the nurse needs to consider that the patient is on a daily dose of 0.075 mg. The ordered dose is equivalent to 75 mcg and is within the usual maintenance dose.

DEVELOPING COMPETENCY (P. 173)

1. 1.5 mL

2. 170 mL

3. 200 mL

4. Yes, the medication is a suspension.

5. No, the nurse can administer the ordered amount (2 tsp).

6. 3 tsp; **a.** medicine cup

7. 2 tablets; **c.** place the tablets under the tongue

8. 2 tablets; **b.** active ingredient is released slowly

9. **c.** Time of reconstitution; **d.** Nurse's initials; **e.** Date of reconstitution

10. **b.** The bottle needs to be shaken well; **c.** 2.5 mL will be administered; **e.** For enteral use only

11. **d.** A conversion is not necessary; **e.** For enteral use only

12. 5 mL; 2.5 mL

13. 24 mL; **a.** The nurse may store the drug in the refrigerator; **b.** The nurse may use this reconstituted drug.

14. 2 tablets

15. 2 capsules

16. **a.** administering one tablet of the 6.25 mg dose. *Coreg 12.5 mg is not a scored tablet.*

17. **c.** calling the pharmacist.

18. 4 mL

19. **c.** Clarifying the drug with the pharmacist. *The order is for Ceftin oral suspension and cephalexin oral suspension is available.*

20. 3 teaspoons

Chapter 10: Syringes and Needles

APPLY LEARNED KNOWLEDGE 10.1 (P. 183)

1. Syringe A. *The TB syringe can only measure up to 1 mL of medication. The 3 mL syringe will accurately draw up 1.2 mL of medication.*

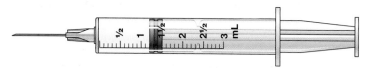

2. Syringe A or B. *Either syringe will accurately draw up 0.4 mL of medication.*

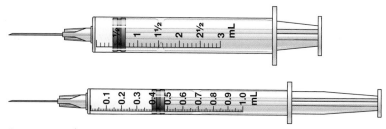

3. Syringe B. *The 3 mL syringe cannot accurately measure hundredths of a mL (0.15 mL). Only the TB syringe can measure to the hundredths of a mL.*

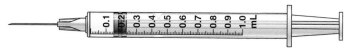

4. Syringe A or B. *Either syringe will accurately draw up 1 mL of medication.*

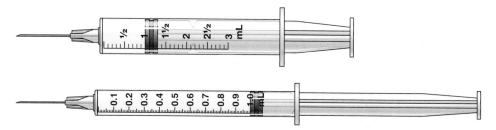

5. Syringe B. *Only the TB syringe can measure 0.25 mL accurately. The nurse never estimates between calibration lines.*

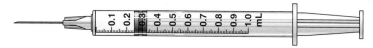

APPLY LEARNED KNOWLEDGE 10.2 (P. 186)

1. False. *The main difference between these two common syringes is that the 3 mL syringe measures tenths of a mL and the 1 mL syringe measures hundredths of a mL.*

2. True

3. True

4. False. *The calibration lines on all syringes measure accurately, regardless of the volume of the syringe (1 mL, 3 mL, etc.).*

5. False. *The 20, 30, 50, and 60 mL syringes measure ounces in addition to mL.*

APPLY LEARNED KNOWLEDGE 10.3 (P. 189)

1. b. 25G 5/8" *This is the standard subcut syringe and needle.*

2. c. 3 mL 23G 2" *The needle on this syringe is the correct gauge for IM injection. The needle is long enough to deliver the medication deep IM in this obese patient.*

3. d. 1 mL 26G 1/2" *This syringe has a short needle with a small gauge. It is a standard ID syringe and needle.*

4. c. 22G 1 1/2" *This is the standard IM needle size.*

5. d. 3 mL 19G 1" *This syringe has a long enough needle to withdraw medication from a vial. The needle gauge is large enough to withdraw the medication easily. The needle will be removed prior to direct IV injection.*

CLINICAL REASONING 10.1 (P. 190)

The nurse has given the wife the correct feedback. The ordered dose is contained in 0.6 mL. The wife has drawn up 0.06 mL into the syringe. The nurse points to the 0.6 mL calibration line and reinforces that each small line measures one-hundredth of a mL.

DEVELOPING COMPETENCY (P. 190)

1. The syringe measures 0.25 mL
2. The syringe measures 2.2 mL
3. The syringe measures 0.2 mL
4. The syringe measures 0.2 mL
5. The syringe measures 4.2 mL
6. The syringe measures 3.2 mL
7. The syringe measures 8 mL
8. The syringe measures 32 mL
9. 0.68 mL
10. 0.5 mL
11. 1.8 mL
12. 2.2 mL
13. 0.33 mL
14. 3.2 mL

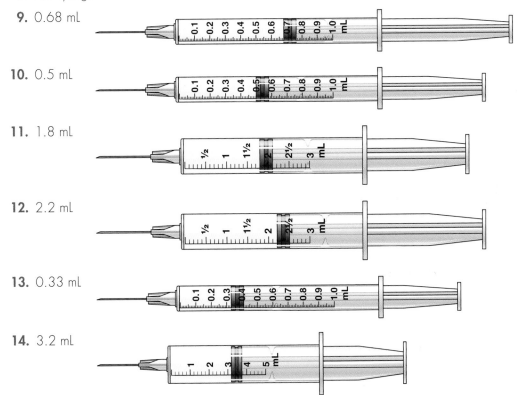

15. 18 mL

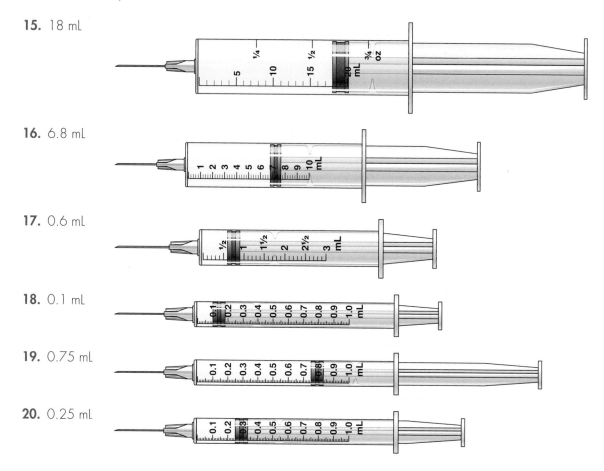

16. 6.8 mL

17. 0.6 mL

18. 0.1 mL

19. 0.75 mL

20. 0.25 mL

Chapter 11: Calculating Parenteral Medication Doses

APPLY LEARNED KNOWLEDGE 11.1 (P. 200)

1. False. *The nurse is most correct to choose a 1 mL syringe and draw up the medication to the 0.95 calibration line.*

2. True. *The space in a prefilled syringe allows the nurse to add another compatible medication. This way the patient will receive two ordered medications with only one injection.*

3. False. *The beyond-use date or discard date, not the expiration date, is used once a multi-dose vial has been punctured.*

4. False. *All single use vials should be discarded after the first dose is withdrawn.*

5. False. *If the opened multi-use vial has no information about the date, time, initials, or beyond-use date, the vial must be discarded.*

APPLY LEARNED KNOWLEDGE 11.2 (P. 207)

1. 0.75 mL

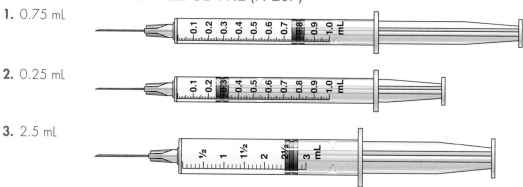

2. 0.25 mL

3. 2.5 mL

4. 0.6 mL

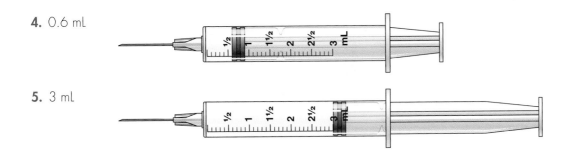

5. 3 mL

APPLY LEARNED KNOWLEDGE 11.3 (P. 214)

1. 0.1 mL

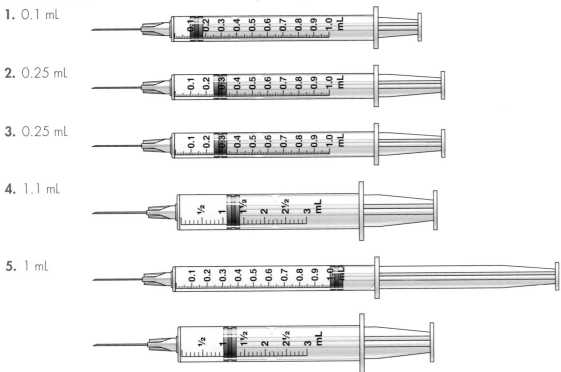

2. 0.25 mL

3. 0.25 mL

4. 1.1 mL

5. 1 mL

CLINICAL REASONING 11.1 (P. 216)

This drug is labeled with three possible dosage strengths: 250 mcg/5 mL, 50 mcg/mL, and 0.05 mg/mL. Any one of these can be used to calculate the dosage. The first nurse's calculation was correct. The second nurse used a correct dosage strength, but made a decimal point error in the calculation. The nurses should recheck their math and consult with a pharmacist if any question about the dosage remains.

DEVELOPING COMPETENCY (P. 217)

1. 1.6 mL

2. 1.5 mL

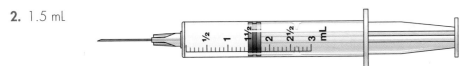

3. 0.5 mL; **a. & b.** The nurse can draw up the dose in either the 1 mL or the 3 mL syringe.

4. 2.1 mL

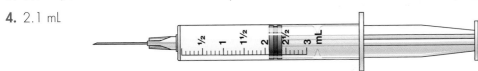

5. **a.** A conversion is not necessary. **d.** The nurse should write date, time, initials, and beyond-use date on the vial after withdrawing the dose. *The ordered dose is contained in 22.5 mL and the 30 mL syringe should be used to withdraw the dose from the vial.*

6. 0.15 mL

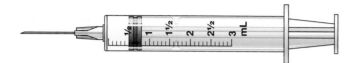

7. Discard 0.5 mL; Administer 1.5 mL

8. 1.5 mL; Label should include the date and time the vial was opened, the initials of the nurse, and the beyond-use date.

9. 0.75 mL

10. 0.5 mL

11. The nurse has calculated the doses of the three medications correctly. The heparin sodium and morphine vials should be labeled with the date, time, the nurse's initials, and the beyond-use date as they are multi-dose vials. The ondansetron vial should be discarded as it is for single use.

12. 2.4 mL

13. Administer 1 mL; Discard 1 mL

14. **a.** A conversion is needed. **b.** Two dosage strengths are listed on the vial. **d.** The 10 mL syringe is the best choice to measure the ordered dose. *8 mL will be administered.*

15. 0.25 mL

16. 0.75 mL

17. Administer 3 mL; There is no need to discard any medication.

18. **a.** The nurse has a choice of dosage strengths to use in the calculation. **b.** There are two possible routes for this medication. **d.** Once opened, the vial can be stored in the refrigerator and used again. *0.45 mL of lorazepam will be drawn up in the syringe, but it must be diluted before administering the medication.*

19. 1.6 mL

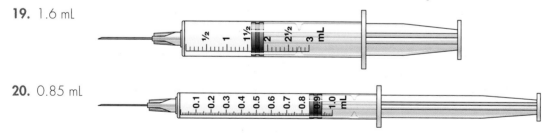

20. 0.85 mL

Chapter 12: Preparing Powdered Parenteral Medications

APPLY LEARNED KNOWLEDGE 12.1 (P. 228)

1. True

2. False. *Sterile Water for Injection is the diluent solution.*

3. False. *The dosage strength is 330 mg/mL. The nurse should not use the total amount of the drug or the volume of diluent as the dosage strength.*

4. False. *330 mg/mL is the dosage strength for the IM reconstitution directions. If the route is IV, the nurse needs to consult the package insert for reconstitution directions and dosage strength.*

5. True

APPLY LEARNED KNOWLEDGE 12.2 (P. 232)

1. a. 250 mg/1.5 mL

2. d. 3 mL

3. c. 2.4 mL

4. c. 1.8 mL

5. c. 1.3 mL

APPLY LEARNED KNOWLEDGE 12.3 (P. 235)

1. *Dosage strength: 250 mg/mL; Administer: 1.4 mL.*

2. *Dosage strength: 125 mg/mL; Administer: 4.8 mL.*

3. *Dosage strength: 500,000 units/mL; Administer: 0.4 mL.*

4. *Dosage strength: 250,000 units/mL; Administer: 0.8 mL.*

5. If 3.5 mL of diluent is added, the nurse will administer 1.5 mL.

   If 6.8 mL of diluent is added, the nurse will administer 3 mL.

CLINICAL REASONING 12.1 (P. 241)

A, B, and D are correct. *The correct dose of Dacarbazine to administer is 17.5 mL IV. The vial is a single-dose vial, so after the dose of medication is withdrawn from the vial, the remaining amount of medication should have been discarded not stored.*

DEVELOPING COMPETENCY (P. 242)

1. *Amount of diluent: 10 mL; Dosage strength: 160 mg/mL; Administer: 6.3 mL (6.25 mL)*

2. *Type of diluent: sterile water for injection; Dosage strength: 500 mg/10 mL; Potency: reconstituted medication can be used for only 4 hours after reconstitution*

3. 0900 on 2/19/xx

4. *Amount of diluent: 10 mL; Dosage strength: 100 mg/mL; Administer: 7.5 mL*

5. *Amount of diluent: 8.3 mL; Dosage strength: 90 mg/mL; Administer: 5.6 mL*

6. *Dosage strength: 125 mg/2 mL; This is a single-dose vial so the mixed medication should be discarded.*

7. Add 6.6 mL diluent; *Administer: 1.6 mL*

8. *Amount of diluent: 5.3 mL; Dosage strength: 100 mg/mL; Administer: 3.5 mL*

9. 5/24/xx

10. *Amount of diluent: 3.2 mL; Dosage strength: 1,000,000 units/mL; Administer: 0.4 mL*

11. *Amount of diluent: 1.8 mL; Administer: 1.6 mL*

12. *Amount and type of diluent: Add 5 mL of 0.9% Sodium Chloride Injection without preservatives to each vial; Dosage strength: 38 mg/mL; Administer: 20 mL; If stored at room temperature, the solution will remain stable for 24 hours, but if a dose is withdrawn, the vial should be discarded as it is a single-dose vial.*

13. *Dosage strength: 500 mg/mL; Administer: 1.5 mL*

14. *Dosage strength: 100 mg/2 mL; Administer: 1.6 mL*

15. 24 hours at room temperature or 48 hours if refrigerated.

16. *Dosage strength: 100 mg/mL; Administer: 5 mL; Reconstituted medication can be stored for 24 hours at room temperature or 7 days if refrigerated.*

17. *Amount of diluent: 75 mL; Dosage strength: 250,000 units/mL; Administer: 4.8 mL; Store in refrigerator.*

18. *Amount of diluent: 2 mL; Volume of displacement: 0.2 mL; Administer: 2 mL*

19. *Dosage strength: 180 mg/mL; Administer: 10 mL*

20. *Amount of diluent: 19.2 mL; Dosage strength: 100 mg/mL; Administer: 10 mL*

Chapter 13: Administering Insulin

APPLY LEARNED KNOWLEDGE 13.1 (P. 259)

1. Humalog Mix 75/25

2. Humulin R

3. Levemir

4. Humalog

5. Novolin N

APPLY LEARNED KNOWLEDGE 13.2 (P. 264)

1. The 50 unit insulin syringe is the most appropriate to measure 7 units of insulin.

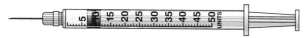

2. The 50 unit insulin syringe and the 100 unit insulin syringes are appropriate to 26 units of insulin.

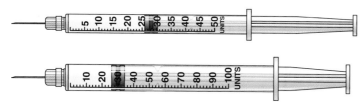

3. The 30 unit insulin syringe is the most appropriate to measure 4 units of insulin. The 100 unit insulin syringe can also measure 4 units but the 30 unit insulin syringe, if available, is easier to read the calibrations.

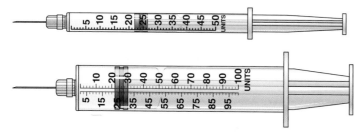

4. The 50 unit insulin syringe and the 100 unit dual insulin syringe may be used to measure 22 units of insulin.

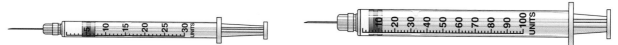

5. The 50 unit insulin syringe is the most appropriate to measure 31 units of insulin.

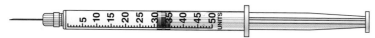

CLINICAL REASONING 13.1 (P. 266)

C. *The insulin available in the refrigerator is not the same as the insulin ordered by the physician. The nurse needs to obtain the correct insulin before drawing up any insulin into an insulin syringe.*

DEVELOPING COMPETENCY (P. 266)

1. Incorrect. *The insulin order includes the number of units of insulin to administer. The nurse will use an insulin syringe, which measures units, to draw the number of units ordered by the physician. A mathematical calculation is not necessary.*

2. Correct.

3. Incorrect. *The nurse may not substitute Novolog for Humalog. The nurse must contact the pharmacist and obtain the ordered insulin.*

4. Incorrect. *Humulin 70/30 is a premixed insulin and should not be mixed with another insulin.*

5. Incorrect. *The 100 unit syringe cannot measure odd-numbered dose of insulin accurately.*

6. Correct.

7. Incorrect. *23 units have been drawn into the 50 unit insulin syringe.*

8. Correct.

9. Incorrect. *31 units have been drawn into the 50 unit insulin syringe.*

10. Incorrect. *44 units have been drawn into the U-100 dual insulin syringe.*

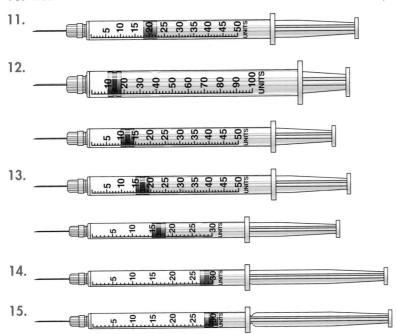

11.

12.

13.

14.

15.

Chapter 14: Intravenous Therapy and Infusion Rates

APPLY LEARNED KNOWLEDGE 14.1 (P. 285)

1. Correct. *This is a primary IV (a large volume continuous IV used to administer fluids and electrolytes). A primary IV infusion set is the correct choice.*

2. Incorrect. *This is a large volume primary IV. When the first liter has infused, the nurse should hang another liter bag of ½ NS.*

3. Incorrect. *An order for an IVPB does not typically include the type or amount of IV solution used to dilute the medication. This is determined by the drug manufacturer if the IV medication is premixed, or by the pharmacist using the available drug reference information.*

4. Incorrect. *This is a primary IV containing the electrolye KCl. A primary IV infusion set is the correct choice.*

5. Correct. *The time in the order (10:00 a.m.) does not provide enough information about the infusion rate of the IV.*

APPLY LEARNED KNOWLEDGE 14.2 (P. 290)

1. 100 mL/hr

2. 150 mL/hr

3. 83 mL/hr

4. 83 mL/hr

5. 125 mL/hr

APPLY LEARNED KNOWLEDGE 14.3 (P. 297)

1. 25 gtt/min

2. 42 gtt/min

3. 42 gtt/min

4. 10 gtt/min

5. 42 gtt/min

CLINICAL REASONING 14.1 (P. 299)

A and C are correct.

The day nurse correctly evaluated that the gravity flow rate of the infusion should be 31 gtt/min:

$$\frac{125 \text{ mL} \times 15 \text{ gtt/mL}}{60 \text{ minutes}} = 31 \text{ gtt/min}$$

When the gravity flow rate was decreased, the IV was correctly adjusted to 19 gtt/min:

$$\frac{75 \text{ mL} \times 15 \text{ gtt/mL}}{60 \text{ minutes}} = 19 \text{ gtt/min}$$

The IV tubing does not need to be changed.

DEVELOPING COMPETENCY (P. 299)

1. a. This IV can be infused by gravity or by an IV pump. No conversion or math is needed as the physician's order specifies the flow rate in mL/hr. If the nurse chooses to run the IV by gravity, the number of gtt/min will need to be calculated, based on the drop factor of the IV tubing. The flow rate of the IV is 13 gtt/min.

2. 100 mL/hr

3. 83 mL/hr
4. 167 mL/hr
5. 15 gtt/min
6. 100 mL/hr
7. 133 mL/hr
8. 33 gtt/min
9. 50 gtt/min
10. 30 gtt/min
11. 13 gtt/min
12. 42 gtt/min
13. 31 gtt/min
14. 63 mL/hr
15. 21 gtt/min
16. 63 mL/hr
17. 16 gtt/min
18. 125 mL/hr
19. 67 mL/hr
20. 125 mL/hr

Chapter 15: Calculating Infusion and Completion Time

APPLY LEARNED KNOWLEDGE 15.1 (P. 309)

1. 8 hours
2. 8 hours 20 min
3. 12 hours 30 min
4. 6 hours 40 min
5. 6 hours 15 min

APPLY LEARNED KNOWLEDGE 15.2 (P. 311)

1. 1515
2. 0825
3. 2330
4. 6:45 p.m.
5. 2:48 a.m.

APPLY LEARNED KNOWLEDGE 15.3 (P. 315)

1.   Start time: 0815
   Infusion time: +0300
   Completion time: 1115

2.   Start time: 2045
   Infusion time: +0800
             2845
   Subtract: −2400
   Completion time: 0445 or 4:45 AM

3.   Start time: 0215
   Infusion time: +1320
   Completion time: 1535

4.   Start time: 1145
   Infusion time: +0830
             1975
   Subtract: −0060
             1915
   +0100 [Add 1 hour (60 minutes subtracted)]
   Completion time: 2015 or 8:15 PM

5.   Start time: 1515
   Infusion time: +0500
   Completion time: 2015

APPLY LEARNED KNOWLEDGE 15.4 (P. 324)

1.

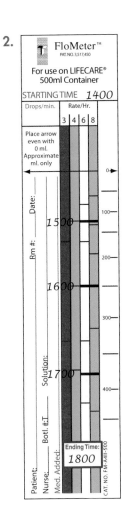

2.

3.

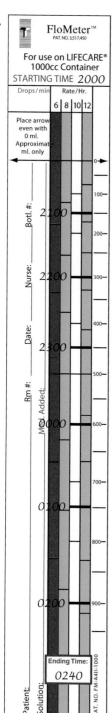

FloMeter™
PAT. NO. 3,517,450

For use on LIFECARE®
1000cc Container

STARTING TIME *2000*

Drops/min	Rate/Hr.
	6 8 10 12

Place arrow
even with
0 ml.
Approximate
ml. only

Botl. #:

Nurse:

Date:

Rm #:

Med. Added:

2100

2200

2300

0000

0100

0200

0 →

100

200

300

400

500

600

700

800

900

Ending Time:
0240

Patient:

Solution:

CAT. NO. FM-A4II-1000

4. Infusion time: 13 hours 20 minutes

5. Completion time: 1120

CLINICAL REASONING 15.1 (P. 327)

The completion time for this IV is 1330 not 1230. The nurse needs to review the line markings on the flow meter to ensure the hourly markings are correct based on the mL/hr and recalculate the completion time.

DEVELOPING COMPETENCY (P. 328)

1. 20 hours

2. 1900 (7:00 p.m.)

3. 8 hours 20 minutes

4. 1520 (3:20 p.m.)

5. 6 hours 15 min

6. 0845 (8:45 a.m.)

7. 1730 (5:30 p.m.)

8. 9:45 p.m.

9. 625 mL

10. 300 mL

11. 350 mL

12. 475 mL

13. 575 mL

14. 300 mL

15. c. incorrect hourly marking

16. c. incorrect hourly marking

17. a. missing the start time

18. a. The hourly fluid level is marked correctly;
    b. The end time is correct; e. By 0730, approximately 375 mL have infused.

19. 1 liter D₅W is started at 150 mL/hr at 1830.

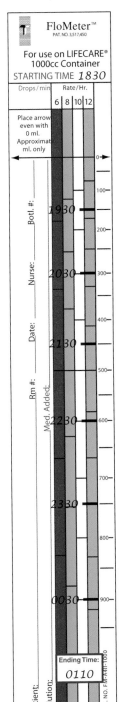

20. 1,000 mL 0.9% NS is started at 125 mL/hr at 1345.

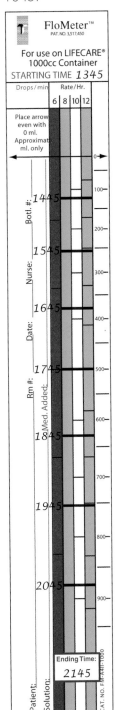

Chapter 16: Administering Direct IV Medications

APPLY LEARNED KNOWLEDGE 16.1 (P. 344)

1. Add 1 mL of diluent to the medication in the syringe.

2. Add 6 mL of diluent to the medication in the syringe.

3. Add 3 mL of diluent to the medication in the syringe.

4. Add 2 mL of diluent to the medication in syringe.

5. Add 0.5 mL of diluent to the medication in syringe.

APPLY LEARNED KNOWLEDGE 16.2 (P. 351)

1. Administer over 30 seconds.

2. Administer over 5 minutes.

3. Administer over 2 minutes.

4. Administer over 1 to 5 minutes.

5. Administer over 2 minutes.

CLINICAL REASONING 16.1 (P. 351)

A. Correct in calculating the dosage of the medication.

B. Correct in calculating the amount of diluent to add to the syringe.

E. Incorrect; the rate of administration should be 2 minutes *to avoid hypotension and cardiac arrest in this elderly patient.*

DEVELOPING COMPETENCY (P. 352)

1. Add 16 mL of diluent.

2. Administer over 4 minutes.

3. Administer over 1 minute.

4. Administer over 1 minute.

5. Add 5 mL of diluent.

6. Administer over 60 seconds or 1 minute.

7. Add 5 mL of diluent.

8. Administer over 5 minutes.

9. Administer over 1 minute.

10. Administer over 2 to 4 minutes.

11. Add 15 mL of diluent.

12. Administer over 3 to 5 minutes.

13. Add 0.25 mL of diluent.

14. The most rapid rate of administration is 1 minute.

15. 8 mg of IV Reglan does not need to be diluted prior to administration.

16. Administer over 2 minutes.

17. The nurse has a choice about whether to dilute the medication or not.

18. Administer over 2 minutes.

19. Administer over 30 seconds.

20. Administer over 7 minutes.

Chapter 17: Verifying Safe Dose

APPLY LEARNED KNOWLEDGE 17.1 (P. 372)

1. 125 mcg IVP daily. Ordered dose is not safe

2. 680 mg PO daily. Ordered dose is safe.

3. 13 to 26 mg IVP q.4h prn. Ordered dose is not safe.

4. 5 mcg IVP bid. Ordered dose is safe.

5. 1.6 g PO daily. Ordered dose is safe.

APPLY LEARNED KNOWLEDGE 17.2 (P. 377)

1. 140 to 280 mg q.8h. The ordered dose is a safe dose.

2. 780 mcg. The ordered dose of 0.8 mg (800 mcg) is not a safe dose. *The nurse will need to clarify the order with the physician prior to administering the medication.*

3. 309.09 mcg. The ordered dose is a safe dose.

4. 270 mg for the initial dose, followed by 135 mg daily for 2 weeks. The initial ordered dose is greater than the recommended dose and the physician should be consulted prior to administration of the medication. The subsequent daily doses, given daily for 2 weeks, are safe doses.

5. 14.5 mg for the initial dose. The initial ordered dose is greater than the recommended dose and the physician should be consulted prior to administration of the medication.

APPLY LEARNED KNOWLEDGE 17.3 (P. 385)

1. 57 mg on the first day of chemotherapy. The ordered dose is more than the recommended dose and the physician should be consulted prior to administration of the medication.

2. 51 mg on days 1, 2, and 3 of chemotherapy. The ordered dose is safe.

3. 2 units for the first two doses of chemotherapy, followed by 21 to 42 units weekly. The ordered dose is safe.

4. 2 units for the first two weekly doses of chemotherapy, followed by 17.5 to 35 units weekly on Tuesdays. The ordered initial doses are safe, but the subsequent doses exceed the calculated recommended dose. The nurse will need to clarify the order with the physician prior to administering the medication.

5. 666 mg after the dose of leucovorin. The ordered dose is safe.

CLINICAL REASONING 17.1 (P. 386)

C. Not correct; the nurse should call the physician because 500 mg is more than the recommended dose and is not a safe dose.
The safe initial dose of medication for this patient who weighs 40 kg is 200 to 300 mg twice a day. (10 to 15 mg/kg/day x 40 kg, divided into 2 doses = 200 to 300 mg twice a day.) The ordered dose is more than the recommended initial dose. The ordered dose would be safe if the patient had been taking the medication for several weeks, but the dose is not safe as an initial dose.

DEVELOPING COMPETENCY (P. 387)

1. a. The recommended adult IV dose of daptomycin has to be calculated.
b. A conversion is needed if the patient's weight is in lb.
c. If the physician ordered this drug for a 15 year old who weighs 50 kg, the usual dose would be 200 mg every 24 hours.
d. If the physician ordered this drug for a 79 year old who weighs 82 kg, the usual dose would be 328 mg every 24 hours.

2. a. The recommended initial dose of diltiazem hydrochloride is a weight-based dose.
c. If the physician ordered this drug for a patient who weighs 110 lb, the usual initial IV dose would be 12.5 mg.
d. If the physician ordered this drug for a patient who weighs 75 kg, the usual dose would be 18.75 mg.

3. b. 0.2 mg

4. The recommended dosage range of cefoxitin for this patient is 199.5 to 400.5 mg q.4h.

5. The ordered dose of doxycycline calcium syrup is a safe dose.

6. The ordered dose of paclitaxel is a safe dose.

7. The ordered dose of cefoxitin is not a safe dose. The maximum usual dose for this child is 1,068 mg q.4h. The nurse would need to contact the physician to clarify the ordered dose.

8. The ordered dose of cefazolin is a safe dose.

9. The nurse would need to determine if the bupropion had been given twice a day for three days. If so, the ordered dose of bupropion, given three times a day, is a safe dose.

10. The ordered dose of DOXOrubicin (0.15 g or 150 mg) is more than the recommended dose for this patient (102–127.5 mg). The ordered dose is not safe. The nurse will need to contact the physician to clarify the order.

11. The usual maintenance dose of interferon alfa-2b is 17.5 million International Units subcut 3 times weekly. The ordered dose is not a safe dose. The nurse will need to contact the physician to clarify the ordered dose.

12. It would not be safe to give an infusion of decitabine 27 mg IV without clarifying the patient's BSA. There is a discrepancy between the patient's recorded height and weight and the documented BSA. For a patient who is 5 feet 9 inches and weighs 130 lb, formula calculation of the BSA would be 1.69 m^2. The safe dose of decitabine for a patient with a BSA of 1.69 m^2 is 25.35 mg. The nurse would need to reweigh and measure the patient and recheck the BSA calculation before determining the safe dose for this patient.

13. The dose of Dilantin is a safe dose.

14. The dose of azithromycin is a safe dose.

15. The dose of amiodarone is a safe dose; however it falls below the recommended guidelines for a patient who has received IV amiodarone for 1 to 3 weeks. The nurse would need to contact the physician to verify the effectiveness of the ordered dose.

16. The ordered dose of doxorubicin liposomal exceeds the recommended dosage range of 62 to 77.5 mg for a patient with a BSA of 1.55. The nurse would need to contact the physician to clarify the ordered dose.

17. The ordered dose of fluconazole does fall within the recommended dosing guidelines for a neonate who is less than 2 weeks old. If 12 mg/kg (dose for older children) is used for the calculation, the recommended dose would be 36 mg q.72h. The ordered dose of 30 mg IV is less than the recommended dose, therefore it is a safe dose for the neonate.

18. The nurse should hold the dose of eribulin and contact the physician to clarify the order. Because of the patient's low platelet count, the recommended dose is reduced to 1.1 mg/m^2. The maximum safe dose for this patient would be 1.61 mg.

19. The ordered dose of clonazepam is a safe dose.

20. The nurse's actions were correct. Both the induction and the maintenance ordered doses of methotrexate are safe doses.

Chapter 18: Titration of Intravenous Medications

APPLY LEARNED KNOWLEDGE 18.1 (P. 398)

1. **a.** This is an order for a primary IV.

2. **b.** This is an order for titration of a drug. **c.** The drug will be titrated per protocol.

3. **a.** Initial dose of infusion rate.

4. **a.** Initial dose or infusion rate. **b.** Titration parameter for adjustment of dose. **c.** Time interval for adjustment of dose. **d.** Patient response or goal. **e.** Maximum dose limits.

5. **a.** Initial dose or infusion rate. **b.** Titration parameter for adjustment of dose. **d.** Patient response or goal.

APPLY LEARNED KNOWLEDGE 18.2 (P. 406)

1. 48 mL/hr

2. 20 mL/hr

3. 6 mL/hr

4. 50 mL/hr

5. 5 mL/hr

CLINICAL REASONING 18.1 (P. 414)

B. Set the infusion rate on the IV pump at 30 mL/hr.

C. Have a second nurse validate the calculation before starting the infusion.

E. Recheck the patient's BP 15 minutes after the start of the infusion.
   A and D are incorrect. The calculation is incorrect and the patient's BP needs to be assessed prior to determining if titration of the dose is necessary.

DEVELOPING COMPETENCY (P. 415)

1. TD: 120 mg

2. HD: 10 mg/hr

3. 50 mL/hr

4. TD: unit of measurement is mg
   HD: unit of measurement is mcg

5. 6 mL/hr

6. 3 mL/hr

7. 6 mL/hr

8. 1 mL/hr

9. 20 mL/hr

10. Keep the heparin at the current rate, 24 mL/hr.

11. 18 mL/hr (17.5 mL/hr rounded to a whole number). (The HD is decreased by 150 units/hr = 350 units/hr)

12. Preliminary calculations:
    (1) Identify the weight-based dose:
        2.5 mcg/kg/min = 150 mcg/min
    (2) Convert the units (mcg to mg):
        150 mcg/min = 0.15 mg/min
    (3) Convert min to hr: 0.15 mg/min = 9 mg/hr

13. 18 mL/hr

14. 36 mL/hr is the adjusted rate. (The initial rate is 18 mL/hr. The increased rate is 18 mL/hr.)

15. Preliminary calculations:
    (1) Convert lb to kg: 176 lb = 80 kg
    (2) Identify the weight-based dose:
        0.3 mcg/kg/min = 24 mcg/min
    (3) Convert the units (mcg to mg):
        24 mcg/min = 0.024 mg/min
    (4) Convert min to hr: 0.024 mg/min = 1.44 mg/hr

16. 7 mL/hr (7.2 mL/hr rounded to a whole number)

17. 2 mL/hr (2.4 mL/hr rounded to a whole number)

18. Preliminary calculations:
    (1) Identify the weight-based dose:
        0.01 mcg/kg/min = 0.7 mcg/min
    (2) Convert the units (mcg to mg):
        0.7 mcg/min = 0.0007 mg/min
    (3) Convert min to hr:
        0.0007 mg/min = 0.042 mg/hr

19. 7 mL/hr

20. 4 mL/hr (3.5 mL/hr rounded to a whole number)

Chapter 19: Calculating Intake and Output

APPLY LEARNED KNOWLEDGE 19.1 (P. 426)

1. True

2. False. *Equivalent to 45 mL. Use the metric equivalent of 15 mL equals 1 Tbs.*

3. True

4. False. *Equivalent to 20 mL. Use the metric equivalent of 5 mL equals 1 t (tsp).*

5. True

APPLY LEARNED KNOWLEDGE 19.2 (P. 428)

1. Incorrect. **Answer:** 60 mL *(Use the metric equivalent: 1 tbs = 15 mL)*

2. Incorrect. **Answer:** 120 mL *(Remember that ice chips melt to one-half their original volume.)*

3. Correct

4. Correct

5. Incorrect. **Answer:** 480 mL *(The nurse gave the patient two feedings of 240 mL each.)*

APPLY LEARNED KNOWLEDGE 19.3 (P. 431)

1. False. *The output has been recorded in the wrong categories.*

2. True

3. True

4. False. *The gastric tube drainage is listed as emesis instead of gastric drainage.*

5. True

APPLY LEARNED KNOWLEDGE 19.4 (P. 435)

1. True

2. False. *The actual urine output is 535 mL. The amount recorded is the amount of irrigant not the amount of urine. (775 mL – 240 mL = 535 mL)*

3. True

4. False. *The actual urine output is 750 mL. Normal Saline irrigation infused for 6 hours (7:00 a.m. to 10:00 a.m. and again from 12:00 p.m. to 3:00 p.m.) at 50 mL/hr = 300 mL of irrigant. (1050 mL – 300 mL = 750 mL)*

5. True

CLINICAL REASONING 19.1 (P. 436)

The nurse will have the patient take 960 mL of tea for the evening shift.

DEVELOPING COMPETENCY (P. 437)

1. 540 mL

2. 420 mL *(Ice chips melt to one-half the starting amount.)*

3. 1,020 mL

4. 800 mL

5. 650 mL

6.

Name R. Patient   Age 87   MR # 899326   Room 108-A

Intake and Output Worksheet

Shift	Oral	Urine	Emesis	Drainage	Other
7-3		180			
		435			
Total (mL)		615			

7.

Name Q. Patient   Age 59   MR # 385248   Room 222

Intake and Output Worksheet

Shift	Oral	Urine	Emesis	Drainage	Other
7-3		325	200		
		175			
Total (mL)		500	200		

8.

Name A. Patient   Age 34   MR # 552681   Room 541

Intake and Output Worksheet

Shift	Oral	Urine	Emesis	Drainage	Other
3-11		300		(NG)	
		175		250	
Total (mL)		475		250	

9. 675 mL

10. 800 mL

11.

Name _M. Patient_ Age _18_ MR # _75412_ Room _125_

Intake and Output Worksheet

Shift	Oral	Urine	Emesis	Drainage	Other
7-3	180	225		(Wound)	
	240	150			
	120				
	240				
	180				
Total (mL)	960	375		30	

12.

Name _S. Patient_ Age _55_ MR # _25610_ Room _131-B_

Intake and Output Worksheet

Shift	Oral	Urine	Emesis	Drainage	Other
7-3	180	(catheter)			
	180				
	270				
	180				
	500				
Total (mL)	1310	550			

13.

Name _J. Patient_ Age _48_ MR # _325487_ Room _327_

Intake and Output Worksheet

Shift	Oral	Tube	Urine	Emesis	Other
11-7		(feeding) 600			
		(H20) 100			
Total (mL)		700			

14.

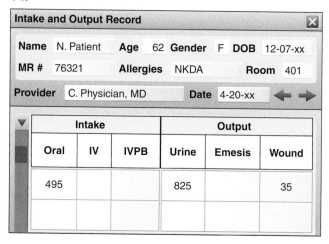

15.

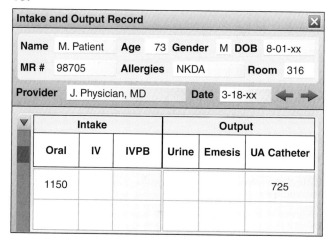

Chapter 20: Parenteral Intake

APPLY LEARNED KNOWLEDGE 20.1 (P. 447)

1. 300 mL (50 mL / hr × 6 hr) from 0800–1400

2. 625 mL (125 mL / hr × 5 hr) from 1700–2200

3. 500 mL (1600–2000 at 75 mL / hr × 4 hr) & (2000–2200 at 100 mL / hr × 2 hr)

4. 300 mL (0100–0200 at 100 mL / hr × 1 hr) & (0200–0600 at 50 mL / hr × 4 hr)

5. 581 mL (83 mL / hr × 7 hr)

APPLY LEARNED KNOWLEDGE 20.2 (P. 451)

1. (A) 100 mL; (B) 100 mL

2. (A) 350 mL; (B) 100 mL

3. (A) 50 mL; (B) 50 mL

4. 150 mL

5. 0 (zero). *An IVPB is not scheduled for this shift.*

CLINICAL REASONING 20.1 (P. 455)

B. The nurse is correct in initially clarifying the documentation of the whole blood since, according to the intake and output record, no entry for the whole blood has been documented.

DEVELOPING COMPETENCY (P. 455)

1. 450 mL (IV started at 1100 and infused until 1400 = 3 hrs x 150 mL/hr)

2. 750 mL (IV started at 1600 and infused until 2200 = 6 hrs x 125 mL/hr)

3. 350 mL (IV started at 0200 at 75 mL/hr until 0400 = 2 hrs x 75 mL/hr = 150 mL; IV rate increased from 0400–0600 = 2 hrs x 100 mL = 200 mL)

4. 900 mL (IV started at 0700 at 150 mL/hr until 1100 = 4 hrs x 150 mL/hr = 600 mL; IV rate decreased from 1100–1400 = 3 hrs x 100 mL = 300 mL)

5. 300 mL (IV started at 1700 at 100 mL/hr until 2000 = 3 hrs x 100 mL/hr = 300 mL; IV is discontinued from 2000–2200 and restarted at 2200 at the same rate. Since the I & O is closed at 2200 no further parenteral intake is recorded for 1500–2300.

6. 300 mL (IV started at 0900 at 75 mL/hr until 1200 = 3 hrs x 75 mL/hr = 225 mL; IV is restarted at 1300. From 1300–1400 = 1 hr x 75 mL = 75 mL)

7. (A) 150 mL (0700–1500 shift); (B) 100 mL (1500–2300 shift)

8. (A) 50 mL (0700–1500 shift); (B) 50 mL (1500–2300 shift)

9. (A) 150 mL (0700–1500 shift); (B) 150 mL (1500–2300 shift); (C) 100 mL (2300–0700 shift)

10.

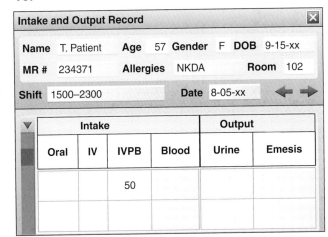

Intake				Output	
Oral	IV	IVPB	Blood	Urine	Emesis
		50			

Intake and Output Record

Name T. Patient Age 57 Gender F DOB 9-15-xx
MR # 234371 Allergies NKDA Room 102
Shift 1500–2300 Date 8-05-xx

11. a. 600 mL

12. b. 550 mL

13. c. 1,000 mL

14. a. 600 mL

15. b. 575 mL

Chapter 21: Considerations for the Pediatric Population

APPLY LEARNED KNOWLEDGE 21.1 (P. 471)

1. True

2. False. *The PO dose of Zofran for children 4 to 11 years is identified as 4 mg and not based on weight.*

3. False. *The IV dose of 4 mg is recommended for post-operative nausea and vomiting for children between the age range of 1 mo to 12 yr and over 40 kg.*

4. False. *The IV dose of 0.1 mg/kg is recommended for children 1 month to 12 years who weigh ≤40 kg. The symbol, "≤", signifies less than or equal to.*

5. True

APPLY LEARNED KNOWLEDGE 21.2 (P. 476)

1. 75 mL/hr

2. 0.9% Normal Saline

3. 50 mL/hr

4. 225 mL

5. 4.5 hours or 4 hours 30 minutes

CLINICAL REASONING 21.1 (P. 476)

D. Obtain the current weight of the child. *The nurse must know the child's current weight to verify if the ordered dose is a safe dose before administering any does of medication. The frequency of administration of the prednisone dose after 48 hours can be clarified later.*

DEVELOPING COMPETENCY (P. 477)

1. False. *The PO dose of Benadryl for antiemetic use is not based on weight.*

2. True

3. True

4. True

5. True

6. False. *The recommended antitussive dose is 25 mg q 4 hr as needed, not to exceed 150 mg/day.*

7. False. *The initial dose is 5 to 10 mcg/kg/day divided BID – TID.*

8. True

9. True

10. True

11. 50 mL/hr

12. D_5/0.45 NS

13. 50 mL/hr

14. 150 mL

15. 3 hours

16. 75 mL/hr

17. 0.9% NS

18. 50 mL/hr

19. 6 hours

20. 2100/9:00 p.m.

Chapter 22: Considerations for the Older Adult Population

APPLY LEARNED KNOWLEDGE 22.1 (P. 485)

1. (A) 7.5 mL; (B) Yes

2. (A) 2 tab; (B) Yes

3. (A) 0.8 mL; (B) Yes

4. (A) 0.5 tab; (B) anise, arnica, chamomile, clove, dong quai, fenugreek, feverfew, garlic, ginger, ginkgo biloba, Panax ginseng, licorice.

5. a. Benadryl is a PIM drug. b. The ordered dose on Librium is less than the usual dose stated in the drug reference.

APPLY LEARNED KNOWLEDGE 22.2 (P. 497)

1. 120 mL

2. 480 mL

3. 60 mL

4. 400 mL

5. 100 mL

CLINICAL REASONING 22.1 (P. 499)

A. The ordered dose is within the usual daily dose.

E. High alert drugs have an increased risk of causing serious injury or death.

DEVELOPING COMPETENCY (P. 500)

1. Yes

2. 2.5 mL

3. 4 ounces

4. No. *Most sodas are carbonated.*

5. No. *Abrupt discontinuation will cause side effects.*

6. Yes

7. No. *Older adults have an increased sensitivity to benzodiazepines, so may experience the side effects even when taking lowerer doses.*

8. Yes

9. b. diphenhydramine (antihistamine)

10. Yes. *Drug effects may last longer in the older adult causing daytime drowsiness/dizziness.*

11. b. 480 mL

12. 360 mL

13. 90 mL

14. 80 mL

15. 79 mL

16. a. 125 mL

17. c. 200 mL

18. 80 mL

19. 720 mL

20. 237 mL

ANSWERS TO UNIT REVIEWS

Unit 1: Safety in Medication Administration

1. **b.** Verify the route of administration.

2. **b.** The route of administration is ordered. **c.** The frequency of administration is missing. **d.** The ordered drug is administered directly into the muscle.

3. **a.** The generic name of the drug is on the drug label. **c.** This drug is for parenteral use only.

4. **a.** The generic name of the drug is on the drug label. **b.** The brand name of the drug is on the drug label. **c.** There are two equivalent dosage strengths.

5. **b.** Digoxin is the generic name of the drug. **c.** The nurse may administer ½ tablet of Lanoxin if necessary.

6. The trailing zero found on the dose (1.0 mcg).

7. mcg

8. 0.5 mcg/capsule

9. The abbreviation "u" in the physician's order should be avoided. The word "unit" should be spelled out to avoid medication errors.

10. 5,000 units/mL

Unit 2: Systems of Measurement

1. Correct

2. Incorrect. **Answer:** 0.1 mg *(Move the decimal point three places from right to left from the "mc" place to the "m" place.)*

3. Correct. *The order 1.0 mg contains a trailing zero and should be clarified.*

4. Incorrect. **Answer:** 2500 mL *(Move the decimal point three places from left to right from the "L" place to "m" place.)*

5. Incorrect. **Answer:** 0.375 g *(Move the decimal point three places from right to left from the "m" place to the "g" place.)*

6. Incorrect. **Answer:** 500 mcg *(Move the decimal point three places from left to right from the "m" place to "mc".)*

7. Incorrect. **Answer:** *The micro symbol (μ) is used in the order and should not be used by physicians or nurses to write drug orders or to communicate medical information. The symbol may be misinterpreted and contribute to medication errors. The nurse needs to clarify the order.*

8. Correct

9. Incorrect. **Answer:** 10 mL *2 tsp equals 10 mL*

10. Correct

Unit 3: Methods of Calculation

1. Correct

2. Correct

3. Incorrect. Administer 25 mL

4. Incorrect. Administer 16 mL

5. Correct

6. Correct

7. Incorrect. Administer 6.5 mL

8. Correct

9. Correct. *However 0.2 mL cannot be measured accurately in a teaspoon. A medication administration device that measures mL will need to be used.*

10. Incorrect. Administer 0.4 mL

Unit 4: Administration of Medication

1. Correct

2. Correct

3. Incorrect. *The warfarin sodium tablets sent by pharmacy are not scored and should not be broken or divided.*

4. Incorrect. *The nurse should have drawn up 5.4 mL in a 10 mL syringe. The dose of medication can be administered after rounding the answer to the tenths place.*

5. Correct

6. Incorrect. *The nurse should have administered 1.8 mL of Oxacillin to the patient. Also, the label did not include the dosage strength of the reconstituted drug, the type and amount of diluent, the time of reconstitution, or the expiration date and time.*

7. Correct

8.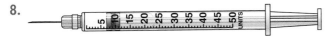

9.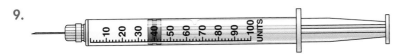

10.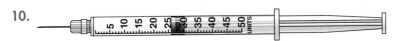

Unit 5: IV Therapy and Administration of Intravenous Medications

1. Correct

2. Incorrect. *The IV pump should be set at 200 mL/hr.*

3. Correct

4. Correct

5. Incorrect. *The IV will be completed at 0500.*

6. Correct

7. Correct

8. Incorrect. *The IV should be discontinued at 1630.*

9. Incorrect. *The start time was not written on the flow meter.*

10. Correct

Unit 6: Verifying Safe Dose and Critical Care Calculations

1. Correct

2. Incorrect. *300 mg/day is the maximum recommended dose for a 78-year-old patient. The nurse should consult with the doctor to clarify the ordered dose.*

3. Incorrect. *400 mg twice weekly is the maximum recommended dose for a patient who weighs 176 lb (80 kg). The nurse should consult with the doctor to clarify the ordered dose.*

4. Correct

5. Correct

6. Correct

7. Incorrect. *The flow rate should be set at 3 mL/hr.*

8. Correct

9. Correct

10. Correct. *The flow rate should be set at 7 mL/hr.*

Unit 7: Intake and Output

1. Correct

2. Incorrect. *The amount output is correct; however, the nasogastric output (475 mL) is recorded as emesis and should be recorded as nasogastric drainage.*

3. Incorrect. *The water needs to be part of the intake for a 24 hr total of 1,400 mL.*

4. Correct

5. Incorrect. *The oral intake is 570 mL (recall that ice chips melt to 1/2 of the starting amount) and the output should be 615 mL (subtract the bladder irrigation for the shift of 360 mL from the total output of 975 mL).*

6. Correct

7. Incorrect. *650 mL*

8. Incorrect. *625 mL*

9. Correct

10. Correct

Unit 8: Dosages for Pediatric and Elderly Populations

1. Correct

2. Incorrect. *5 hrs 20 min using the additional 30 mL/hr to replace the fluid loss.*

3. Correct

4. Correct

5. Incorrect. *The weight-based dose range for the IM dose for children is 0.1 to 0.15 mg/kg.*

6. Correct

7. Incorrect. *The midazolam dose must be individualized based on the patient's weight. A reduced dose may be required for certain patients.*

8. Correct

9. Correct

10. Correct

Credits and References

References

Kliegman R., Stanton, B., St. Geme, J., Schor, N., & Behrman, R. E. (Eds.). (2011). *Nelson textbook of pediatrics* (19th ed.). Philadelphia, PA: W. B. Saunders.

Vallerand A. H., & Sanoski, C. A. (2015). *Davis's drug guide for nurses* (14th ed.). Philadelphia, PA: F. A. Davis Company.

Venes D. (Ed.). (2013). *Taber's cyclopedic medical dictionary* (22nd ed.). Philadelphia, PA: F. A. Davis Company.

Index

Note: Page numbers followed by "b," "f," and "t" indicate boxes, figures, and tables, respectively.